PRAISE FOR THE PARENTING YOUR PAR~~E~~... ~~SERIES~~

Parenting Your Parents is a very valuable addition to the bookshelves of any families who are caring for aging relatives, as well as for physicians and other health professionals who care for older people. The book is a unique mixture of personal wisdom, case examples, and practical information that will assist caregivers of frail older people with the approaches and resources they need to deal with the everyday realities of a most difficult and challenging role.

> — *Joseph G. Ouslander, MD, Professor of Medicine and Nursing, Emory University School of Medicine; Director, Emory Center for Health in Aging; Director, Division of Geriatric Medicine and Gerontology, and chief medical officer, Wesley Woods Center*

The use of case vignettes to discuss the complexities of parent care works very well. It is easy for caregivers to find a vignette that matches their current dilemma and read a well-balanced discussion by experts in geriatrics…. It is a great resource to read cover to cover and to refer back to as new situations evolve.

> — *Jane F. Potter, MD, Harris Professor of Geriatric Medicine, University of Nebraska Medical Center; President, American Geriatrics Society*

Parenting Your Parents is about caring for aging loved ones. Through vignettes of family interactions, sons and daughters and friends and clinicians grapple with relationships, survival, and finality. This book is highly recommended as a valuable and readable resource providing us with insight, wisdom, and reassurance.

> — *Dr. Richard Neufeld, Vice President of Medical Services, Jewish Home and Hospital; Associate Clinical Professor, Dept. of Geriatrics and Adult Development, Mt. Sinai Medical School*

As I was reading this new edition of *Parenting Your Parents*, I was reminded of the extraordinarily influential book *The Common Sense Book of Baby and Child Care* by Benjamin Spock. His book brought about a major change in attitude toward the care of children. This immensely readable work has many of the characteristics of Spock's work. Perhaps the greatest achievement of *Parenting Your Parents* is its global appeal to a broad spectrum of family members and health care providers…. The personal experiences described by the authors reflect the stresses that even experienced practitioners can have in coping with difficult situations. The "Resource" section is thorough and practical. The authors fill a vital need to optimize quality of life for our aging population and ease the burden on their caregivers.

> — *Dr. Jerome Kowal, Professor Emeritus of Geriatric Medicine, Case Western Reserve School of Medicine*

Everyone who has aging parents should read this exceptionally sensitive, clearly written, highly informative exploration of the often vexing, emotionally challenging task of providing the care and dignity that aging parents deserve. Illuminating, touching case examples and insightful commentary about them provide extremely important lessons that help readers identify and cope with the salient psychological issues involved. In addition, the authors provide an exhaustive guide to invaluable resources and a system for identifying all pertinent financial, health-related, and personal information required to plan properly for the care and well being of one's aging parent(s).

> — Steven R. Sabat, Ph.D., Professor of Psychology, Georgetown University, Washington, D.C., Author of The Experience of Alzheimer's Disease: Life Through a Tangled Veil (Blackwell, 2001) and co-editor of Dementia: Mind, Meaning, and the Person (Oxford University Press, 2006)

Whether your aging parent is weighing the risks of major surgery, becoming romantically involved with another resident of her nursing home, or resisting moving to assisted living despite progressive frailty, you will encounter another family in the throes of a similar dilemma in Parenting Your Parents. As you read the more than twenty rich narratives in this compelling guide, you will come to understand the older person's perspective, the struggles of his family, and the health care professional's point of view.

> — Muriel R. Gillick, MD, Associate Professor, Harvard Medical School; Author of The Denial of Aging: Perpetual Youth, Eternal Life, and Other Dangerous Fantasies

Parenting Your Parents is not just for family caregivers. I recommend it to all social service and health care professionals who work with seniors. This thorough book articulately presents aging challenges and solutions in a family context … a perspective too often ignored by practitioners.

> — Gail Reisman, Ph.D., Geriatric Care Manager and Educator, RSCR California, Inc.

This book offers a unique and sometimes moving blend of information, insight, compassion, advocacy, and humor. It should be a valuable resource for families needing to help frail parents who have many things wrong at once, but who must deal with health care systems that largely prefer people to get sick with one illness at a time.

> — Kenneth Rockwood, MD, FRCPC, Professor of Geriatric Medicine, Dalhousie University, Past President, the Canadian Society of Geriatric Medicine

PARENTING
YOUR PARENTS

Straight Talk about
Aging in the Family

THIRD EDITION

BART J. MINDSZENTHY
DR. MICHAEL GORDON

Foreword by Alexis Abramson, Ph.D.

DUNDURN
TORONTO

Editor: Britanie Wilson
Design: Jennifer Scott
Printer: Webcom

Library and Archives Canada Cataloguing in Publication

Mindszenthy, Bart J., 1946-, author
Parenting your parents : straight talk about aging in the family / Bart J. Mindszenthy and Dr. Michael Gordon.
-- 3rd edition.

Issued in print and electronic formats.
ISBN 978-1-4597-1061-0 (pbk.).--ISBN 978-1-4597-1062-7 (pdf).--ISBN 978-1-4597-1063-4 (epub)

1. Aging parents--Care. 2. Parent and adult child. 3. Adult children of aging parents--Family relationships.
I. Gordon, Michael, 1941-, author II. Title.

HQ1063.6.M55 2013   306.874   C2013-903909-0   C2013-903910-4

1 2 3 4 5   17 16 15 14 13

 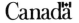 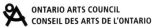

We acknowledge the support of the **Canada Council for the Arts** and the **Ontario Arts Council** for our publishing program. We also acknowledge the financial support of the **Government of Canada** through the **Canada Book Fund** and **Livres Canada Books**, and the **Government of Ontario** through the **Ontario Book Publishing Tax Credit** and the **Ontario Media Development Corporation**.

Care has been taken to trace the ownership of copyright material used in this book. The author and the publisher welcome any information enabling them to rectify any references or credits in subsequent editions.

J. Kirk Howard, President

The publisher is not responsible for websites or their content unless they are owned by the publisher.

Printed and bound in Canada.

Visit us at
Dundurn.com | @dundurnpress | Facebook.com/dundurnpress | Pinterest.com/dundurnpress

Dundurn
3 Church Street, Suite 500
Toronto, Ontario, Canada
M5E 1M2

Gazelle Book Services Limited
White Cross Mills
High Town, Lancaster, England
LA1 4XS

Dundurn
2250 Military Road
Tonawanda, NY
U.S.A. 14150

*To our parents, who gave us limitless love and helped us focus;
to our spouses, who bolster our spirits and add clarity;
to our children, who bring us the light of life and strengthen our purpose;
and to all of you who, like us, live the circle of
family beginnings, life, love, and endings.*

CONTENTS

FOREWORD

Parenting Your Parents may sound peculiar to those who have not been there — by 'there' I mean having been the child of an aging parent. In many cases the tables appear to have turned for adult children, who are now faced with the complex health problems and life situations that interfere with the well-being of their older parents. For those family members who are dealing with all the issues that occur, and who have raised their own children, they know that *Parenting Your Parents* is not exactly the same thing as parenting your children … but as many have said along the journey — "it sure feels the same."

In many ways the growing aging population is one of the miracles of the modern world. With these blessings have come issues, concerns, and roadblocks that were not part of the dynamics of families and communities generations ago. Prior to many of the advances and medical breakthroughs in society, it was more common for older parents to die without the toll of long, drawn-out illnesses that previously were relatively rapid and fatal. But now, they can be treated and controlled, if not cured, thereby extending life way beyond what was the experience of previous generations.

Coupled with the aging population are social issues unlike those experienced in bygone years: many families are now separated by work, marriage, and geographic distance. Being as mobile as people are now, both in the United States and Canada, it is often taken for granted. Now it's common for children to live far removed from where they grew up, whether in a different part of the state or province, or a different country altogether. As a consequence, the aging population may become increasingly isolated from the family support systems, which in the past were the backbone of family cohesiveness and care in the face of medical problems.

With this third edition of *Parenting Your Parents: Straight Talk about Aging in the Family* the authors, Bart Mindszenthy and Dr. Michael Gordon, have added a new level of insight and sensitivity to the issues encountered by families as they try to unravel the various problems that they will inevitably face as their parents age and gradually decline. By incorporating case histories that readers can relate to, and insights into the many narratives and situations that the authors have experienced within their own families, they have truly captured the essence of what it means to be the child of an aging parent. In addition, Dr. Gordon brings to the discussion his vast clinical experience as one of Canada's first certified geriatric medical specialists. *Parenting Your Parents* weaves together these compelling vignettes in a seamless and inspiring manner.

As a PhD gerontologist, having worked in the field of aging for over 20 years in the United States, I have been engaged in dilemmas comparable to those described so eloquently by Mindszenthy and Gordon — both professionally and personally. These co-authors have citizenships in both countries and have been exposed to many situations on "both sides of the border" with friends and family members. In the case of Dr. Gordon, he has also dealt many patients whose families come from either country — most frequently the parent in question lives in Toronto, Canada, where Gordon works at the internationally renowned Baycrest Geriatric Health Care System.

Having worked with Dr. Gordon over the years on various projects dealing with older members of the population, I can attest to his sincerity, knowledge, passion, and commitment as a geriatrician and educator. The previous editions of *Parenting Your Parents*, first published in 2002, with subsequent editions in 2005 and 2006, were, like the current edition, co-authored by Bart Mindszenthy. The books are a tribute to two very caring authors who want to support family members, who like them, have experienced the personal and often painful (as well as joyful!) experiences of helping to navigate aging parents through the turbulent and troubled waters of their later lives. I am pleased, and honored, to recommend this book to the children of aging parents. It is they who almost invariably carry out their responsibilities with compassion, commitment, humour, and humanity. This book is meant to pay homage to them and all their family members who share in this journey — one that is often full of predicaments, doubts, misgivings, and then exquisite moments of deep satisfaction.

— Alexis Abramson, Ph.D.
Atlanta, Georgia, June 4, 2013

Alexis Abramson, Ph.D. is the author of the *The Caregivers Survival Handbook*, a guide to help caregivers balance the responsibilities of caring for others and for themselves, and *Home Safety for Seniors*, a room-by-room reference and idea book for making independent senior and home-bound living easier. Visit her website at: *http://www.alexisabramson.com.*

INTRODUCTION
Caring for Aging Loved Ones *Is* a
Major North American Social Issue and Challenge

We were sitting in a restaurant some months ago discussing the changes and new case histories to be added to this latest offering in the Parenting Your Parents series. We were pretty animated because this is a subject not only close to our hearts, but because we were pumped by how the book was shaping up.

Suddenly a woman was standing next to our table. She said: "I was sitting at the table behind you and I couldn't help but overhear what you were talking about. I want you to know I'm living it right now with my aging mother. A lot of my friends are. And I want to tell you how import-ant what you're doing is for all of us. I want to just thank you, and tell you I'll be buying the book as soon as I see it."

Once she left we realized how many times in the past dozen years since we'd been collaborating on various editions of *Parenting Your Parents* we had shared this exact kind of experience either together or individually.

It seems that the challenges and issues surrounding family caregiv-ing for aging parents and other elderly loved ones has finally moved from the side street of social consciousness to the main street, whether it be in New Brunswick or New Mexico.

Eldercare in the family is getting to be where childcare was half a century ago. Demographics and longevity are major drivers. The new family compact most North Americans are embracing of more accept-able distances between parents and their offspring is a contributing factor, and the state of the health care systems in the United States and Canada exacerbates the situation.

Unfortunately, it's the same around the world. Aging and its conse-quences are a global reality, and knowing how to deal with this reality at the family level is something too many choose to ignore, neglect, or avoid until it's too late. Waiting too long opens a Pandora's Box of unwanted and unwelcome surprises that tax the ability of any family to deal effectively with the issues and uncertainties that arise with aging and elderly parents. All the more reason to face a certain family future head-on now and build agreements, plans, and procedures that will minimize the painful impact of what otherwise surely will come to be.

So welcome to *Parenting Your Parents: Straight Talk about Aging in the Family.*

Our goal is to help you think about, better understand, plan for, and to some extent more effectively navigate the roller coaster ride you'll face.

This 2013 revised new edition includes an expanded set of twenty-four case studies; a new Vulnerability Index to help you gauge how your parents are right now; an updated resource directory; and an updated financial primer. We also bring you up-to-date on our own personal experiences. Why? Because caring for our aging parents and other elderly loved ones is now a major familial and societal issue in the United States, Canada, and around the world, and we feel that relating our personal experience could potentially help you navigate your own similar experiences to come.

THE AMERICAN STORY

The numbers speak for themselves. According to the year 2000 figures from the U.S. Census Bureau, there were nearly 36 million Americans 65 years of age or older. By 2011 the numbers changed dramatically, with more than 41 million people now 65 years and over (male: 17,745,363/ female: 23,377,542). Some are doing remarkably well for their age, some are in line with statistical expectations, and many are in failing health — physically, mentally, or both. They all need, and most expect, our care and concern.

And consider the implications of this amazing advancement: in 1900, the average life expectancy in America was 47 years of age; by 2000, it edged to 77. By 2011 the average life expectancy was 78.4 years, with 75.9 years for men and 80.9 for women.

As they become more frail, our elderly parents and other loved ones will require us to commit more of our time and patience to ensure they'll live their closing years in as much comfort, dignity, and safety as possible.

Physicians acknowledge that eldercare is extremely demanding on their professional time and on the health care system in general. They point out that the elderly, especially those over 80, usually require more time for an appointment because they tend to have more complex medical issues that must be addressed, and as a rule they usually move more slowly. Frequently children visit the doctor with their parents to assist, and that too requires extra time for explanations. As well, the elderly generally have doctors' appointments more often than healthier young or middle-aged persons. If hospitalized, elderly patients more often need a higher level of care and treatment and longer periods for recovery.

The National Institutes of Health (NIH) estimates that by 2030 there will be at least 72 million Americans 65 years of age or older. And right now, the fastest growing segment of the American population is the age group of 85 and up.

In the year 2004 there were more than seven million older adults in America who needed some level of long-term care, and that number will leap to 10 million by 2020. Right now, there are at least 22 million households across the nation providing care for a family member or loved one.

Today, more than 96 million Americans are between the ages of 35 and 59, and the majority of them have living parents and in-laws who will increasingly need their help and support in some way. An estimated 36.3 million Americans aged 45 to 65 already provide informal care to those aged 65 and older who are experiencing long-term health problems. In 1997, the National Alliance for Caregiving (NAC) and American Association of Retired Persons (AARP) said that many women spend more years caring for a parent than they did raising a child. In 1990, *Newsweek* reported that the average woman spent 17 years raising children and 18 years helping aging parents.

An October 2005 study by Opinion Research Corp. showed that millions of American women and men are experiencing serious workplace consequences as a result of providing what is termed "informal" parent and eldercare. They've reported impacts ranging from reduced hours of work to lost income; some people have turned down job opportunities or actually quit work. The study also demonstrated that there are very real and tangible negative consequences for their social activities, holiday plans, actual expenses, and even sleep patterns and personal health.

For example, an NAC-AARP study found that 15% of those caring for someone else said their own health suffered, and 35% reported emotional stress and strain. The same study estimated that people who provided care and as a result went from full-time to part-time jobs or left the workforce entirely ended up losing more than $650,000 in wages and Social Security benefits over their lifetimes.

And it gets even more challenging with new projections of what will be the growing demands on families and the health system in the years ahead. The February 2013 edition of the medical journal *Neurology* reports a new study that predicts nothing short of an epidemic of Alzheimer's and other dementias by 2050 as Boomers continue to age. The study estimates that in 37 years the number of those living with dementia will soar from the current 4.7 million people to 13.8 million of those afflicted with the condition. About one in three of those aged 85 will have the disease and one in six between the ages 75 and 84 will be diagnosed with dementia. The implications for the individuals, their families, and the health care system are hard to fathom when even now, with much lower numbers, so many struggle to facilitate proper care.

So the implications are clear and imperative to address: as baby boomers start to retire they become the next and greatest wave to challenge the health care system and the family structure.

There is even more data that drives home the scope of the issue. The 2005 Opinion Research study found that about 66% of the population — more than 138 million Americans — believe they will need to care for someone in the future.

To exacerbate the challenges facing us, about 44% of Americans between the ages of 45 and 55 have children under 21 living at home as well as having eldercare responsibilities. All this underscores the point that caring for our aging parents is a major personal and social issue. There isn't a shortcut. There aren't any easy answers.

Yet, given our social structure, there should be more government recognition for what we do in the home for our parents, which actually relieves the pressure on the health care system. Family caregivers provide unpaid services valued at an estimated $257 to $306 billion a year, an amount comparable to the total Medicare budget less than a decade ago.

THE CANADIAN STORY

As in the United States, the numbers tell the story. For example, according to the 2011 Canadian census there were 4,945,060 people aged 65 and older in Canada, an increase of more than 609,810, or 14.1%, between 2006 and 2011. This rate of growth was more than double the 5.9% increase for the Canadian population as a whole. Of all five-year age groups, the 60- to 64-year-old group experienced the fastest increase, at 29.1% with a substantial increase as well in those over 85 years. This suggests that population aging will accelerate in Canada in the coming years, as the large baby boom generation, those born between 1946 and 1965, reach 65 years of age. The first baby boomers reached 65 years old in 2011. As for the so-called "old-old," that group will increase in numbers as well with demand for care needs from families and increasing challenges to the health care system.

This is reflected by the fact that the 2011Census counted 5,825 people aged 100 years and older, up from 4,635 in 2006 and 3,795 in 2001. Between 2006 and 2011, the number of centenarians increased 25.7%. Of those categorized as elderly, including those who are very elderly, many do remarkably well for their age, some are in line with statistical expectations, and many are in failing health — whether physically, mentally, or both. They all need, and most expect, our care and concern.

Population aging in Canada is expected to accelerate between now and 2031, as all people in the large cohort of baby boomers reach their senior years. Projections show that seniors could account for more than one-fifth of the population as soon as 2026 and could exceed one-quarter of the population by 2056.

As of July 1, 2010, there were 1,333,800 people aged 80 years and over in Canada, representing 3.9% of the total population. The number of people aged 80 years and over could double by the year 2031 and by 2061 — the end of the assessment period of the most recent projections — there could be 5.1 million people in this age range. There were roughly equal proportions of men and women in each age group under 65 years; however, the disparity grows throughout the senior years. As of July 1, 2010, of the total population of people 65 years and over, 55.6% were women, increasing to 63.0% for those aged 80 years, and to 79.6% for centenarians. Much of this gender difference is due to the higher life expectancy of women compared to men. In recent years, though, gains in life expectancy have been more rapid for men than for women, resulting in a narrowing of the gap between the sexes.

As in the United States, physicians acknowledge that eldercare is extremely demanding on their professional time and on the health care system in general. They point out that the elderly, especially those over 80, usually require more time for an appointment because they tend to have more complex medical issues that must be addressed.

Meanwhile, according to the 2009 Special Senate Committee on Aging Final Report, about 25% of all Canadians 45 years of age or older are providing in-home care to a family member or close friend with some form of long-term illness.

A 2011 Desjardins Financial Security Canadian national health survey found that just slightly less than 20% of respondents have worked with their parents to develop a plan for ongoing care. Put another way, more than 80% of those interviewed have never managed to candidly discuss and agree with aging parents on a sound, helpful course of action for when tough decisions need to be made — and, made when that parent might not be able to offer a view or preference because of a health condition.

The same study found that the majority of people who provide daily support to their aging parents totally or somewhat agree that their assistance impacts their mental health (67.3%), the wellbeing of their family (62.4%), their physical health (60.1%), and their professional life (58.2%).

WHAT WE ALL CAN LEARN TO GUIDE US

The fact remains, as research shows, that we're generally opting to avoid the very critical discussions we should have while our parents are well because those kinds of discussions are uncomfortable and usually downright difficult. However, those are precisely the kinds of discussions we must have if we're to do the right things, the right way, when the time comes.

After all, as they become more frail, our elderly parents and other loved ones will require more of our time, patience, and commitment to ensure they'll live their closing years in as much comfort, dignity, and safety as possible.

All this underscores the point that caring for our aging parents is a major personal and social issue. There isn't a shortcut. There aren't any easy answers.

Yet, given our social structure, there should be more government recognition for what we do in the home for our parents, the result of which is a relief of pressure on the health care system.

The lesson to be learned: we need to be more open, more involved, and able to more easily access the kinds of support and services we need for our aging parents and other loved ones, as well as for ourselves.

So, welcome to the wonderful new world of parenting your parents.

It's a world of tingling emotions, stress, and fear, and, very often, of finding new bonds and levels of love and affection. It's a journey of discovering conflicting personal weaknesses and strengths. It's all about recognizing that we are extensions of our parents, whether we like it or not, and understanding that the needs they have as they age and decline are heartfelt weights we must carry. It's a new, uncharted path in the process of discovering how human we really are.

Bart Mindszenthy and Michael Gordon
Toronto, Ontario, Canada, 2013

FAMILY CASE STUDIES

CASE STUDY 1
Control: Laying on the Guilt Trip

For whatever reason, some parents find it necessary to induce a sense of guilt in their children, and sometimes even their grandchildren, making relations difficult and at times strained. Careful planning is necessary to defuse these very delicate situations.

THE CHALLENGE

Beth and Lloyd Thurmont are 83 and 86 years old, respectively. They have three children — Darrin, who is 58; Donna, 56; and Cameron, 54. Beth and Lloyd live in a retirement home on the outskirts of Orangeville, Ontario.

Darrin, a chartered accountant, lives with his family in Brampton (a 45-minute drive away). He and his wife, Betty, have four children: 30-year-old twin sisters Tracy and Tammy; Tom, who is 28 and lives in London, Ontario, with his wife, Angela, and their four children; and 26-year-old Terry, who lives in Toronto with her lesbian partner.

Donna's marriage fell apart two years ago when her husband announced he was leaving for another job in Vancouver and wanted to start life over again. They have one child, Arthur, who at 38 goes from job to job and city to city, still looking for a career path that suits him. Donna lives in a downtown Toronto bachelor apartment and works as a paralegal at a large law firm.

Cameron lives in Berlin, Germany, where he's been working as a freelance artist for the past five years. He enjoys his work and where he lives immensely. Single and unattached, Cameron loves roaming around Europe and has been back to Canada only twice to visit family and friends. He does call his parents about twice a month, and he sends them email messages through his brother, Darrin.

Lloyd has been in failing health for some years and is visited regularly by a nurse arranged through Ontario's Community Care Access Centre services, as well as by a physiotherapist who helps him exercise his severely arthritic legs and arms. Beth is in relatively good health, except for Type 2 diabetes, controlled by medication, and a weight problem she's had for decades.

Beth longs to have her children pay more attention to her and for Lloyd to see more of their grandchildren. No matter how much attention her family pays to her and Lloyd, for Beth it's not enough. She believes that in their old age she and her husband are entitled to as much of their children's and grandchildren's time as they want and need.

In fact, in the past few years Beth has been exerting a steadily increasing level of control over her family by playing on their fears and instilling feelings of guilt in them. This has led to instances of both capitulation and confrontation among her children. Sometimes they've given in to the pressures placed on them, and sometimes they've had violent verbal battles. But most often, they've acquiesced in order to keep the peace and because their father always asks them to bear their mother's insecurities and to put up with her needs.

But now Beth's claims and attacks are more frequent and her needs more intense. She often calls with pleas for a quick appearance by one of her children because, she claims, Lloyd is desperate to see Darrin or Donna — usually a surprise to Lloyd, who is content to watch movies and read magazines most of the time. And every so often she attacks Donna for failing in her marriage and causing embarrassment and grief for the whole family. Meanwhile, she alleges that Cameron rarely visits because he is selfish and has elected to escape his family responsibilities and that he lives a decadent life far away while everyone else is close to home and willing to help. And Darrin, she says, is guilty of putting his family before his parents because he visits only for an hour or so once or twice a week.

Beth is scathing in her views of her grandchildren, who, she alleges, are only waiting to inherit the small fortune she and Lloyd have managed to save through years of back-breaking work. (The truth is that Beth and Lloyd are not very well off, and their three children actually contribute to offset the cost of their living in the retirement residence.) She often tells her children that they, like her grandchildren, would be smart to be nicer to her and Lloyd or they may lose their inheritance in favor of some worthy cause. And ever since Beth discovered that Terry was a lesbian, she's regularly harassed Darrin and Betty about it, telling them that if she were Terry's mother, this would never have happened. Terry, not surprisingly, has refused to see her grandmother for several years. Beth's other grandchildren tend to avoid any interaction with her, although they do confess to their parents that they would like to visit Lloyd alone, if that were possible.

No matter what responses her children give, Beth counters all of them with emotional outpourings and claims of feeling unwell or rejected. She works very hard at making all her children feel guilty in different ways.

For Beth's birthday in January, Darrin came to collect her and Lloyd and took them to his Brampton home, where Betty had prepared a lavish dinner. All four of Darrin and Betty's children attended, as did Donna. But by midway through dinner everyone was miserable, as Beth spent considerable time telling stories about how during the past year she and Lloyd had been disappointed and hurt by their children's insensitivity and their grandchildren's poor behavior. The event turned into a painful experience for all of them, and at one point Donna got into a bitter exchange with her mother that left all of them hurt and embarrassed.

When she hasn't slept well for a couple of nights, or when she's feeling especially lonely and depressed, Beth calls her children and becomes agitated and confrontational, and the content of her message is almost always the same: "What are you doing for me today?" Now, it's reaching the point where her children want to rebel and find ways to contain her outrageous claims, accusations, and anger.

Meanwhile, Lloyd continues to distance himself from the tension the family is feeling. For whatever reason, when he does talk to his children, it's always in a remote way that seems to imply his lack of interest in his wife's needs and intensity. Lloyd, when he does see one of his children or talk to one of his grandchildren, usually discusses some movie or television special he's seen, or an article he's read in *Reader's Digest*. And when he talks about Beth and her behavior, it's usually in a very passive way, simply asking the family to be understanding and to ignore her accusations.

But the reality is that Darrin and Donna are having an increasingly difficult time coping with their mother's attitude and outbursts. And since they can't detect any certain signs of mental illness or any other problem, they are confused and frustrated. They relay their impressions to Cameron, who says he just isn't close enough to be able to pass judgment.

Darrin recently spoke to his parents' family physician, who said that there doesn't seem to be anything wrong with Beth. In fact, she seems relatively well — generally upbeat and positive about her life, but she has expressed concerns that her children and grandchildren are ignoring Lloyd, and this she finds hurtful and wrong. She told the doctor that Lloyd suffers as a result, which is stressful for her. The doctor told Darrin that Beth did volunteer that she misses more interaction with her children and grandchildren, and that she believes all of them would just as soon see her and Lloyd dead and gone so they wouldn't have to worry about them.

Darrin, in sharing this information with Donna and Cameron, also tells them that he feels their parents' doctor sympathizes with their mother's sense of being wronged. He tells them he's concerned that the doctor is, for whatever reason, biased in her favor, and that, as a result, he's not being as helpful as he should be in assessing her and possibly prescribing some kind of medication to manage her moods.

THE GERIATRICIAN'S POINT OF VIEW

This is the kind of difficult family dynamic that can either lead to further family disruption, with a permanent legacy of hurt and guilt, or bring a family together and demonstrate how robust they are in dealing with difficult situations. Most families have to face trying situations that may test the very fabric of their ties. Whether the issue involves illness, death, terrible financial situations, or complex family dynamics, there are ways of reaching resolutions so that irremediable damage does not occur.

We will work on the assumption that there is nothing wrong with Beth medically that can account for her increasing need for family attention and that, therefore, her behavior is merely a manifestation of her underlying personality. Even though the family physician may not believe there is anything wrong with her, it may be worthwhile for a family spokesperson to speak to the doctor and question whether, indeed, something underlying might be going on. Sometimes conditions such as depression or early dementia result in peculiar exaggerations of personality. The family physician can address this possibility by probing for symptoms and conducting mental-status tests. If the physician is sure that what is going on is not related to an underlying clinical condition, then Beth has to be dealt with as a full participant in whatever process might be developed to help resolve this increasingly tense and potentially destructive situation.

To assist the family and Beth and Lloyd, a two-part process can be implemented. First, the children, especially the two who are relatively close by, need to get some help in sorting through this very challenging situation. If this is not done in some cohesive fashion, the result could be terrible alienation of the various members of the family that is likely to have long-lasting effects on the family structure. It is important that the grandchildren who live in the vicinity also take part in the process, as the patterns of family interaction, the value put on relationships, and the ability to deal with difficult situations are often measures of a family's strength for the present and the future.

One approach is to find a social worker (or some other family counselor) who is experienced in dealing with issues of family dynamics. It is important to define who the key players will be in any family meetings that take place initially to try to provide a framework for the issues, problems, and options. But, even for those who do not actually attend family sessions, there must be consistent communication so that everyone is on board with the approach. This is an opportunity for all the children to address the issues and, if at all possible, to be consistent with the approach to their parents (and grandparents).

Assuming that such family counseling takes place, the second part of the process is to have a clear discussion with Beth and Lloyd about what is going on. There are a number of ways of doing this, including having the key members of the family meet with Beth and Lloyd alone (not too many in the first meeting, but clearly representing the consensus of the family) and explain the enormous difficulties that everyone is facing.

It makes sense to begin a meeting of this sort with a clear statement of the love, devotion, and commitment the family members have for their parents or grandparents, and to explain that it might not be possible to participate in their own complex lives and at the same time respond to Beth's every whim and need.

Of course at this point, it is possible that Beth may become very upset or angry at being "ganged up on," and she may not want any further part of the discussions. If this happens, it would be time for one person, perhaps Darrin, to speak to his mother again and continue with the same message: "We love you and Dad, and we want only the best for you, but … ", and continue by laying out the difficulties that everyone is facing. It must be made clear to Beth that insulting her children and grandchildren has the opposite effect to the one she hopes to achieve.

It might be suggested to Beth and Lloyd (or to Beth alone if that seems preferable) that she join a few of the family members to meet with the counselor. If she agrees, that is a major step forward. If she rejects that offer, it may still be possible to work with her and Lloyd to find an acceptable and agreeable common ground.

Arrangements that sometimes work in such situations include developing a rotation system of who will visit or communicate with whom on a regular basis. There may be some need to increase the interaction of the family with Lloyd and Beth, but rather than that interaction being on an on-call basis, the family could put together an outline of what can and cannot be done reasonably within clearly defined limits.

Someone should make it clear that there are no financial expectations from Beth and Lloyd, and if, indeed, the children are paying for some of the expenses, this can be pointed out. Most important, it must be related to Beth, either by a family member (or two) or by a counselor, that her recriminations and accusations are disruptive and may ultimately cause the family network and ties to unravel. That would be the worst outcome possible, because eventually Beth and Lloyd may have needs that require a great deal of devotion and time, and an enormous sense of guilt may follow the family members for years to come if they are not involved in this process.

Family dynamics is among the most difficult issues to challenge. But the children and grandchildren have to come to terms with the long-haul implications of the decisions they make. Families are not replaced by other entities, and it is worth the investment to try to salvage whatever relationships exist for the immediate situation and for the future. There are ways of learning how not to react to hurtful words when it is clear that in the ways that really count, her family really loves her but that she must find better communication methods to help them carry out their love than trying to bully them into it.

CASE STUDY 2
Surgery: Weighing the Odds

Surgery at any age can be traumatic, but for the elderly there are special issues and considerations. Weighing priorities and planning recovery is a complex and demanding process that requires careful consideration.

THE CHALLENGE

Lee Ann Bowater is 76 and a widow. Her husband, Martin, died four years ago after suffering several heart attacks. She lives alone in a one-bedroom apartment in Portland, Maine, and while she still mourns Martin's death, she has moved on with her life. Lee Ann has several friends, and they try to get together at least once a week for tea and talk.

Lee Ann's daughter, Sylvia, is an elementary school teacher. She's 52 years old and lives in Westbrook with her husband, Gerry, who works long hours managing a car rental outlet in downtown Portland. Sylvia and Gerry have two children: Jay, age 28, and Linda, age 19. Jay moved to Yarmouth three years ago to work in a call center, and Linda lives at home as she continues her education at a local college.

Lee Ann's son, David, is 47 years old and lives in Houston, Texas, where he works as an analyst for an oil company. He divorced two years ago and lives in an apartment with his common-law partner, Mary, whom Lee Ann has never met.

Both children are in close contact with Lee Ann, especially Sylvia, who lives only ten miles away and visits her mother every other day. As well, once every two weeks Gerry picks up Lee Ann to take her to their home for dinner. David calls from Houston at least once a week to talk to his mother for a few minutes, and he tries to visit at least once a year.

Lee Ann relishes visits from her daughter, and she tries hard to be a loving, non-intrusive grandmother to Jay and Linda, although she considers both to be somewhat spoiled. However, she strives to keep those feelings to herself, and she spends most of the time during Sylvia's visits asking about her teaching and Gerry's work.

Lee Ann is relatively sound in body and mind. She is short and a bit overweight, but not so much that it's a problem. In fact, since Martin's death, she has shown a surprisingly strong sense of independence and has learned to manage her finances so that Gerry needs to spend only an hour a month reviewing her bank statements.

Five years ago Lee Ann had surgery for cataracts in both eyes. This was a low-risk, high-benefit proposition that allowed her to see well again and resume a relatively normal lifestyle. In fact, she found she could once again play pinochle with her friends.

Now, however, Lee Ann has developed a malignant tumor in her colon that is still relatively small but has the potential to grow and spread. Her doctor believes surgery will be required at some point. As well, she is in constant pain because of severe osteoarthritis in her left hip, and a hip replacement operation is the only certain way to help her with that condition.

Lee Ann's doctor is cautious about the prognosis, noting that while the operations are fairly routine, Lee Ann will need substantial support for a prolonged period of time afterward. The hip operation is not critical, but it would allow Lee Ann to walk and function more easily and would probably eliminate the pain she's currently living with. The colon surgery, on the other hand, is more urgent because of the risk of the tumor spreading.

Lee Ann understands that she needs the colon surgery, and she also wants the hip replacement, but she is fearful of the two operations and the period of convalescence that would follow each. It's clear that if either operation is to proceed, Lee Ann will require close, ongoing help and support during her recovery.

Sylvia knows that her mother would like to live with her and Gerry during her recovery. Gerry is against this idea because they live in a small house with two bedrooms, and they both work full-time. While he hasn't said no to the prospect of Lee Ann living with them, it's not an option he would happily embrace.

David has said that he wants to be supportive but that distance prevents him from doing much in terms of hands-on help.

Given Lee Ann's limited income, as well as the limited incomes of both Sylvia and David, there is no clear resolution to the question of how the family will support her.

The challenge for the family is how to help Lee Ann face two surgical procedures, both of which are necessary to give her a chance of survival and an improved quality of life. How can they help without disrupting their own equilibrium in an unacceptable way? The family faces several important issues. Should the colon surgery be performed first? If so, Lee Ann would require at least two or three weeks of in-home care. But where should she stay for that period of time? If she were to remain in her apartment, she would require professional home care services, as well as someone to live with her during her convalescence. Or could Lee Ann stay with Sylvia and her family, or with David and his partner? Could David take a few weeks off and stay with his mother?

If the colon surgery is performed first and Lee Ann has a good recovery, then should the orthopedic surgery be undertaken to replace her left hip? And if so, when? Rehabilitation work would be necessary after the hip surgery, and that would mean Lee Ann would have to be taken for rehab sessions at least twice a week for some weeks.

Sylvia and Gerry have talked about what they could and should do. Their daughter, Linda, has made it clear that she won't have time to help because of her school and social commitments. Their son, Jay, is relatively independent but works long hours. Sylvia is concerned about any surgery taking place during the school year because she won't be able to take the kind of time off that would probably be required. And Gerry, given the nature of his job, can't be counted on for any extended level of support.

Sylvia has discussed the situation with her brother during the course of several telephone conversations. She's even suggested that David take his holidays and spend two weeks with their mother after the colon operation to help her. David listened to the case Sylvia presented but responded by saying that Mary was really counting on having their holidays together for a long-planned drive to tour the Grand Canyon and to spend time in Las Vegas. This has irritated Sylvia, but the siblings have stayed very polite with each other.

Lee Ann's doctor, in a recent telephone call with Sylvia, advised that while he wants to do some further tests, he believes the colon surgery will be imperative based on the steady growth of the tumor. He tells Sylvia that "sooner than later" is the way they should think about it.

THE GERIATRICIAN'S POINT OF VIEW

Lee Ann and her family have a few things to figure out, and a real examination of relationships and priorities is necessary in order for this situation to work well. It is worth dividing the issues into those that are mainly clinical and those that are related to the way family members feel they should and can support Lee Ann, who wants to remain independent but who is facing some difficult challenges during the course of the next number of months.

When considering the clinical issues, the priority is likely going to be the removal of the colon tumor. Based on the information provided, it appears that the tumor is still at a stage where if it is removed surgically, a good outcome is likely and Lee Ann should be able to function independently.

It is worth asking the surgeon if the surgery can be done in such a way that bowel function will be maintained and a colostomy (exit of bowel through the skin) will not be required. The answer will have a big impact on the type of care required immediately after the surgery and for the longer term following.

Also, the assumption is that the tumor will be contained and will not spread (metastasize) to other organs, so that the outlook over a longer period of time would be good. However, until the surgery is done it is hard to know whether further treatments, such as radiation therapy, might be required.

The family must understand that there is some urgency to the decision about the colon surgery and that they must find ways to support their mother through this emotionally and physically trying situation. Although Lee Ann may be holding herself together in the face of what is probably a very frightening prospect, it appears that she does not want to be a burden to her family. This is the time for her children to find the means to rally around and support their mother with the resources, human and otherwise, that they have available.

They can look at the challenges in a few stages. The first is the immediate preparation for surgery, with its emotional and physical impacts. This is the time for everyone, including Jay and Linda, to find at least some time to, in a cooperative fashion, be there to bolster their mother and grandmother.

Assuming that all goes well, the stages following surgery will be divided into the immediate post-operative phase and then the period of Lee Ann's reactivation and return to a normal functioning lifestyle. It is important for the family to explore what assistance is available for Lee Ann's post-surgical care to help all of them cope in terms of time limitations. Although such assistance often does not completely replace the need for family, it can provide proper care for the patient while families carry on with their other responsibilities. Reactivation programs in sub-acute care and some long-term care facilities may be available in some jurisdictions, and home care options, providing nursing care and some homemaking, may be available as part of their hospital, local community-based, or insurance-supported health care program. These services may have to be supplemented through paid help in addition to whatever the family can weave together to support their mother and grandmother in getting over the immediate post-operative and return-to-home period.

It would be worth exploring whether there are friends and neighbors available to give a little help. In fact, such help may very well be readily forthcoming and may pleasantly surprise the family and Lee Ann. Although the family may not want to impose on others, often neighbors and friends feel that helping out is one of the ways to demonstrate affection and caring, so the idea of asking for help should not be dismissed out of hand.

It's a real challenge to families when they have to interrupt their busy lives to deal with a family crisis. But everyone in the family has to step back and ask, "Do I want my mother [grandmother, mother-in-law, etc.] to survive this ordeal?" After all, family should take priority in times of difficulty, and major cancer surgery is just that kind of challenge.

Lee Ann's moving into Sylvia's home is probably not ideal given the cramped space, but if another arrangement cannot be made for the immediate period after surgery this option should be reconsidered. Families can usually find ways to come together during times of crisis, and Lee Ann's surgery should be considered to be precisely that: a crisis in the making. Most employers understand when there is a family illness, and it may be necessary for family members to get some extra time off to help look after Lee Ann at Sylvia and Gerry's home until she feels secure enough to return to her own home with some home care, in addition to what her family can provide.

As for David, this is a time to test his relationships. It would seem reasonable to expect one's significant other to compromise on vacation plans if a family member's health is at stake. David's moving in with his mother for a week might make all the difference, with a little supplement from home care professionals and homemakers, and input from other family members, including the grandchildren, in helping Lee Ann get over this difficult time. The way everyone comes together in this time of need will be a reflection of the fabric of this family. Anyone can be constructive and positive when there are no demands. It is during difficult times that a family's true strength is tested, and for Lee Ann's family, this is such a time.

If Lee Ann gets through the colon surgery without much difficulty, the issue of her hip should be a lesser challenge. First, if the colon surgery goes well, that experience should help Lee Ann and her family understand the steps necessary to negotiate the health care and home care systems. Second, there are often programs in place to assist in the rehabilitation process following major orthopedic surgery.

It would be wise for Lee Ann to wait at least three months after the colon surgery to have the hip operation. This should give her ample time to regain her emotional and physical strength and her independence. If more time for recovery is required, then the hip surgery should be done later, as the urgency for it is not great.

Lee Ann's family should inquire whether or not in-patient rehabilitation exists. Many hospitals do have rehabilitation in-patient programs or are affiliated with other organizations that provide such programs. If it does exist, plans should be made after discussions with the orthopedic surgeon and, if appropriate, the social service department of the hospital to make certain that post-operative care will include admission at an in-patient rehabilitation unit. If such an arrangement is possible, then Lee Ann's concerns about being a burden to her family and disrupting their lives change considerably. Following anywhere from four to six weeks at a rehabilitation unit, Lee Ann will in all likelihood be able to return home with minimal assistance.

Most rehabilitation programs provide some evaluation or make a referral to an outside agency to evaluate the home setting and recommend or arrange for modifications to accommodate the patient's ability to function. If the hip replacement will make Lee Ann more independent than she was prior to surgery, it is likely that little, if anything, will have to be done to the home to meet her needs. However, some safety measures might be recommended, especially in the bathroom to make sure she can bathe safely with minimal risk of falling.

If Lee Ann and her children are concerned about Lee Ann being alone in her home, they can look into an emergency response system, such as Lifeline®, or some other medical alarm system that allows individuals to call for help should they fall or injure themselves, providing a sense of security to clients and their families.

Illness poses a great challenge both to those affected by the illness and to their families. This is a special time for families to enrich their relationships and to demonstrate what they are willing and able to do for their loved ones. It has to be a cooperative affair so that there is no lingering resentment that can cause hard feelings later. What better way to demonstrate affection to a parent in special need, even the most independent parent, than to help as an act of love and devotion? That's what families are all about.

CASE STUDY 3
Eldertravel: Balancing Risks and Benefits

Traveling distances can be difficult these days even for the middle-aged, and all the more so for the elderly. Good intentions aside, any significant travel plans for the elderly must be carefully considered and, if they're to proceed, thoughtfully planned.

THE CHALLENGE

Raul Rodriguez is 80 years old. Born in Costa Rica, he moved to Canada in the early 1960s, and after two years married Kate, a Canadian woman he met a year earlier. They lived for some 20 years in Dartmouth, Nova Scotia, where Raul worked in the shipyards until he retired in 1984.

Kate gave birth to a daughter, Mandy, in 1966. They always were a close-knit family, and Kate's sudden death in an automobile accident 10 years ago devastated both Raul and Mandy.

Raul has a son, Ramon, from a previous marriage, who remained in Costa Rica and over the years built a successful restaurant business. They have always stayed in close touch; Raul would visit his homeland and son every two to three years, and Ramon has been coming to Canada three or four times a year to see his father the past decade, when Raul's health started to decline and after Kate had died. Ramon had never approved of his father's marriage to Kate, and although he'd met her only a few times, he'd always elected to dislike her, feeling strongly that his father never should have remarried.

However, Ramon felt closer to Mandy. While he didn't consider Mandy a part of his true family, he did acknowledge that she worked hard and cared a great deal for his father. Yet whenever Ramon visited, he tended to dominate the relationships. Whether staying in his father's apartment or in a hotel during his visits, Ramon would make it clear that for the duration of his stay he would look after his father and that Mandy's presence wasn't necessary.

During the winter of 2004, Raul slipped and fell on an icy patch of sidewalk while walking to a nearby grocery store. He suffered what was diagnosed as a mild concussion, broke his right arm, and fractured his right pelvis. For weeks following his release from the hospital, Mandy spent several hours every day at his apartment caring for her father and spending time with him. She did all his shopping and prepared all his meals, while helping Raul adjust to using only his left arm and hand. Since Raul also was relatively immobile because of the fractured pelvis, Mandy helped him get out of bed in the morning and into bed at night until he was able to function again.

At her father's urging, she had called Ramon to report the incident and his condition. Ramon paid a hurried visit the following week and spent two days with his father. During the visit, he urged his father to return to Costa Rica. Ramon told Raul that his business was starting to prosper and that he would look after him much better than Mandy had been. He also reminded his father that in Costa Rica he could speak his native tongue, and assured him that he would find many new friends there. Raul appreciated his son's concerns and thoughts but told him that, for the time being, he felt he should stay in what had now been his home city and homeland for some decades.

Meanwhile, Mandy continued to look after her father. She arranged for special support services and physiotherapy sessions. She asked for and got a flex-hour work schedule from her employer, which made it easier for her to manage the added caregiving responsibilities she'd assumed.

For months following his fall, Raul seemed to be making real progress with his recovery. Then one morning, he lost his balance getting out of his bathtub and fell. While he was diagnosed with nothing more severe than some bruises and a twisted ankle, somehow Raul seemed less able to recover. In fact, he required more attention and support.

Mandy arranged for in-home support and more physiotherapy sessions. But walking was now much more difficult for Raul, and he relied more and more on using a walker. Whenever Mandy took him outdoors, he was now in a wheelchair. His family physician ordered a battery of tests, and while the results were inconclusive, the doctor felt that Raul's initial fall could have caused more damage than originally suspected.

Over the following year, Raul became more and more reclusive and less and less certain of himself and his ability to walk.

During Ramon's last visit in January, he pressed his father to come to Costa Rica, at least for a few weeks' visit. He predicted Raul would enjoy and benefit from the warm weather and change of scenery and that the visit would be good for his health. He insisted that any medical needs could be arranged easily and quickly.

Raul was more receptive this time. After a long winter and feeling depressed about his condition, Raul told Mandy that perhaps a few weeks in his homeland would be good for him. Mandy couldn't disagree more. She challenged her father and Ramon, telling them that her father needed special care and that she had worked hard to arrange for him to get that care on a regular basis. She said that while the climate might be wonderful, there were just too many unknowns, and the possible risks outweighed the benefits.

While her father wavered and became indecisive, Ramon became all the more adamant. He argued passionately that his father had a right to go home and enjoy himself. He told Mandy that there was nothing she did that he couldn't do for his father, and that he was now financially well off and could arrange for anything that might be needed.

Mandy didn't know what to think or do. On the one hand, she loved her father and worried about his health and well-being. On the other hand, she started to wonder if she might be overreacting, and questioned herself about how much of her feelings were driven by Ramon's domineering behavior. She was now confused and uncertain, but she felt a nagging concern about the dangers of such a major trip for her father at his age and in his condition.

THE GERIATRICIAN'S POINT OF VIEW

Traveling can present many problems and challenges for an older person — even when for a simple vacation. When the travel situation is more complex, as it is in this case, it is important to examine all the issues and implications of the travel itself, as well as the stay in the faraway place.

In this particular situation, the issues go way beyond the trip and revolve around the relationship between Ramon and Mandy and the way each sees the relationship to his/her father. The child who flies in periodically from a faraway place often has a very disruptive impact on the family that is struggling to keep things together, especially when a frail parent's immediate caregiver is struggling to find ways to meet his many medical and psychosocial needs. Whether from a true sense of devotion or from the need to be seen as being important and to be "doing something," these fly-in-and-fly-out children may cause havoc to arrangements carefully put together for the ailing and needy parent.

The first thing that has to happen before Raul goes on a trip to Costa Rica, for however long, is for Mandy and Ramon to find a way to agree on how Raul's long-term needs will be met by the two of them. Only then should the trip to Costa Rica be contemplated. It is also very unfair to try to direct the decision to Raul, who clearly is caught between his two children and would like to please both of them in addition to wanting to feel better. Mandy and Ramon have inadvertently put an unnecessary burden on their father and they should be taking steps to eradicate that uncomfortable experience. Their mutual priority should be the care and well-being of their father. They must put aside their own needs, even the ones couched as concern for their father. Ramon would like his father in Costa Rica for a number of reasons, but one might very well be so that he can demonstrate to his friends and family just how much he cares for his father — something he cannot do from afar.

Mandy may be acting in an overprotective manner, but much of that is probably based on suspicions of her stepbrother's motivations and of his ability to take care of Raul should things not go smoothly. The real challenge for Mandy is to approach Ramon on general terms regarding their mutual care of their father. It probably would be worthwhile for Mandy to find a way to speak to Ramon openly and tell him that she is not necessarily opposed to Raul visiting Costa Rica for a short period, but that the trip must take place within a framework of a plan for the present and future of which they are both a part. The benefits would be that their father could finally feel comfortable knowing that the two of them had found a way to bridge their differences, which is something that a parent always wants. Ramon may not be aware of just how trying their lack of closeness has been for Raul, and anything that might make him feel better would be very important to him in these waning days of his life.

It might even be worthwhile to pursue whether Mandy could join her father on the trip to Costa Rica and be involved in his time there. That would probably be very meaningful for Raul and also possibly improve the relationship between Mandy and Ramon. It would then frame the trip differently — going from Ramon's arrangements for his father to his children's attempt to improve Raul's state of mind. Even if Mandy cannot stay for the whole trip, going on the flight and staying a few days to help get things settled would be beneficial if it could be arranged.

As for the trip itself, there are certain basic principles that should be kept in mind when frail seniors undertake longer trips, especially by air. Some of the factors that should be considered include the medical implications of traveling and being far away from the normal professional caregivers, the need for adequate insurance that can be counted on to cover unanticipated illness, the actual travel itself and its trials and tribulations, and the expected benefits of being in another place for a period of time.

THE MEDICAL CONDITION

One should not travel if a medical condition exists that requires frequent monitoring and has resulted in repeated, unexpected admissions to hospitals or emergency rooms. Most insurance companies will not cover individuals with such uncertain medical conditions. One guide insurance companies often use, sometimes erroneously, is whether changes to medications have occurred during a previously defined period (often 90 days). This guide sometimes does not make medical sense, as in the case of the discontinuation of a medication that is no longer necessary, or a decrease in dosage because of better outcomes of an already established treatment. The reasons for any changes, especially positive ones, should be documented by the physician to make sure that, should something happen, there is a good, sound explanation available that would not imply increased risk during the trip.

The risk of not being covered is potentially huge medical bills, especially, but not exclusively, from illness that occurs while outside the country. In Raul's case, considering his fragility and instability, it is very likely that adequate medical insurance to cover the trip will not be available. To travel without such insurance is financially very risky. Whatever decision is made about the trip, it is imperative that the necessary medications be brought along for the trip in the hand luggage and not checked in, in case there is an accidental loss of luggage. Having copies of the prescriptions is also worthwhile even though they might not be valid in another country — at least another physician would be able to see them and decide if there was a basis for renewing them based on a new assessment of the patient and the situation.

THE TRAVEL ITSELF

The trip itself might pose many problems and barriers, especially with the very long waits at airports due to heightened security. This might be a problem for frail, elderly, individuals such as Raul. Problems with behavior or potential agitation may also be reasons not to attempt to fly, as they are difficult to deal with on a plane and not fair to other passengers. For someone who has severe urinary urgency or incontinence, it's probably best not to fly at all; we all know how long the wait can be to use a washroom on an airplane. If there are problems in walking and falls might occur, it would be best to let the airline know beforehand so that arrangements can be made to provide shuttling from the check-in counter to the gate to avoid long walks. If Raul needs a wheelchair, for instance, that has to be arranged in advance with both airports. It is important to make sure that all necessary supplies, including medications, continence supplies, and, if there is a risk, a change of clothes, are easily accessible.

BENEFITS OF DESTINATION

The benefits of the trip should be weighed carefully. There are several important factors to consider: Will the trip be a vacation that will improve the person's sense of well-being? Can the trip be arranged so that it is safe? Will it relieve the person of having to face a bad winter? Will it reunite the person with a loved one? It is always necessary to make sure that there will be appropriate support and supervision to decrease potential danger. How necessary medical services will be provided and by whom, as well as who to contact in case of an emergency, must be determined before travel. In Raul's case, Ramon may be able to make many of these arrangements, because rather than the trip being a vacation in an unknown destination, it is in some ways a visit to a place of friends and family who should be able to provide the necessary support once Raul arrives.

Travel is not as easy as it once was. With good planning many people can travel safely and enjoy the benefits of warmer climates, especially during our harsh Canadian winters. If the warmer climate is part of the rationale for this trip, Ramon has to find a way to discuss openly with Mandy and, if possible, Raul all the implications of the trip. Maybe it can work, and indeed it might provide a lift to Raul's spirits and result in some improvement in the relationship between Mandy and Ramon. If there is such a chance, it might be worth the effort and potential risk. If not, and the trip might lead to further conflict and put Raul at unnecessary risk, perhaps it should be rejected as a viable option.

CASE STUDY 4
Independence: Helping Parents Live Their Lives

Sometimes in their zeal to help and protect their parents, children add to their discomfort by making decisions that may be well intentioned but actually serve to disrupt tried-and-true lifestyles. The result is increased family tension and parental angst.

THE CHALLENGE

Ivan and Sophie Bogdonovich immigrated to the United States in 1948. Their eventual arrival is a story in itself. During the depths of the Second World War, Ivan, who had been unwillingly conscripted into the Soviet army, was injured and judged unfit for further service. Instead, he was assigned to work in a factory several hundred miles from his village. Two months before the end of the war, after nearly a year at the factory, he managed to escape, work his way back to his village, and reunite for one night with his family and his young wife, Sophie.

Under the deep cover of the next night, he and his wife left their native village in the Ukraine with only the clothes on their backs and a satchel full of food. They managed to reach the Austrian border just as the war ended, and they were two of the first few to be accepted into an Austrian refugee camp, where they were interned for two years. They applied to the United States for refugee status and were eventually linked through the Red Cross with a sponsor in Bismarck, North Dakota. The sponsor was a distant relative who agreed to help them settle in Bismarck.

Ivan is now nearing 80 and Sophie is in her mid-seventies. (No one is certain of their ages, and no birth record has ever been found.) They're in fairly good health but starting to show signs of forgetfulness.

They have two sons: Boris, in his mid sixties, who was born in the Austrian refugee camp just months before the family came to the United States, and Bob, in his late-forties, who was born in Bismarck. Both brothers left home some 20 years ago and now live in Minneapolis/St.

Paul, Minnesota, about a seven-hour drive away. Because the brothers are close to each other and comfortable with their lives in Minneapolis/ St. Paul, they decided that to best help their parents, they should move them into a neighbourhood apartment so they can be close to them.

At the time of this decision, neither parent really wanted to leave Bismarck, where they had a number of friends and an active social life. They were well known in the community because, from the mid-1950s to just two years ago, they had operated a popular diner known for its spicy cabbage rolls, various potato soups, and other ethnic dishes. But Boris and Bob were persistent. During their annual visits and weekly telephone calls, the brothers made their case and finally convinced their parents that they should move to Minneapolis/St. Paul.

Nine months later, Ivan and Sophie sold their home, shipped their belongings ahead, and a week later were driven by their sons to Minneapolis/St. Paul. They had been to the Twin Cities a handful of times during the past 15 years to visit their sons, but they knew only a little about the city, which they considered to be somewhat intimidating in comparison to comfortably sized Bismarck. But as they got older, they also longed to be closer to their sons, and they knew of no other way than moving to make that possible.

Boris and Bob, who really are close to each other, very fond of their parents, and proud of what they have done with their lives, were determined to make the move a good one. After considerable searching, they found a small but attractive one-bedroom apartment for their parents, the cost of which they agreed to subsidize.

To surprise their parents, Boris and Bob arranged to have some of their parents' furniture, clothing, kitchenware, and all other belongings shipped and delivered to the apartment. They spent a full day putting the place in some kind of order that they thought would please their parents.

When Ivan and Sophie arrived, Boris's wife, Janet, Bob's wife, Adele, and Bob and Adele's two children, Jennifer, 19, and April, 17, met them at the apartment. Initially, there was much joy, and Sophie cried when she met her family and saw the new apartment, which was about equidistant from both sons' homes. She cried even more when she saw most of what was in her old home crammed into the small apartment. And so began a new life in a new place for Ivan and Sophie.

Now, months later, the euphoria of being reunited and living in the same city has waned. The first negative experience was when Ivan discovered that he was very intimidated driving in Minneapolis/St. Paul. The volume of traffic scared him, and in contrast to Bismarck, it was complicated to get around the city. Yet driving was important to him; having a car and being able to drive was, for Ivan, an important symbol of his independence. Now he was hardly driving at all.

Both Ivan and Sophie have found getting around the city without the help of their sons to be difficult, if not impossible. They find the city's public transportation complicated and confusing. There are buses, but it is sometimes necessary to change buses to get from one place to another. In short, Ivan and Sophie feel lost and confused by Minneapolis/St. Paul's size and its rather cosmopolitan culture. They miss their friends and the city that for so long was home and that they knew so well.

But worse for them is that they have a strong sense that Boris's and Bob's wives are resentful of the time their husbands spend with their parents. Neither Janet nor Adele call or come to visit very often, and when they do, or when Ivan and Sophie go to their homes for a visit or a meal, there is always a feeling of tension and discomfort. But, just as hard to bear for Ivan and Sophie is that their two granddaughters are completely alien and show no interest in or respect for them. When they spend any time at all with Jennifer and April, it's strained and unsatisfying.

After nearly nine months in Minneapolis/St. Paul, Ivan and Sophie are miserable, lonely, dejected, and depressed. They see their sons less frequently and are certain it's because the wives are exerting pressure on Boris and Bob — which, in fact, is the case.

Meanwhile, Janet and Adele continue to lobby their husbands for more of their time and for more time with their own parents. It's now become a subtle battle of wills to see whose parents will get what level of attention.

Boris and Bob are confused; they thought they'd done the right thing, for all the right reasons. They're further agitated by the behavior of their wives, which they'd never anticipated and can't fully understand.

Then, when their parents tell them they would rather return to Bismarck, the brothers are frustrated and angry. In their minds, they've been very responsible and logical, and they can't understand why their parents aren't content and, in fact, grateful. Nor can they understand why their parents don't go out on their own more often and meet people in the Ukrainian community. Both Boris and Bob have taken them to the Ukrainian Orthodox church in Minneapolis/St. Paul and to a Ukrainian social club, where they thought their parents would find some new friends.

But their parents are adamant about their unhappiness and their desire to move back to Bismarck. Even though their health is slowly deteriorating, Ivan and Sophie are still capable of independent living, and they tell their sons that while they love them dearly, this arrangement isn't working out at all.

THE GERIATRICIAN'S POINT OF VIEW

Nothing is as disappointing as disappointment. We often have ideas of what people are like and how we can create situations that will ensure their happiness or at least contentment. But these fantasies are often very different from the actualities of everyday life. That is why everyone is disappointed in the outcome of Boris and Bob's plans for their parents and the reality of Ivan and Sophie's day-to-day lives in Minneapolis/St. Paul.

Moving is hard for anyone, and a new situation is often fraught with unknown experiences and unanticipated responses. Whether a move is for work, study, or personal obligations, most people adapt out of necessity. And sometimes a move means immediate success — perhaps a better job, a nicer house, new challenges, and often new friends. But when a move happens later in life, it can be much more difficult. Most people's dearest friends are from the earlier years of life, and such bonding is not easily duplicated in later years. The shared memories and reference points for collective reminiscing, such an important part of social activity, are lost as the fabric of friendship is torn by death or by a move away.

So what happened here with this clearly caring family that might have been averted, and is there any way to salvage the situation?

First of all, a decision to move an older relative must be made with careful thought. A family can rarely be a sufficient substitute for a social network. Families may care for loved ones more in the deepest sense, but they cannot replace the normal social activities of a familiar circle of friends in a long-accustomed environment.

Before considering the move, Boris and Bob should have discussed with their parents what it was that they thought they would need in order to be reasonably satisfied, if not happy, in Minneapolis/St. Paul. If all the answers were focused on the closeness of the family, everyone might have stepped back and asked, "Is that going to be enough?" Also, some frank discussion with spouses and children should have taken place in order to avoid feelings of hurt or abandonment. Spouses or children can easily feel that their usual family time is lost when so much time and attention shifts to the care of elderly parents.

It might have been worthwhile to try out the arrangement, perhaps giving it a chance with a three- or four-month visit, using a rented apartment or house and not moving almost everything out right away. This would have given Ivan and Sophie an opportunity to figure out what there is in the new community that might be attractive enough to make the move worthwhile, separate from the anticipated need to be with family as their faculties decline and health becomes compromised.

If, after a prolonged visit, Sophie and Ivan felt that they would likely be isolated, perhaps a permanent move would not have been contemplated. Some families choose to have a number of prolonged visits to provide an opportunity for the parents to explore and make some acquaintances that might form the nucleus of new friendships should a permanent move be undertaken. The sons could not possibly fill the void left by the loss of the network that Ivan and Sophie had in Bismarck. Children are rarely friends with their parents, and the child-parent role is hard to change, even in mature years.

For their part, Ivan and Sophie should have had a heart-to-heart talk with each other to understand why they decided to make the move. They needed to understand that while they would be losing some of their present happiness in Bismarck, they would at least be with family and feel secure should something go wrong. There is nothing wrong with that choice, but when they made it, they needed to decide to dedicate themselves to finding ways to make it work, rather than comparing their new situation to what they had had before. Such a move could never result in their having the same milieu that existed with their friends in Bismarck. But if they felt that the modest amount of loneliness and lack of social network was worth the investment in the future, then they might have come to terms with the trade-off. Clearly they had the strength during their younger years to make such a choice, but in later years it was less easy to do.

Finally, Boris and Bob need not feel that they failed. They also cannot blame their families for letting their parents down. It would be an extraordinary family that could accept a major shift of attention from their lives to the needs of parents now living in the community without some feeling of resentment. This would be true even when coupled with great filial dedication to care for one's parents and those of one's spouse.

Because things are not working out, the family needs to explore the alternatives, the last one being that Ivan and Sophie be allowed to move back to Bismarck, either temporarily or permanently. A frank discussion with everyone in the family, without any blame or suggestion that anyone is at fault, might help clear the air. A counselor might help the discussion, but one is not necessary for this situation to be fully explored among everyone involved.

Sometimes people imagine the past as being better than the present. Maybe, indeed, life would be better if Ivan and Sophie moved back to Bismarck. But perhaps not; they may not be able to realign themselves with their previous network. They could try moving back for a few months, renting a suitable place that would not require them to move all their belongings again. Or they could decide as a family that the future is so risky for Ivan and Sophie that everyone is going to have to sacrifice a bit for things to work out.

Ivan and Sophie are going to have to discard their illusion that their life in Minneapolis/St. Paul is going to be as good as their life in Bismarck. They need to figure out what they can do to make it as good as possible. They clearly had the strength to make difficult moves in the past, and now they have to draw on their strength to do it again. They need to decide to force themselves to join activities or centers that might provide them with a new network of acquaintances and activities, even if they aren't ideal. The attitude with which they undertake that task will go a long way in determining their success. I have seen many of my patients resist joining a club or taking on a volunteer position only to thank me later because of the successful outcome they had when they finally took a chance.

The wives and grandchildren have to come to some agreement about how they will deal with Ivan and Sophie living nearby. This should include a commitment to spend a reasonable amount of time with them, knowing that in all likelihood things will improve with time if everyone is very caring and supportive in the beginning. It is not too late to salvage the situation.

Boris and Bob should admit to their parents that they made some mistakes moving them to Minneapolis/St. Paul, but tell them that there is a time to try to turn things around. And they should remind their parents that the reason for the decision to move in the first place was the concern that Ivan or Sophie, or both of them, might need help in the near future because of failing health. Bob and Boris would not be able to provide that help in Bismarck, and Ivan and Sophie could end up quite isolated in that community. Ivan and Sophie should agree to give the move another try for about four months. During this time they could join some social groups and really make an effort to see what might happen if they attempted to meet people and develop a new network of friends.

The agreement might be that if, after four months of everyone trying their best to explore the relationship, build on its strengths, and understand the long-term benefits for the future, things are not better, Ivan and Sophie will move back to Bismarck. If so, Boris and Bob will not have failed, nor will have their families.

In due course the situation may resolve itself, if, for example, Ivan and Sophie need medical care in Bismarck and receive it there, or if they progressively deteriorate so that they cannot look after themselves but find somewhere to stay in that community. Or perhaps after one parent dies, the one who survives will accept that there are no real choices but to rejoin the children in Minneapolis/St. Paul.

No matter what decision is made, it is important to remember that this experience was not a failure, but merely a human attempt to be a loving family. Plans don't always turn out the way we would like them to, and that is just the way things are, even when those plans are made with the best of intentions.

CASE STUDY 5
Breaking the Mould: The Rebellious Grandmother

Sometimes we make assumptions about our parents that are wrong, and that can lead to negative consequences, as in this case of an elderly woman whose daughter mistakenly decides what her mother would like to do.

THE CHALLENGE

Fatima Campenello is a 76-year-old widow who never mastered English, despite living in Canada for nearly 50 years. She and her husband, Julio, moved to Canada from their native Italy in 1964, the day after her twenty-seventh birthday. On arrival, they landed in Toronto's large Italian community, where for the first few years they lived in a one-bedroom apartment and started life anew.

Julio's cousin, who had come to Toronto several years earlier, already had a relatively good job in a bakery, and he helped Julio and Fatima settle in. While Julio soon landed a job working as a shipping dock hand at the city's food and produce terminal, Fatima found nothing after considerable searching. Eventually, though, she started cleaning homes in the area. She also spent a lot of time babysitting for neighbors and even for some of the clients for whom she cleaned. And so cleaning and looking after young children became her full-time work for many years.

In 1974, when Fatima was 37 and Julio 42, Fatima became pregnant and gave birth to their only child, Angela. While both were delighted at the arrival of the child, it was a surprise coming fairly late in their lives.

Fatima lavished time and attention on her daughter while still working five days a week cleaning homes and babysitting. If she had to babysit in the evenings, she'd often take Angela along so she could spend time with her daughter and her daughter could play with new friends.

Eventually, the Campenellos moved into a two-bedroom unit of a four-plex, still in Toronto's Italian community. Twice they made the pilgrimage back to their old hometown in southern Italy, and over the years a few relatives came to visit them.

Angela thrived in school and reveled in her cultural heritage. She learned to speak fluent Italian and to read and write in the language. Her English was also flawless. She graduated with honors from high school and went on to earn a university degree in psychology with top grades.

Once she finished her schooling, she found a job in a teen counseling center. In her late twenties, Angela married Frank Combriani, a hard-working chartered accountant whose parents had also emigrated from Italy in the early 1960s. For the first few years of their marriage, Angela and Frank lived in a downtown apartment; later they bought a small house in suburban Scarborough. When Julio retired at age 66, Fatima continued to babysit a few half-days a week. The extra income was welcome and she enjoyed the work. Over the years she had gained a strong reputation for her skill with children. In fact, she was babysitting the children of some of those she had babysat years earlier. In their increasing free time, Julio and Fatima socialized, still staying for the most part in their Italian community.

Four years ago, Julio, who'd complained with increasing frequency about headaches but had refused for the longest time to see a doctor, was diagnosed with a brain tumor. Surgery was determined to be too risky, and his age further compounded the situation. Julio died two years ago.

For a period of time after his death, Fatima continued to live on her own in their small home, but found it increasingly difficult to manage. She explored the option of finding another woman to share the house with, but that seemed complicated. She considered moving into a retirement home, but because she was in relatively good health, the notion of being around so many "old people" left her thinking that wasn't such a good idea.

That's when Angela and Frank suggested to her that she move in with them. By this time they had a five-year-old son, Frank Jr., who was about to start kindergarten, but they had a large house that included a small, self-contained apartment in the basement. After much discussion and a lot of thinking, Fatima decided that perhaps it would be a good move. She loved her daughter, and she was very fond of Frank. A month later, she made the move.

Generally, the transition was good. Fatima liked her little room and her privacy, and she also liked spending time with her grandson. She especially liked her time with her daughter and son-in-law because they could speak comfortably in Italian. She would also watch a considerable amount of Italian television programming, and every few weeks Frank or Angela would take her to visit friends in her old neighborhood.

Then Angela became pregnant again and delivered a healthy, beautiful daughter, Gabriella — which soon became "Gabby." Angela took six months off work to be home with Gabby, and life seemed to be good for all. When it was time for Angela to go back to work, she asked her mother to babysit Gabby, since she was living with them anyway and it was clear she liked spending time with her. Fatima seemed reluctant, but she did agree, and so Angela didn't give it any further thought as she resumed her work life.

As the months passed, both Frank and Angela noticed that Fatima seemed more withdrawn and, as they saw it, depressed. But whenever they asked Fatima if there was a problem or if she felt well, the response was always the same: a firm denial that anything was wrong, end of conversation. Yet neither Frank nor Angela could accept Fatima's protests, as they could see that her day-to-day behavior was becoming ever more inwardly focused.

Finally, Angela called a nearby geriatric clinic to arrange an assessment and then broke the news to her mother. She told her mother that she was simply worried about her, and disguised her true concern by explaining that, given her age, Fatima needed to be seen by those specializing in the health of the elderly.

Mother and daughter went to the clinic for the appointment. The geriatrician first met with Fatima and Angela together, and Angela explained that her mother seemed increasingly depressed. She shared that her mother was withdrawn and preferred to spend more and more time in her room, whereas just months ago she seemed to really enjoy family interaction and playing with her grandchildren. Fatima did not contradict her daughter's depiction of the situation.

Then the physician started his examination of Fatima alone, during which time he asked her what was going on from her perspective. He noted that he could not find anything physically wrong with her but was concerned about her mood. He told her she seemed down and "blue." Although her English was not perfect, Fatima was able to express herself adequately enough to explain that she didn't want to babysit her new granddaughter. Fatima explained that she'd been looking after people's children and homes for most of her life, and that she was tired of looking after others — whether they were children or adults. She said she loved her grandchildren, but she wanted to enjoy them and not feel like she had to work at it five days a week.

The geriatrician told her that she had to be honest with her daughter about her feelings, but Fatima initially balked, saying she did not want to hurt her daughter, whom she loved very much. The doctor said he would help her explain and that everything would be all right.

When the geriatrician told Angela what Fatima had said, Angela was shocked. She and Frank had assumed that because her mother had spent so much time babysitting over the years that she'd be very comfortable continuing to do so with her own grandchildren. Plus, they trusted Fatima with Gabby and Frank Jr. And, truth be known, the arrangement helped them reduce expenses. But mostly, Angela said, they had believed that her mother would thrive in looking after her grandchildren; this, after all, is what both remembered seeing so much of in their old Italian neighborhood in their youth.

Angela expressed regret that she had put her mother in this unfair situation and said she wanted to help resolve the situation in any way suitable to Fatima. With this freedom bestowed on her, Fatima generously offered a few days a week to act in her loving grandmotherly role while knowing that she had the other days for herself, to explore and grow in areas that appealed to her.

THE GERIATRICIAN'S POINT OF VIEW

The experience of Fatima, Angela, and Frank is a perfect example of wrong assumptions that may lead to family strife and, in this case, an almost pathological emotional state on the part of one member of the family. Almost any family situation can result in misunderstandings, and if they aren't addressed in an open and honest way, they can lead to family dysfunction and disruptions that last for many years and, if not dealt with, become irreversible.

Sometimes stereotyping of traditional gender-based roles may interfere with a family member's ability to fulfill his or her personal goals and expectations. Many older women recall their childhood experiences when they were directed to choose a career path or personal direction based on assumptions of what was right for a girl. Of course, nowadays that is less common, and most mature women feel they have the right and personal obligation to fulfill their own interests and aspirations. We may forget, however, that our parents may feel the same way, even though they have never had the chance to act that way in the past.

An important key to mature and respectful relationships is open and honest communication. When we feel thwarted or unable to address an important personal issue because of fear of rejection or anger or disappointment, we may turn in to ourselves and develop the kind of symptoms that Fatima manifested; in this case, what appeared to be a depressive state.

She felt trapped by the assumptions made by her daughter and her own true devotion to her child and her grandchildren. She was even willing to make the personal sacrifice of not addressing the issue with her daughter, but her deep emotional strife manifested itself in her behavior. It is fortunate that Angela, being a caring and sensitive daughter, sought to help her mother without realizing the source of her emotional problem.

Fatima did not have the courage or perhaps the practice of expressing her own wishes or needs and accepted the situation rather than disappoint her daughter. This is where a knowledgeable and sensitive physician can play a crucial role in helping to solve a family problem. The trust that most people feel toward their doctor allows the physician to use his or her experience and knowledge to influence the decisions that families may make. In this case, giving Fatima the opportunity to express herself privately to the doctor, away from her daughter, was key to figuring out what was going on. All older patients, when visiting a doctor, especially a new one, should have the opportunity to speak to the doctor alone and in confidence, if they are able to do so. Many doctors structure their interview to include all family members during the initial history-taking and then examine the patient alone, thereby allowing the person to express his or her own feelings in private. Doctors should try to structure their visits to accommodate this need to speak to the patient privately and confidentially.

Once the issue is recognized it is important to discuss it with everyone involved, and here again the physician can play a role in helping the different players in the situation understand that there is no blame involved but rather a misunderstanding that led to an unfortunate decision. In this case, Angela's response was most crucial. Had she berated her mother for not being a caring parent and grandparent, or made her feel guilty by saying that she had decided to go back to work based on knowing that Fatima would be looking after the infant, Fatima may have changed her mind, acquiesced, and then been resentful for many years to come.

This situation worked out well because of Angela's willingness to be open and respectful and the physician's insight into discerning that there was something wrong that did not fit into the usual picture of clinical depression. The result is likely to be fruitful and satisfying for everyone, with the possibility of Fatima expanding her free days or contracting them, depending on which of her activities gives her the most satisfaction. Or she may continue with the same mix of time, thereby enjoying both her family and her own new achievements and personal growth.

CASE STUDY 6
Culture Clash: Pitting Values against Needs

When hard, pragmatic decisions are required, the differing views and values of parents, their children, and those who influence them can lead to new challenges when trying to decide on the right thing to do.

THE CHALLENGE

Moshe and Miriam Greenberg were born in Poland. They were teenagers when they met in Warsaw, and both they and their families became very good friends. When the Nazis invaded their country, Moshe was 19 and Miriam had just turned 16.

As Poland crumbled under the onslaught of the Germans' massive war machine, both Moshe's and Miriam's families wanted to flee, but by then the options were few and far between. Trapped, like hundreds of thousands of other Jewish families, they tried to live their lives as normally as possible. However, that didn't last long at all.

For the first year of German occupation, Moshe and Miriam and their families remained in their homes, although day by day their world kept deteriorating until it was shattered completely when the Nazis announced they would be moved. That move, of course, was to a concentration camp. Two days before they were herded into trucks, Moshe and Miriam were married in a secret ceremony because they wanted to be together forever — whatever "forever" would come to mean for them.

What followed was almost five years of unimaginable personal terror and horror for each of them. They watched in anguish and anger as family members and friends died before their eyes or simply vanished, never to be seen again. Sometimes, Moshe and Miriam didn't know for weeks on end whether the other was even alive. But because they were young and in good health at the outset, and because they both had a fierce will to live, at war's end both were still alive — barely. It was weeks after their camp had been liberated that Moshe and Miriam were reunited, both of them mentally and physically scarred.

They slowly recovered their health, and once the emotional pain had subsided to a manageable level, Moshe and Miriam knew they had to get on with rebuilding their world, which was now empty of all their family members and most of their friends. Fortunately, Moshe had a cousin who lived in Los Angeles who sponsored them to come to America.

Moshe and Miriam adjusted to their new world with remarkable agility. Thanks to some helping hands and their own sense of drive and purpose, the young couple soon had good entry-level jobs: Moshe learned the tool and die business, while Miriam, who had a special skill with numbers, learned to be a bookkeeper in a small import-export company.

They worked hard, saved money as they could, and forged ahead. In 1952 they bought a small house in North Hollywood, and a year later Miriam gave birth to their first child, a son they named Seth. Two years later she had another son, Isaac. Helen was born 18 months later.

As the years moved on, the Greenberg family remained very close-knit. Moshe and Miriam were very traditional in their religious beliefs and practices, and carefully and thoughtfully observed all the Jewish holidays. Moshe took his sons to synagogue every Friday night and often talked to them about the importance of their heritage and the huge pains inflicted on their family and their people during the course of history, and especially during the Second World War.

Eventually, Moshe and Miriam's children reached adulthood and each went off in search of his or her own destiny. Seth became a chartered accountant and landed a good job with a San Diego-based firm specializing in the lucrative field of forensic accounting. Isaac, who had always loved music and was an accomplished pianist, studied business in university and ended up managing a number of rock groups, bands, and singers. Helen studied physiotherapy and started a small but successful clinic with three partners that grew into a real going concern.

As the children moved ahead with their own lives, Moshe noted that Seth, Isaac, and Helen and their families spent less and less time with their parents, and they seemed to drift away from the strong religious grounding he and Miriam had instilled.

Several years ago, Moshe and Miriam moved into a retirement home that had an adjacent long-term nursing facility. They continued to live fairly independently, with daily support services. Their three children and their spouses and grandchildren visited regularly and phoned often to check on them and discuss their needs.

Moshe's health has been steadily failing over the past five years. First, he was diagnosed as a diabetic. A year later, he suffered a mild heart attack that left him weakened and tentative because he was afraid of another, more severe, attack. But instead of another heart attack, Moshe suffered a stroke, and then another. Since his second stroke, Moshe has been unable to speak or move his left arm or leg. He's lost control of his bowels and is having a very difficult time chewing his food. Late last year, Moshe was transferred to a nearby Jewish-affiliated long-term nursing facility, while Miriam moved to a smaller apartment in the retirement home.

At 88, Miriam is still vigorous and mentally alert. She visits her husband at least twice a day and sometimes sits with him for several hours at a time.

Seth, Isaac, and Helen have discussed their father's health, acknowledging that he is on a course of steady deterioration. They have talked with their mother about the future, urging her to consider allowing him to pass on if there are any further complications.

Miriam was very upset about her children's suggestion and turned to her rabbi for advice. Rabbi Rubinfeld was very clear and firm in his counsel to her: the sanctity of life is more important than any other factor, he told her. He said that was true in Judaism and every other religion, and that no matter what, every effort must always be made — with no exceptions — to keep any living being alive. Miriam accepted his wisdom totally and told her children how she felt.

What her children saw, though, was a father who was a shell of the man they knew and whose life was barely liveable. But their mother made it clear that she was in charge of the situation, and that as long as she was of sound mind her first priority was to keep her husband alive. Besides, she told them, there were new medicines and treatments coming on the market almost every day, and she knew that people in their father's condition did improve sometimes, so that couldn't be ruled out, either.

In what they thought might be a good step to take, Seth, Isaac, and Helen decided that Seth should meet with Rabbi Rubinfeld and ask for his support. Seth explained to the rabbi that he and his brother and sister were worried about their father's quality of life, and he asked the rabbi to help prepare their mother for a difficult decision that was bound to have to be made sometime. The rabbi, however, was steadfast and told Seth that he couldn't help, given his own strong convictions.

Meanwhile, Moshe contracted pneumonia and required treatment with antibiotics and oxygen. He recovered, but it was clear to the physicians and nurses that he contracted pneumonia because of the difficulty he has swallowing. They felt that he would need a feeding tube to provide nourishment and fluids to maintain him and to reduce the risk of further episodes of pneumonia. The doctor at the nursing home asked Miriam what she would like to do. He said they could try feeding him again, but that if he developed another bout of pneumonia he could die from it. On the other hand, the feeding tube had some risks, although for the most part it was a fairly safe procedure.

The doctor also explained the situation to Seth when he came to check on his father. Seth called his sister and brother to tell them about the choice they had to make. One of the nurses caring for Moshe indicated to Seth in private that she thought it would be cruel to prolong their father's suffering by putting in a tube and that she could never understand families that made such a decision even though she was aware of some of the religious imperatives. On a different occasion two nurses spoke to Helen and said that Miriam was so devoted that even with a tube her father could still have some meaningful and comfortable life ahead of him.

The three siblings then arranged to visit their mother, and they pleaded with her to let events take their course without putting in a feeding tube, which they felt would just prolong their father's suffering. Only Helen was ambivalent about not feeding her father — not so much for religious reasons, but because of the idea of "starving" him, especially with her knowledge of the symbolic meaning of food for her parents because of the Holocaust experience. Seth and Isaac told their mother that while they loved their father, watching him like this was very painful for them, and they wondered if he would have wanted a feeding tube had he been able to make such a decision himself. They felt he would not.

Miriam was furious. She told Seth and Isaac that she felt they were betraying their father and their faith. She appealed to Helen for support. She said that since she was the decision-maker she simply wouldn't talk about it anymore because she believed Moshe, as an observant Jew, would want to follow Rabbi Rubinfeld's advice about the feeding tube. She reminded them of the terrible ordeal she and Moshe had experienced so many years ago and said that was evidence that one should never, ever give up on living.

Now, there is a high level of tension between Seth, Isaac, and their mother, with Helen not quite sure if her mother is right in making this decision. They would like the rabbi to be more "realistic" in the advice he is giving to their mother.

THE GERIATRICIAN'S POINT OF VIEW

Conflicts over cultural, ethnic, and religious perspectives are common in any multicultural society. In the health care profession, we usually think of the conflict as being one in which a patient and family have their own peculiar perspective which is not understood or shared by the health care team, thereby leading to unnecessary conflicts. In fact, many health care organizations and health care professionals seek ways to get advice about and assistance with cultures they do not fully understand. This is usually less so if the facility in which care is being provided is strongly affiliated with the religion in question. But even under those circumstances, there may be a range of opinion and options on what is believed to be necessary, and as a result conflict between family members or between families and staff often occurs.

Therefore, it is not that unusual for the health care staff, because of a failure to fully appreciate the nuances and interpretations of the underlying values and beliefs that determine a family's decision, to end up in situations of terrible conflict.

There are even cases, although fortunately this is not one, that have made their way through the court system because, for example, a family's belief in the sanctity of life persuaded them to demand that the patient be kept on a respirator following a severe motor vehicle accident, even though the health care team felt that the there was no chance of a good recovery and that it was a waste to continue with intensive care treatments. In other cases, some health care team members might be so intent on allowing the patient to have the final say that they fail to recognize and appreciate that in some cultures it is the accepted practice for the eldest son to make a decision and protect the parent from the pain associated with such a step.

All religious, cultural, and ethnic groups have beliefs and rituals with special meaning and importance to those who follow the tenets of the particular group involved. It is important for health care providers to understand where decisions come from so that they can best support the decision-makers.

In this particular case, the problem appears to be an estrangement of underlying values between Miriam and at least two of her children, coupled with different health care team members providing some discordant advice to family members. It is often the case that different generations with different life experiences have incongruent value systems when facing difficult end-of-life situations. As for the staff, they should avoid whenever possible providing advice based on their own personal values to a family in turmoil. Rather, they should limit their advice to the factual level of whether feeding tubes could safely provide nourishment to Moshe and decrease the risk of aspiration pneumonia or other negative clinical outcomes to his present state.

What is the best way to support this family and do everything possible to help them through a difficult period so that after Moshe dies they will still be a loving and caring family?

First of all, the children have to accept that their mother is the rightful surrogate decision-maker, whether they agree with her values or not, and that she appears to be acting in a way that is consistent with Moshe's religious beliefs. From their past actions, it is clear that Miriam and Moshe take pride in their Judaism and have expressed a commitment to follow its tenets. For most observant Jews, this would mean that when there is a difficult situation and a rabbi's advice is sought, that advice must be followed.

For Miriam, the concept of sanctity of life is very important, and its importance was emphasized to her by the rabbi she consulted. He also would have told her that providing food is an obligation except when doing so causes harm, and so giving Moshe a feeding tube would be an extension of that obligation to feed.

If Moshe was not likely to survive the pneumonia and was in fact dying, the rabbi might very well have given different advice to Miriam. For most religious Jews, the obligations concerning the care of a dying person are different; comfort becomes paramount, so a feeding tube might not be inserted.

For Miriam, it is clear that the religious rules and obligations are important to her husband, as they are to her. She would likely take great comfort after Moshe dies knowing that she assured his care was in the religious tradition of Judaism, even if the outcome was not what she wanted. If, on the other hand, she were to ignore what she believed his wishes would be, she would likely carry the guilt with her for the rest of her life and blame herself for not doing the right thing. The children, who are no longer committed to Jewish tradition and law (known as *Halacha*), may fail to appreciate that certain rules exist that may not make sense to them in a secular world. Similar value systems are shared by Muslims and many of the Catholic faith. On the other hand, people from Southeast Asia may approach the same situation differently from someone from South America and still differently from someone from the Caribbean.

Seth and Isaac may have difficulty understanding why Miriam is so intent on trying to keep their father alive when he appears to have such a poor quality of life. Helen appears to be in a better position to support her mother's wishes, whatever they may be, and that will be very important for Miriam as she struggles through this difficult period. It is terrible to feel alone when making difficult decisions and the support of a parent's children is often key to his or her ability to survive emotionally during trying situations.

It might be worthwhile for Seth and Isaac, if they have forgotten the basic tenets of Judaism when it comes to decisions such as these, to meet with the rabbi privately for an explanation of the basis of the decision. Even if they long ago abandoned their own Jewish religious beliefs, they are likely able to project sufficiently to understand the basic underpinnings of the faith and how it affects decisions. If they could successfully bring themselves to see the situation from their mother's perspective, they could likely be a great support to her. Even if in their own hearts Seth and Isaac disagree with the decision, if they can accept that it is consistent with their parents' belief system and embrace it and its possible consequences (i.e. Moshe being kept alive for a period of time with a feeding tube in place), it would go a long way to restoring family peace.

For families in which the value-based ties have been splintered, it is important that the children step back a bit and try to imagine the values of their parents. By doing this, they should be able to understand the importance of following through in the practice of the religion or culture that they hold. Many people who appear to have abandoned their religion during their adult years find comfort in the traditions and practices as they approach death. There is nothing inconsistent or hypocritical in this shift, and everything should be done to support people who need to revert to previously held beliefs, even those they may have ignored for years, if that is what makes them comfortable during their remaining days.

Seth, Isaac, and Helen should try to find a way to gather around Miriam and tell her that whatever decision she makes is the right one and that they understand the Judaic reasons for the decision and support her in that difficult choice.

If Moshe lives for many months, even if he does not improve at all, they must not waver in their support of her decision. If, on the other hand, a tube is inserted and Moshe succumbs, they can feel comfort in the fact that they supported their mother's decision to do the right thing according to Judaism. That support will give her comfort for the days, months, and years ahead when she thinks about what transpired during those terrible days of Moshe's last illness.

CASE STUDY 7
Substance Abuse:
Drinking All Day Keeps Reality Away

Parents who are unwilling or unable to cope with their lives sometimes resort to excessive drinking or taking too many medications. It is especially dangerous if drugs and alcohol are mixed, which can lead to dire consequences and to huge concerns for the children.

THE CHALLENGE

Gilles Ducet is a 78-year-old widower who lives in a small two-bedroom home in Trois Rivières, Quebec. Gilles was a construction worker from the time he left school when he was 17 until he retired at age 67. Over the years, Gilles worked hard; he was physically strong because of the type of work he did. He always liked to have a few beers with his buddies at the end of the day, followed by several shots of whiskey in the evenings after dinner. When Gilles retired, he kept drinking but began putting on weight because he wasn't nearly as physically active.

His wife, Hélène, died six years ago of cancer. They were very close and her death was a terrible blow for Gilles. He retreated into his house, and further into himself, for several years. And he drank more, although he denied it to his twin 52-year-old daughters, Eva and Estelle.

Two years ago, Gilles was in a minor car accident late one night and was charged with impaired driving. His license was suspended, and although he can now reapply for a license, he has not done so. The fact is that Gilles rarely leaves his house since the accident; the most he does outdoors is mow his small lawn in the summer and sweep the snow if it's not too deep during the long winter months.

Estelle, who is divorced and lives alone, works as a real estate broker in Trois Rivières. She visits her father once a week for an hour or two, but because she often finds him tipsy, argumentative, and moody, she rarely enjoys the visits.

Eva lives in Montreal with her second husband; they have no children and are financially secure, which in their case means they often enjoy traveling to distant destinations for several weeks at a time. Eva visits her father about once a month and calls weekly, although, like her sister, she doesn't derive much pleasure or satisfaction from the encounters.

About a year ago, Gilles met and became friends with Claudia, a widow who is ten years younger than Gilles and lives in a nearby apartment building. Claudia now spends most of her time with Gilles at his home.

In comparing notes, Estelle and Eva agree that Claudia seems to tolerate their father's drinking. In fact, they believe Gilles gives Claudia money to buy his beer and whiskey. They also find that Claudia is not particularly open or friendly with either of them, and she usually defends Gilles in any discussion about his lifestyle or drinking. As worrisome to the daughters, they believe that their father is lavishing gifts on Claudia, and that Claudia is under the misguided impression that, despite his meager lifestyle, Gilles has a lot of money.

Both Estelle and Eva have noticed over the past few months that their father's tolerance for whiskey has declined, but not his consumption. This, of course, results in his being inebriated most of the time. And recently Estelle discovered that her father is also taking tranquilizers prescribed by his doctor.

Although she didn't like doing it, Estelle called the doctor to ask him about the tranquilizers and whether he knew about Gilles's drinking. The doctor acknowledged that he knew Gilles was an occasional drinker but not that he drank as much as Estelle claimed. The doctor also confided that he gave Gilles the prescription because at his last visit Gilles said he was still very depressed about Hélène's death and about his own deteriorating condition. It was clear to Estelle from this conversation that Gilles had never talked to his doctor about his drinking and that the doctor hadn't picked up on the problem.

Estelle then called Eva, and the two of them went to visit their father. They confronted him about the drinking, but he denied that he drank too much and was very defensive. They also told him that they were worried about what to them appeared to be memory lapses and poor judgment during recent visits and telephone calls, and they wondered if mixing the liquor with the tranquilizers was wreaking havoc on his mind and body. If anything, they told their father, he seemed more depressed than ever.

Gilles was adamant in his rebuttal of his daughters' allegations and dismissed their concerns. He got quite angry and told them that his life was much better now that Claudia was part of it, how she looked after him with much more care and attention than his own daughters, and how much that meant to him. Then he told them that he'd asked Claudia to move in with him. They would both benefit, their father explained, because Gilles would always have someone around, and Claudia would be able to save the money she paid for her apartment. It was at this point in their heated exchange that Claudia arrived, and a strained, polite, and inconsequential conversation followed before Estelle and Eva left.

The sisters both went home. Later that night they had a long telephone debate about what to do and how to do it. They agreed that most worrisome for them was Claudia's move into the house with their father. Not only didn't they particularly like or trust Claudia, but more importantly they felt certain the woman would continue to supply their father with all the beer and whiskey he wanted. In addition, they feared Claudia had a self-serving agenda: to save her own money and live off Gilles's limited savings.

The more Eva and Estelle talked, the more other fears surfaced, like the thought that Claudia would somehow manipulate their father into assigning ownership of the house to her, or talk him into giving her power of attorney and then having him institutionalized, selling the house, and walking away with what was left of his modest savings. They also worried about their father's failing health and mental capacity, but they didn't know what to do next because they weren't sure Gilles's doctor was paying close enough attention to the real needs of his patient.

THE GERIATRICIAN'S POINT OF VIEW

This is a difficult situation for Gilles's daughters. They should have many concerns, the first being the psychological and physical well-being of their father.

Gilles is on a path to the almost certain severe consequences that result from consuming excessive alcohol combined with tranquilizers. The risk is twofold: first is the negative effect of alcohol on his neurological function and the potentially serious damage to other organs such as his liver, and second is the effect of his depression on his health. Alcohol and tranquilizers aggravate depression, and if no intervention takes place, Gilles will be at risk for doing something extreme such as committing suicide.

Older men have a very high suicide rate, and when they decide on the act they often succeed, using rather violent methods such as hanging or guns. If Gilles is indeed depressed over his wife's death, he might benefit from medical treatment of a combination of antidepressant medication coupled with counseling or psychotherapy.

Another confounding aspect to this situation is the role of Claudia. The children may be suspicious of her intentions, but she may, in fact, have true affection for Gilles with no ulterior motives. Whatever the situation, the daughters will likely require her co-operation in their attempt to help their father. If they find that she is an obstacle to his well-being, the situation is more complex and may require some legal action to protect their father.

Assuming that Claudia cares for Gilles but does not realize the risks of his drinking and use of tranquilizers, Estelle and Eva must discuss the situation with her. They will need Claudia's assistance to achieve their goals of getting Gilles to stop drinking and taking tranquilizers, and of getting proper treatment for his depression. They will also need the assistance of Gilles's family physician, with whom they should have a meeting.

The sequence of meetings depends on whether Claudia is in agreement with them about Gilles's condition or is part of the problem. If Claudia proves to be an ally, she might join them when they meet with the doctor. Or she might prefer to defer to the daughters to outline the situation to the doctor and confirm that she is willing to co-operate in any fashion required to assist Gilles if she indeed cares a lot for him.

At the meeting with the doctor, the daughters must impress upon him that they are observing serious changes in their father's mood and cognitive function. They must use words and examples that describe sufficiently their observations so that the doctor can understand that Gilles is doing his best to hide the extent of his drinking and is not adequately expressing the degree of his depression. If the physician agrees to assist Estelle and Eva, an appointment should be made for Gilles to see the doctor. This can be arranged either by the daughters or at the initiation of the doctor.

The daughters should explain to Gilles that they have concerns about his drinking and that they really believe a visit to the doctor would be helpful. If he refuses, the doctor might be able to assist by calling Gilles and asking him to visit to make sure that he is all right. Subterfuge in such situations does not usually work because the whole process should be based on trust, and if Gilles begins to not trust his daughters' dedication to him, it will be very hard to resolve this complex situation.

If Gilles agrees to visit his physician, and if Claudia agrees with and supports the goal of decreasing Gilles's alcohol consumption, Claudia should accompany the daughters on the visit. Then, together, they can express their love and devotion to Gilles and their desire to help him.

The physician can be extremely helpful in how he approaches Gilles's drinking problem. It is well known that people who abuse alcohol and other drugs that effect mood usually deny their problem. An approach by the physician that is non-judgmental, but that focuses on the effects on Gilles's mental function, is likely to have the best impact. People like Gilles are more likely to listen to a straightforward explanation that continuous exposure of the brain to alcohol can lead to a condition of dementia similar to Alzheimer's disease. Few people are willing to risk the loss of their cognitive function when the implications are laid out (e.g., loss of independence, loss of memory and judgment, inability to perform simple tasks such as dressing and going to the toilet). A discussion about the negative effect on sexual function may also be effective. Gilles may already be aware of this phenomenon but not realize the connection to alcohol use. This discussion should include the potential benefits of using a proper combined therapy for depression with antidepressant medication and counseling.

One visit to the doctor may not be sufficient. The physician should be willing to initiate a process by which to assist Gilles in the very challenging process of recognizing that there is a problem and then taking the steps to address it. The physician may suggest counseling from a social worker or psychologist if there is someone with that expertise available. There may be a special program in the community available for people dealing with substance abuse (the term often used for excessive use of alcohol and medications that affect the brain's function). If so, the physician may recommend that Gilles should access such services.

The most important part of the process is a commitment to help Gilles even if he does not follow through exactly as everyone would like. Sometimes an agreement to cut back gradually on the amount of alcohol consumed is a reasonable first step. This type of arrangement is important to consider because alcohol abusers usually can't imagine completely discontinuing their drinking. Also, when alcohol consumption is suddenly discontinued there is a potential danger of seizures occurring, which can be very frightening and sometimes cause serious injury. So a gradual approach with the support of everyone who cares for Gilles is necessary to achieve the goal.

If things go well, Gilles will gradually decrease his alcohol intake and the tranquilizers will be discontinued also in a gradual fashion to avoid rebound effects. At some point a decision will likely be made to undertake treatment with antidepressants. It is preferable to discontinue using alcohol before starting these drugs, but sometimes, if small doses are started and the results carefully monitored, antidepressants can be introduced while alcohol intake is reduced. Sometimes antidepressant therapy improves the patient's mental state so that the commitment to stop drinking becomes stronger and is more readily implemented.

If these steps are followed through, there is a good chance that Gilles can cease his alcohol abuse and respond properly to antidepressant therapy. He can then have a full relationship with his daughters and, if it proves appropriate, with Claudia.

If the situation proves to be more difficult — with Gilles denying there is a problem and Claudia ignoring the concerns of his daughters — the approach is more complex and may require legal intervention. If Claudia is acting in a malicious manner and taking advantage of Gilles, then Eva and Estelle are faced with finding a way to have her influence on Gilles diminished or removed altogether. This will not be easy and may result in Gilles and his daughters becoming alienated. If Eva and Estelle are convinced that no alternative is possible, they may have to pursue a legally based course of action. If this is necessary, Gilles may not be amenable to the course of action that is best for him in terms of his alcohol use.

The last option for Estelle and Eva is to let things go and not do anything until some crisis occurs, which may allow them to intervene without causing an affront to Gilles. Such a crisis might be a severe medical consequence of his drinking, such as bleeding from his stomach, a seizure, or severe loss of mental competence that forces decision-making upon the daughters. This is not the way anyone would want the situation resolved, but it may be the only viable option to avoid severe alienation and disruption of the family's fabric and integrity.

CASE STUDY 8
Sexuality, Romance, and the Family: When Children Worry about Their Parents

What do you do when your elderly mother or father becomes romantically involved at a stage of life when you think such relationships are no longer appropriate?

THE CHALLENGE

It wasn't easy for Sandra and Denise. On one of their recent visits to the nursing home they were told that their 87-year-old mother, Margaret, experiencing moderate Alzheimer's dementia, was becoming romantically involved with Gerald, a gentleman in the same unit. Sandra and Denise had been feeling quite comfortable during the past year or so since Margaret had moved into the home, as they saw that rather than appearing lonely — which had been the case when she was living at home, even with all kinds of community supports — she seemed quite happy in her new environment. They had heard from the staff that she was attending arts and crafts activities and social events and had perked up since her admission, even though her memory was still quite poor.

Both the head nurse and social worker told Margaret's daughters that Margaret was showing signs of becoming quite attached to Gerald, who had moved into the home about five months ago and had a mild degree of cognitive impairment. The social worker, for reasons of confidentiality, could not reveal to the daughters that Gerald had been admitted because he had sustained a stroke from which he made a good recovery. He had been living more and more in isolation, and his family felt that it wasn't safe for him to be on his own anymore, so the nursing home seemed to be the best option. He required, in fact, relatively little nursing care, and he participated in all the creative and social activities of the nursing home in general and his unit in particular. One of his favorite activities was dancing, and he started to attend the weekly social event that had dancing, to which Margaret often went. They had started dancing together and were already recognized as very good dance partners.

The two sisters heard from the unit staff that Margaret and Gerald were spending more and more time together, and that their relationship seemed to be taking on a romantic flavor.

Gerald's two sons, Ralph and Phillip, and his daughter, Brenda, were also aware of the growing relationship but didn't seem to be upset by it. They'd mentioned that following their mother's death four years previously, Gerald had a female companion for a while, but after that faded he expressed loneliness, and then the decision was made to move him into the nursing home. They see the new relationship with Margaret as having a very positive effect on their father and heard that the staff thought the same about the effect on her. The three children indicated that they'd be happy to meet with Margaret's children, but Sandra and Denise have rejected that offer. Since they visit at different times due to work schedules, they haven't yet bumped into each other even informally. But it's just a matter of time before that happens, and the staff is concerned about how they may interact with each other if a formal meeting to discuss the issue is not arranged.

The social worker and one of the senior nurses explained to Denise and Sandra that they have spoken to Margaret about her relationship with Gerald and she seems to be able to express her feelings and enjoyment of their romantic relationship. If anything, they say that she likes to talk about it and at times expresses very acceptable insights into the relationship, such as, "He makes me laugh," "He makes me feel good," "He reminds of my days with my late husband, Larry, and the fun we used to have," and "I feel like a young girl again." Sandra and Denise discount such comments as being irrelevant to the discussion and revert back to the diagnosis of Alzheimer's disease and their understanding of her incapacity for decision-making.

Sandra and Denise are concerned about what the relationship might lead to, as they have recently observed their mother acting very affectionately with Gerald and believe that she might end up in a sexual rather than just a romantic relationship. In fact, they asked for a formal meeting with the social worker and head nurse. "You have to stop this relation-ship from going any further. Our mother is not able to understand what is happening to her and she could end up in a difficult position if we do not protect her," they said at the meeting.

"It's not really possible to stop them unless you were to remove her from the unit, or if Gerald is transferred, but his children are very happy with where he is," the social worker explained.

Sandra replied, "We are very happy with the unit as well, and until this happened we'd never have thought of moving her. She was here first, so we don't understand why he can't be moved so that our mother is protected."

The staff suggested that maybe further discussions should take place with the facility's ethicist in attendance. There were, according to staff observations, many issues involved for which an ethics perspective might be worthwhile. One of the concerns they discussed among themselves was what would happen if the relationship were allowed to progress: Where could Margaret and Gerald go for privacy, since the unit had only double rooms and each of them had a roommate? Also, the structure of the unit didn't facilitate privacy in general, and staff members expressed concern that should the relationship become overtly sexual, it might dis-turb other residents of the floor or lead to a degree of discomfort among other residents and for Margaret and Gerald.

THE GERIATRICIAN'S POINT OF VIEW

Sandra and Denise's concern about their mother is understandable. But before they take it upon themselves to force the nursing home to try to separate their mother from Gerald, they should really step back a bit and look at the situation through their mother's eyes.

Margaret was always a very warm and affectionate woman, they both admit. She adored their father, and after his death often talked about how lonely she was. She was an attractive woman, and her daughters won-dered for the first few years after their father died if she might connect with another man, especially at the senior's club or the bridge group she belonged to where there were some eligible men. But she never mentioned that she had any interest.

There was once a neighbor who seemed to be interested in her, but Margaret told her daughters that he was "just being a good and helpful neighbor," and then he connected with a woman a good deal younger, and that stopped any musings about a possible relationship. When she started becoming forgetful, she would sometimes appear to lose some of her natural inhibitions and become a bit flirtatious with men, but they did not take it seriously and believed it was just part of her charm that endeared her to everyone.

But now they are concerned. Although Sandra and Denise admit that she seems very happy and acknowledge intellectually to the social worker that the romantic relationship might be responsible for that sense of well-being, they cannot accept that it could lead to physical sexuality. Even though they consider themselves liberal when it comes to sexuality, the sisters exclude their mother's case from their views, since because of her Alzheimer's disease they do not believe that she really knows what she is doing. They have tried to give her the opportunity to be involved in many decisions about herself, such as choosing which furniture she has in her room and the clothes that she has recently bought and whether or not she wants new glasses, but both Sandra and Denise are adamant that a romantic, and possibly a sexual, relationship is beyond Margaret's mental capabilities.

The social worker asked them again if they would discuss the situation with Ralph, Phillip, and Brenda, but the daughters made it clear that the issue is too sensitive for them and that they never discussed sexuality with their mother even during their younger adult years. They admit that they would not even know how to broach the subject without being excessively embarrassed.

One of the problems that children of those suffering from Alzheimer's disease often encounter is determining how much decision-making they can leave up to their parent. Years ago it was believed that a person with Alzheimer's dementia who was deemed incompetent could not be left to make any personal decisions. During the past decade or more, that view has changed considerably.

It is now believed, and clinical practice supports the premise, that competency (often called "capacity") for making decisions relates to the nature of the task under consideration. Therefore, there has been a move to engage and permit many more personal decisions to be made by individuals with Alzheimer's disease, including some of a serious nature related to health care. Some Alzheimer-afflicted individuals appear to be able to accept or refuse serious medical treatments, or to accept or refuse the need to move into a nursing home. Often, they can decide which family member they would like to have make decisions for them should they not be able to do so at some future date. The issue of romance and sexuality very well may be an area where those with mild or even moderate dementia are able to make reasonable and appropriate choices, and depriving them of this option would undermine the important principle of respecting their decision-making and personal dignity.

We know that even when there is no problem with memory or cognition, families may find it difficult when an elderly single parent develops a romantic relationship. There are all kinds of reasons for such feelings, including guilt for the deceased parent, concerns about what other family members and friends might think, and sometimes concerns about money and property should the relationship result in marriage and what is perceived as an interloper enters into the family structure. Not every child is able to look beyond these issues and focus on the well-being and apparent happiness of a parent, just as parents often try to protect their children when they think they are not in a good relationship. Many of us have had such an experience and use it as the basis when we respond to a new stage in the romantic situation of a parent, even a well one.

With concerns about dementia, and perhaps the fear of exploitation and possible harm, it is understandable that Sandra and Denise are reacting the way they are toward Gerald and the nursing home, which they feel may be complicit in the blossoming of this romance by not impeding its further development. They fault the nursing home for not telling them sooner or trying to separate Margaret and Gerald at social events. They even think the nursing home should have told Gerald's children that he would have to be moved to another floor, although they realize that he has just as much a right to stay on his current floor and that his children are very content with where he lives and the fact that he has found a female companion who seems to make him happy.

As for the nursing home staff, they are of two minds. Some who are very sensitive to the need for interpersonal relationships among their residents think that what is happening between Margaret and Gerald is a very nice development. They feel that both have the mental capacity to be involved with each other and that no one is being exploited. They have witnessed the good feeling between the two of them and know of previous situations where such relationships have developed and have been very positive. Staff members are even trying to figure out how they could provide Gerald and Margaret with adequate privacy should their relationship become sexual, so that other residents of the floor and staff members are not embarrassed. They know that some organizations have privacy rooms for this very purpose and wonder if the administration should be asked to make some renovations to the rather large day room so that a small privacy suite could be built for Margaret and Gerald and any other couple that may want to be alone together from time to time.

Other members of the staff are mortified. For personal and what they perceive to be ethical reasons, they think the nursing home should take steps to stop further development of the situation, "before it goes too far." They support Sandra and Denise in their concerns and discount the arguments to respect the relationship made by the social worker and by Philip, Brenda, and Ralph, who are happy that their father has become involved in such a way.

Sandra and Denise must consider the repercussions if they act forcibly to end the relationship between their mother and Gerald. They cannot in all likelihood force the nursing home to move Gerald from the floor to another unit against his will and for no clinical reason, and they know that his children would not agree to it. They do not want to move their mother if they can help it, because they acknowledge that she is flourishing on the unit and that the staff really like her. They would not consider moving her to another facility for the same reason, and because they recall Margaret's reluctance to move into the facility in the first place. The sisters believe a move to another facility might be devastating for their mother.

They want the best for their mother, but they also want to protect her. They may have to go along with the development of the relationship and try to assess whether it is doing more good than harm. Although this might not be easy for them, it is probably the best thing they can do to protect Margaret's dignity while trying to look after her best interests.

In addition, rather than maintaining what has become a somewhat adversarial relationship with Brenda, Philip, and Ralph, they should try to engage them so that together they can look at what is happening to their respective parents and agree to common goals and measurements to assure themselves that the relationship is providing more good than harm for both parties. This way, should interventions be necessary, they can be carried out in a cooperative rather than an adversarial way. Since it is likely that everyone wants the same outcome — the well-being of their parent — each family can agree to respect and support the other in this common goal. Such an arrangement would also make it easier for the staff of the nursing home to assess and respond to this budding romance without fear of alienating one family while pleasing the other. This way, everyone involved can deal with the situation in a manner that above all maintains love, respect, and dignity.

CASE STUDY 9
Tapping the Human Spirit: It's Never too Late to Create

An elderly parent is losing a sense of purpose, having no driving ambition and few interests. The challenge is to stimulate and invigorate that parent so there will be a regained sense of discovery and satisfaction.

THE CHALLENGE

Lisa called the clinic secretary again: "I'm really worried about my father. He's begun to say that life is not worth living again, which he hasn't done for more than a year," she reported. The secretary said she would try to arrange for someone to speak to Sam, Lisa's father, an 86-year-old retired family doctor who's been an occasional patient of the geriatric clinic for more than five years.

There already was an appointment scheduled to see Sam in three weeks as a follow-up to a previous appointment two months ago. Since he moved into a retirement home, Lisa reported, Sam's mood has become much more subdued, and, in fact, more passive in general.

An appointment was made with the outreach psychiatry team while the staff at the retirement home was asked to make sure that Sam was managing and safe, given his negative attitude. Over the ensuing few days, a social worker from the outreach team spoke with Sam and Lisa, as well as the nursing director of the home, who was able to discuss the issues with Sam. It appeared that although he was very sad, there was no indication that Sam was experiencing a major depression at a level that would endanger him. Sam told the nursing director that he was looking forward to the appointment, because he had "lots to talk about."

Arriving for the appointment, Sam, as usual, was very well dressed and looked quite well, according to the secretary who signed him in on his arrival at the geriatric clinic. The medical resident, who talked with him as part of the educational experience with the consultant geriatrician, saw Sam first. "He expresses some despair over his life and that he has nothing much to do, which seems to have been exaggerated since he moved into the home, with all of the 'old folks,'" noted the resident in his report. The resident added, "He continues to eat and sleeps pretty well, and takes his medications as prescribed for his high blood pressure and diabetes and high cholesterol and the last laboratory results that were sent to us were quite good."

The geriatrician and the medical resident then met with Sam; he had come without his daughter, as was his usual habit — he liked the privacy of the interactions but agreed that the geriatrician could speak to his daughter about the visit if she called, which he expected she would do; being his only daughter, he knew that she often worried about him. He also admitted that he was in the habit of expressing his feelings to her. Sam acknowledged that sometimes it might worry her, but he also knew that if she were involved she would help get things done.

He had agreed to move into the retirement home, partially at her prodding, because Sam recognized that he could no longer manage in the house that he had lived in alone since his wife's death eight years ago. Although he felt he could manage in his home, it was becoming clear that he needed lots of help; he no longer drove and was becoming dependent on Lisa for all kinds of ordinary activities and admitted that he was also becoming very lonely.

Sam began to explain how he felt to the geriatrician and the medical resident. "Since I moved into the home, I feel that this must be the last stage," he said. "I've lost my independence and the place is full of 'old' people, at least people who are needier than I am. But in the last two weeks, since I received all those calls, I've started looking at what I might do at the home to make things a bit better. I feel a bit bad that Calvin Able, who was my psychologist and friend for many years, has moved away so I don't really have the kind of support that I really needed during the past few months with the move and everything else that happened to me."

The geriatrician and medical resident reviewed the medical issues and felt that everything was quite well controlled and the medications taken properly. Previous attempts to control his mood with antidepressants hadn't been successful mainly because of side-effects, and it was felt that the present situation was not a manifestation of a true and deep depressive illness, but rather an existential feeling of worthlessness and lack of meaning, which could be put into perspective considering his past professional life and his gradual losses, culminating in the move into the retirement home, which Sam saw as the end, with little to look forward to, especially with evidence of aging all around him.

It was agreed that the geriatrician and medical resident would explore options with Sam when they went in to visit him together.

THE GERIATRICIAN'S POINT OF VIEW

It is fairly common for older people to feel a loss of meaningfulness and experience various physical illnesses as they age, and in response they do not see any real positive aspect of their future lives. Their reaction depends a great deal on personality and previous experiences and how they have dealt with the many losses of life and the challenges of inter-personal relationships in the past. It seems that men who have been focused during their adult years primarily on their work or profession often suffer the greatest sense of loss when they can no longer participate in those activities that once gave them purpose and a sense of impor-tance. For whatever myriad reasons, women appear to cope better with late-life challenges. Perhaps it is because women are often more involved in family-related activities, even if they have had work or professional responsibilities as well.

In the world of retirement planning, one of the recommendations to people to help them avoid feelings of emptiness and loss of purpose is to develop interests and activities while they are still working which they can develop further and enjoy when the work part of their lives is over. I recall visiting one elderly gentleman whose house was full of won-derful woodworked cabinets and furniture. He explained that after he retired, he realized that he would go crazy if he did not have something to do. He had some previous experience with woodworking and decided to enhance his skills with some adult education courses and started redoing his house, resulting in a marvelous dwelling with beautifully crafted items that added not only to the beauty of the house but also to its resale value.

Sam, who had been a practicing doctor for almost 50 years, retired ten years ago, against his desires but at the request of his daughter and the advice of his own physician, who felt that it was time for Sam to hang up his shingle. He had very little in the way of outside interests, and when his wife died three years later Sam was quite devastated. For the first few years of retirement, Sam tried to attend medical meetings and see old friends and younger colleagues, but that gradually became very disappointing, as after the few pleasantries about how he was doing and how retirement was treating him he could not really participate in the world of medical practice, which was often the underlying focus of the meetings. It was clear he liked being called "Doctor," which was understandable, and he enjoyed telling anecdotes, often with great vividness, about his practice and the history of medicine during his time.

The geriatrician and resident during their interview asked him if he liked to write. He answered "Why did you ask me that? I was actually thinking that maybe I should try doing a bit of a diary, but am not sure who would read it." The geriatrician recounted a story of one of his patients from some years ago who had retired from being the CEO of a large company he owned, and after he stopped working he just fell apart. His wife brought him to the geriatrician because she was sure he was "losing it," when in fact it was his sense of loss that was giving him the appearance of depression. He had expressed a feeling of worthlessness, and at the age of 70 said he felt it was too soon for it all to be over. Although he liked visiting his children and grandchildren, that family time and the few trips he took with his wife failed to provide much excitement and challenge in his life. He did not like golf very much and, in any event, could not see playing it more than once or twice a month.

As the geriatrician and that patient discussed possible options, the patient looked over the geriatrician's shoulder at the computer, which was sitting on his desk and said, "I have thought about getting me one of those."

When the geriatrician asked him, "One of what?" as he turned around and realized that he was pointing to his computer. "Why is that?" he asked.

"You know" the patient said to the geriatrician, "I was in the British merchant navy during the Second World War. I crossed the Atlantic many times from '41 to '44 and lived through some harrowing times. I was torpedoed, abandoned ship, dealt with U-boats and aircraft attacks, and managed to survive even in situations where I lost a lot of my friends from the ship. I have always wanted to tell my story."

"So what is keeping you from doing it? Can you type?" the geriatrician asked.

He said that although he could not type fast, he could peck on the keyboard because he had worked himself up in his company and at one time did a lot of his own typing when he could not afford a secretary, and his wife, who usually helped him, was busy with their growing family. And then he said, "I am sure I can learn if I really wanted to."

The geriatrician responded, "I am sure you can, and I think it's a great idea."

A few months later the retired executive returned with his wife for a follow-up visit. The geriatrician hardly recognized him when he came into the clinic area, as he appeared engaged and animated while registering with the secretary. The geriatrician looked at his wife, who smiled and nodded in a way that seemed to be positive. When the patient came into the office, the first thing he said was, "I am up to 1942 and I have been torpedoed for the first time. We haven't been rescued yet. We're still in life boats."

The geriatrician asked him to elaborate. "I told you I was going to do my memoirs of the merchant navy and the war and my experiences. I've written quite a lot and have reached the first time I was torpedoed. Ships I served on sank twice, and once we were hit but the damage didn't keep us from continuing the trip, sort of limping along. I think I'm capturing it all."

He no longer had that sense of having no direction and indicated that he did not care if the book got published, as long as it was there for his family to see whenever they wanted to know more about his life. The geriatrician wished him well and told him how much he admired him, not only for his war service, but also for putting it all down on paper.

After that story, Sam looked at the geriatrician and the resident and said, "You think I should do that as well?"

The geriatrician nodded yes and told him that he would be happy to look at what he wrote, as it would teach him a bit about the history of local medical practice. The geriatrician, as it were, grew up elsewhere and did most of his training overseas and much later in time than Sam did his. Sam left the office and agreed to think seriously about his new goal and how it might give him something meaningful to do.

Finding meaning in life is very important to every one of us. Family members often recognize when their loved one acts in a way that reflects a loss of self-worth: the way they speak, the absence of spark, and the negative commentaries. During our younger and mature adult years, it is the very common and mundane things, mixed with little jewels of insight, delight, and a sense of accomplishment, that make up our lives. When we cook a meal, we want to know that it is good and hope that someone will tell us so. When we get a haircut, we want to hear that our new look is pleasing. These are the kinds of simple but important things that connect people.

There are many ways to bring meaning back into the lives of those we love who, for one reason or another, seem to have lost their spark of interest and excitement. Writing is just one of the many creative ways to excite the mind.

Art, whether painting or sculpture or silk-screening, can do the same, and recognition of this fact has resulted in many artistic activities being offered to seniors, drawing on innate talents and arousing interest in creativity. Outside the office of the geriatrician in question there are two paintings by a woman who in her late seventies began to draw and became an acknowledged late-age artist with pictures hung in many parts of the geriatric facility in which she lived, the two near the geriatrician's office being full of life and spirit and color.

Music is another way to express one's joy and interest in life and its potential for delight. It is common to observe music programs for seniors who have significant cognitive impairment and yet can respond very well to sounds, rhythms, and melodies that evoke wonderful feelings from their past. There are choirs in which seniors excel, and the need to be at a place for rehearsal and performance can be a very strong, motivating force that gives excitement and a sense of satisfaction to an older person.

Roz, the mother of Dr. Gordon, whose story is told later on in the book, continued to participate in dance until just before her final illness.

Involved in dance since her adolescent years, she always found a way to dance at any gathering where it was possible. She joined groups of folk dancers and, if given a chance, was happy to perform to bring joy to others. During her final days, after her devastating stroke, one of the first ways she showed any movement of her paralyzed leg was to move her toes to music that was provided to her through earphones and to point her toe in the way she would when she demonstrated a ballet step.

There are many ways to be creative besides participating in the arts, music, and writing. For some, gardening might do it, and for others photography or flower arranging. It does not matter what one chooses to do, as long as it draws on one's sense of creativity. It should also be something that one can share with family and friends and evoke the kind of feedback and encouragement that gives meaning and satisfaction.

One man known to Dr. Gordon loved to make small wooden toys and items for his grandchildren. Nothing gave him more joy than seeing them play with something he made or hearing one of his granddaughters tell a friend that the little chairs they were sitting on were made by her grandpa. Dr. Gordon's mother started making kitchen aprons in her seventies and would bring one to every household she visited when she wanted to give a personal gift. Years after her death, her relatives to whom she gave aprons long ago continued to wear them, and continued to extol the beauty, usefulness, and love that came with those aprons because they were made by someone for whom they cared.

Children can help their parents find their creative spirit in many ways. When possible, they should provide opportunities for their parents to participate in creative activities and share their joy of accomplishment — that is all any of us want from our lives: to do things that have meaning and thereby give meaning to our lives.

CASE STUDY 10
Siblings: In Charge and On the Attack

When brothers and sisters vie for attention and favor from an elderly parent, the inevitable outcome is sibling rivalry and mutual distrust. If ever there is a time for siblings to pull together, it's when a parent is in failing health.

THE CHALLENGE

Edna Delaney lives in a retirement home in Seattle. She's a vigorous, high-energy 84-year-old, but she is showing early signs of dementia that her doctor says is likely Alzheimer's disease. She's been highly independent since the death of her husband, Frank. From the time he suffered a massive heart attack, Edna blossomed in terms of managing his care and their family finances. Three years after his heart attack, and after steadily declining health, Frank died. Edna grieved greatly, and then she seemed to put Frank's death, but not her ongoing love of him, behind her, and decided she wanted to live what was left of her life to the fullest.

Edna has four children: Frank Jr., 57, a lawyer who specializes in estate planning and lives with his family in nearby Tacoma; Joan, 53, a housewife who lives with her family in Olympia, about 60 miles away; Roger, 51, divorced and living in Los Angeles where he works as an on-again, off-again scriptwriter for various television shows; and Heather, 50, who lives with her second husband and their three children in Chicago, where she sells real estate.

When their father died, there was some discussion among the four siblings of the best way to help their mother. It was agreed that Frank Jr. and Joan would take lead roles, since they were in closest proximity to their mother. Both Roger and Heather pledged to help as needed.

About six months after his father was buried, Frank Jr. talked with his mother about what help she felt she really needed and what other help she wanted. In that discussion, Edna made it clear that she wanted to remain as independent as possible and not rely on her children. However, she also made it clear that she wanted to stay in touch with them on a regular basis. She said she favored none over the others and that she felt that they were all equal in terms of her affection and attention.

Financially, Edna is in extremely good condition. Her husband was very successful in real estate and in the stock market, and Edna's net worth is somewhere in the area of $3.5 million. The greater concern — at least on the surface — is her health and well-being.

All four Delaney children have a pretty good idea of their mother's financial worth. Frank Jr. has a high income that he's invested wisely, and he is the least concerned about any possible inheritance. Roger, in contrast, is the most financially insecure, because his work is sporadic while his lifestyle is pretty expensive, and he's very aware of what a good inheritance could do for his life.

During the past year, Edna has become increasingly confused, uncertain, and forgetful. She's fallen several times in her apartment, lying on the floor until either the maid service found her or it was noticed that she wasn't present in the dining room for a meal. Although she has been given a panic button to wear around her neck to use in precisely such situations, Edna — either in her stubborn wish for independence or because of her forgetfulness — more often than not leaves the button in her night table drawer.

Because of these experiences, the administrator at Edna's retirement home called Frank Jr. a few weeks ago and explained that his mother required more attention than the home could offer. He suggested that Frank consider how to ensure she gets the level of attention that she increasingly seems to need. They discussed increasing the care provided on-site with some in-home supplementary services and even a move to the assisted living level in the home or alternatively to a nursing home, although the latter option is one they both believe she would strongly resist.

In addition, a few weeks ago during Edna's annual physical examination, her doctor surmised, based on her movements and a slight tilt to one side, that she may have had a mild stroke. The doctor has scheduled her for a CT scan to see if there is any evidence to support the observations.

But the doctor did tell Edna — and also called Frank Jr. to advise him — that there could be other smaller strokes and that there is a potential for a more serious stroke to occur because of Edna's weight, eating habits, and past history of heavy smoking.

Frank Jr. shared this information with his brother and sisters. They all agreed at the time that he should take the lead in ensuring their mother has the care that she needs. Based on this collective decision, Frank Jr. has decided that his mother needs more in-home help. He has arranged for her to be moved to a larger apartment in the retirement home and has hired a caregiver, with backup support. In all, Edna's accommodation, meals, and care are now costing nearly $8,000 a month.

Edna has been prescribed medications to improve her function and decrease the likelihood of further strokes, and Frank Jr. has arranged for the pills to be dispensed in such a way that Edna will be more likely to take them correctly. The increase in help is imperative now that her medication regimen is more complex and her care needs are increasing.

Roger, who seldom called or visited his mother in the past, now calls her every other day. He has visited her twice in the past six months. Edna confides to Frank Jr. that Roger has suggested that she should move to California to be near him. Roger has also impressed on his mother that the weather there would be better for her. Plus, in all his calls, Roger has probed about her will — again, something Edna tells Frank Jr. — and has urged her to consider which of her children needs and deserves more of her money when she passes away.

Frank Jr., having reflected on all he's learned and been told, urges his mother to think through what she wants to do with her will, which hasn't been revised since before her husband died. But he's reluctant to give advice. Despite his vocation, it's an uncomfortable situation for Frank Jr. since this isn't just a client — it's his mother. Heather, in her weekly telephone call, urges her mother to write a new will and plan her life to suit her own level of comfort and needs, pointing out that all her children are adults and can and should look after themselves without depending on her. Finally, Joan, who visits her mother once a month, is subtly lobbying her mother by reminding Edna that she's always there for her and that she comes to see her regularly.

When Frank Jr. conducts an inventory of the state of the family affairs, he realizes that none of Edna's children are really talking to the others about the situation and how best to manage it. He's troubled by this, but not quite certain what to do about it. While Frank is busy with his day-to-day work and thinking about how to talk with his mother, Roger arrives for another visit. During that weekend, Roger applies great pressure on Edna to move to Los Angeles and to give him power of attorney over her financial affairs and her health needs. He vows to look after her, telling his mother that he's the only one who doesn't have family to support and, therefore, he can devote his time and attention to her well-being.

Edna tells Frank Jr. about Roger's thoughtful suggestion. But she's already confused, and when Frank Jr. tells her to think about what's best for her, she confides that Roger made it clear that he was the one who could care for her best.

A week later, Roger calls his brother and sisters and makes his case for being the prime caregiver and moving their mother to Los Angeles. He's adamant in his position and pleads for support. Heather is concerned; worried that Roger has a self-serving agenda. Joan doesn't know what to think, except that Roger is going to end up with a lot of money. And Frank Jr. is worried that his mother will give in to the pressure being exerted by Roger.

None of the siblings feels comfortable with the others, or with the way things are shaping up. Nor do any of them know what to do, or how to do it, except for Roger, who the others believe has a clear agenda.

Suddenly, there is growing doubt and concern among them and a sense that perhaps they must jockey for their mother's attention and favor.

THE GERIATRICIAN'S POINT OF VIEW

The primary focus of all of these deliberations must be Edna. If any of the children forget this, there must be a way of reminding them clearly, while things are still reasonably stable and before there is a crisis in Edna's care needs or a breakdown in the relationship of the siblings. This may require a family meeting, even if it means that all of them have to visit Seattle. If that is impossible, they should plan a conference call in which they all can participate. If their basic relationship prior to Edna's decline has been good, they can build upon that foundation to take the steps that will assure Edna's well-being for the present and the future.

There are a number of issues that must be aired during the family discussion. With the necessary information from the doctor (a family meeting with the doctor could be of great value, but might not be logistically possible), it should be possible to get a prognosis and likely timeline of the progression of Edna's medical condition.

If she has Alzheimer's disease and also suffers from some small strokes, it is pretty clear that there will be continued deterioration of her mental and intellectual functioning. This is the case even if she is considered a suitable candidate for one of the more common drugs used in combating Alzheimer's disease (e.g., Aricept®, Exelon®, Reminyl®, or Namenda®) that might decrease the rate of decline but will not offer anything like a cure for her condition.

With the knowledge that there will be a progressive decline, the next question that must be asked is whether, in fact, Edna has the mental capacity to make the kinds of decisions that she is being asked to make, such as changing her will or moving to California. It is likely that if formally tested, she would be found not to have the capacity to change her will in any substantive way. If she were to make changes now, they would likely be open to legal challenge after she dies if one of the siblings is not happy with the changes.

If she is not mentally capable of making a new will, it is also unlikely that she can understand and appreciate the implications of a move to California or of making what would be considered a legally capable decision. Also, it should be made clear to all the siblings, especially Roger, that as their mother deteriorates her care needs will increase and she will need a lot of family support, which is unlikely to be available from Roger alone in Los Angeles. Even though the children are spread out, at least two of them live in close proximity to Seattle if that is where they decide to look for appropriate accommodations, or perhaps one could be found in the same community as Frank Jr. or Joan, as they do not live that far away from each other.

As for the quality of care that Edna may eventually require, she should be able to get as good long-term care in Seattle or Tacoma or

Olympia to be closer to at least one of her children. Comparative costs between the various cities for the same type of care should be considered and looked into if there is concern about her having the funds to sustain her over a long period of decline and perhaps leave a legacy for her children, which seems to be her wish.

With these factors taken into consideration, the siblings' discussion should include who is going to be the formal spokesperson for the family so that decisions about Edna's health can be made. Unless they agree to a spokesperson to represent them (with, of course, reasonable consultation with the others), they could end up in a situation in which the courts appoint a guardian in the absence of a defined decision-maker.

If the family decides, as most families do, that it is better for them to find a way to cooperate than to have an outside person make decisions without their consultation, they will eventually agree to designate one of them, likely Frank Jr., to be the decision-maker or surrogate. It would have been better if, prior to Edna's losing her capacity, she and her children had discussed the possibilities for the future should she become ill. At that time they could have agreed on this process and structure, rather than leaving it open to potential conflict that may result in resentment among the children as Edna deteriorates.

Assuming that, after hearing the facts and implications of the various options, the children agree that the best arrangement for Edna is to have her stay in Seattle at whatever level of care facility that is sufficiently supportive of his needs. Frank Jr. will take on the primary care-provider role with some appropriate backup arrangements in place. They should agree that when Frank Jr. needs time to go on a vacation or travel on business, someone else will be able to visit Seattle frequently to ensure that Edna continues her social visits and outings. This might be less of a concern as they would continue with the previous arrangement in which she has a full-time companion to provide support and whatever back-up plan as was previously made should be continued. This should ensure the greatest likelihood of social interaction that might be available from the facility's own programming.

With this agreement in place, it is possible that Frank Jr. will be able to carry on with the main responsibility. Rather than challenging his role, his siblings should be grateful that they have him as a strong support for Edna and not someone who is likely motivated by a future inheritance. In addition to all the other responsibilities that Frank Jr. would have if the plans work out as suggested, he and his siblings may want to do everything to assure Edna's safety. There are all kinds of arrangements and devices that are being developed that can assist in fulfilling such responsibilities. For example, there are devices that have been developed to help families looking after their loved ones with Alzheimer's should they become lost. Using one of these GPS-related instruments, which can be as small as a wristwatch, might give peace of mind to the siblings, especially if Edna shows evidence of having an inclination to wander.

If the situation is not resolved happily, and Roger or one of the other siblings challenges the status quo, it might be necessary for Frank Jr. to go to court and ask that he be appointed the formal surrogate and power of attorney for Edna's financial and personal needs. It is likely that he would be successful in such a request, but the repercussions in terms of family structure and resentment could be so great that the fabric of the family would be irrevocably destroyed. If the children feel inclined to pursue the matter through legal channels, they would be wise to get some impartial advice and perhaps pursue some mediation and to avoid the short- and long-term potentially disruptive and destructive implications for them, for Edna, and for their family relationships.

If the family agrees to Frank Jr.'s role as primary caregiver, they can all focus on making sure that Edna receives the best possible health care as she continues to decline mentally and physically. This will be provided through the cooperation of a loving and devoted family who do their best to make her comfortable and to visit as often as possible, considering that some of them live far away. Whatever financial legacy might be left to them, the most important legacy is the knowledge that they cared for their mother, taking into account her best interests rather than their own.

CASE STUDY 11
The Conflicted Single Child:
A Confusing Battle of Priorities

What does a young, single, upwardly mobile woman do when her mother is in the early stages of dementia and rejects all attempts to offer support? The emerging frustration has the potential to harm both the relationship and her career.

THE CHALLENGE

Maria Pontes is 33 years old. She is single and lives in an upscale down-town apartment building. Maria has been with a large, multinational public relations/public affairs firm for four years and is considered a shining star with high potential.

A political science graduate from Carleton University, she completed an MBA at York University five years ago. She is ambitious, asser-tive, articulate, and knows a bright future is in her grasp. Maria works extremely hard, putting in long hours on weekdays and at least five to ten hours most weekends. She also has a fairly active social life and is an avid squash player, trying to get in three or four hits a week, usually early in the morning.

Maria's most significant current challenge is her mother, Camilla who is 67 years of age. She moved to Canada from Portugal when she was 31 with her husband, Manuel. They settled in Hamilton, where Manuel worked at one of the steel mills and Camilla worked at a small fabricating shop. She had difficulty conceiving and had almost given up when she finally became pregnant. Maria was born, and no other pregnancies fol-lowed, which was a bit of a disappointment for both Manuel and Camilla.

When Maria was 15, the family took a trip to Portugal, where she got to meet her grandparents and relatives for the first time. The trip left a lasting impression on Maria; she learned all about her family and discovered they were very warm and caring. She was a hit with her aunts and uncles and found the basis for what would be a strong long-distance relationship with them and her six cousins.

In fact, from that visit on, she has corresponded in English with her cousins, first by mail and during the past few years by email, since their broken English was and remains much better than her fractured Portuguese.

When Maria was 17 years old, her father died of a brain aneurysm. She and her mother grieved for Manuel deeply and for a long time. Both loved him very much. Maria had been actually closer to her father than to her mother. No matter how tired he was after a long shift at the plant he would spend time with Maria, teaching her all he knew and always encouraging her to strive for an education as the means to success. He often reminded Maria that they were immigrants to Canada from poor but very decent, honest, and hard-working families. He told her that she would be the first generation to break through the barriers they all had lived with for generations and challenged her to study hard, to have high goals, and never indulge in self-doubt. Maria valued her father's convictions and truly cherished his vision of what she could do with her life.

Maria and her father also shared a passion for hockey. Throughout her childhood and until his death, watching Saturday night hockey on television had been a ritual for them. Two or three times a season, they would go to Toronto to see the Maple Leafs play.

So when Manual suddenly died, it was crushing for Maria. She faltered at school and became withdrawn. Her mother, while also in pain, sometimes became agitated with Maria's behavior and admonished her for being so hard on herself.

Eventually, Maria came to terms with her father's death and plunged full steam into her schoolwork. She graduated with honors and won two scholarships, and the rest, as she likes to say, is just life playing out as it should.

When she landed her current job, she commuted for the first year and lived with her mother. Then she moved to Toronto, explaining to her mother that the demands of her job meant that the daily travel time was simply too much. Camilla was upset, and after six months, Maria encouraged her to move closer. Her mother did part-time work as a salesperson at a department store and could find a similar job in Toronto.

Camilla resisted for another six months and then decided to move to Scarborough, at the eastern end of the city. She found a small but suitable apartment with Maria's help, moved, and within two months got a full-time job at a new big box outlet.

Maria tried hard to see her mother two or three times a week, at least one of those times being for a home-cooked meal. The relationship, though, was strained. Her mother wasn't very happy with the move because most of her friends were in Hamilton, and there was no easy way for her to get there and back. More than that, while Camilla never articulated it she was, in fact, unhappy that Maria didn't spend the same kind of time with her now that she remembered Maria spending with her father. And she had a hard time understanding exactly what Maria did, or why she worked such long hours.

Two years ago, Camilla seemed to start changing in ways Maria didn't understand. The changes were very subtle at first: her mother would call to ask for something and then, when Maria did what she had asked, her mother would act surprised and deny asking in the first place. Sometimes when Maria arrived for dinner and a visit, her mother wouldn't have any dinner prepared. But Maria was busy with her work and personal life and never thought much about it.

However, about six to eight months ago, Maria noticed more worrisome changes that started to concern her. Her mother seemed to be both more withdrawn and more combative. Camilla started asking for more help, yet whenever Maria tried to be helpful, her mother would berate her or deny asking. She stopped calling Maria at the office, and while they used to speak for at least a few minutes most evenings, now it was only once or twice a week. When she visited, Maria noticed that her mother's apartment wasn't as neat and tidy as it used to be, and she seemed somewhat more confused when speaking. Plus, Camilla was now working part-time, only about a dozen hours a week. Maria also noted that some bills were not paid on time, and one month the phone company called a few times to question what was going on with the late bill payment.

Maria got worried. She finally insisted that her mother have a full medical examination, and even went with her. The physician's conclusion: Camilla was physically well, but she was exhibiting symptoms of early Alzheimer's disease. Camilla denied that there was anything wrong with her.

The doctor explained that there were a number of drugs that could help Camilla. He prescribed a new medication for her, and while she got the medication, Maria discovered her mother wasn't taking it. During one visit, she looked in the medicine cabinet and saw the container was still full.

The doctor also recommended that her mother attend a day program a few times a week that helped people with Alzheimer's understand how to cope with their disease and served as a mutual help network. Camilla flatly refused to attend.

Meanwhile, Maria was finding she had less and less time for her mother, or anything else except work. While she used to be able to squeeze in time to take her mother for doctors' appointments and shopping, it was becoming more difficult to get away at a reasonable time.

Now, Maria is conflicted. The president of her company's Canadian operations met with her and said a promotion was in the works. Her new position would require extensive travel across Canada to manage a major account and would probably mean that she'd be reassigned to Amsterdam within the next year or two to work on the global team managing the strategy and hands-on support at the client's head office.

Maria wants to help and support her mother, but she is also eager to take on the new position; it fulfills the dream her father had and instilled in her. She's considered all the possible options and decided that perhaps getting her mother back to Portugal would be the best solution, especially if she would be working in Europe anyway; after all, she could find time to visit her there more easily than in Toronto. And, her mother would be with her family, with all the support that offered. She even phoned her cousins to talk about this option, and the word back was that the family would be more than pleased to have Camilla return home and to help her.

But Camilla flatly rejected the idea of a move back to her hometown. She lashed out at Maria, accusing her of wanting to get her out of the way. She also accused Maria of wanting to take her money and started withdrawing substantial sums of money from the bank; Maria knew because the account is a joint one and she can access it online. She has spoken to the bank manager about her concerns.

Meanwhile, when Maria visits Camilla, she notices yet more evidence that her mother seems to be neglecting her home and herself. And she experiences more strain in their relationship — more tension, more terse words and accusations. Maria wants to do the right thing, for her mother and for herself, but all she sees is conflict, confusion, and uncertainty.

THE GERIATRICIAN'S POINT OF VIEW

Doing the right thing for one's parent is not always what neatly fits into one's personal or professional aspirations. There is always a balance, and depending on many factors, a child may move in one direction rather than another. Despite the difficulties with the relationship between Maria and Camilla when she was growing up, and especially after her father died, Maria does not sound like she is willing to abandon her mother for her career or personal life.

The challenge, then, is how to provide for her mother in a way that can assure some semblance of safety and security while she tries to pursue both a personal and a professional life. The fact that her mother refuses to acknowledge her illness is very common in diseases such as Alzheimer's. But until such time that she is clearly a threat to herself or others, it would be very difficult to take over or force care on her mother. Some simple steps can be taken to make sure that bills are paid — Maria can arrange automatic withdrawals for utility and other necessary payments — even though Camilla may resent Maria's appearing to take over.

As for Camilla's withdrawing money from her bank account, that may be a bit more complicated and touchy. Since it is a joint account, Maria can likely put a limit on how much money can be withdrawn at any given time, although Camilla might get upset with the bank teller who refuses to give her whatever amount she demands. Maria will then have to explain the reason for the limit and deal with Camilla's anger.

If the account were not a joint one, it could be necessary for Maria to take the step of using the legal system to verify that Camilla suffers from dementia and requires Maria to be a surrogate for some decisions, including financial ones. This may be necessary eventually, but since in this case the account is already joint in nature that legal step can probably be avoided for now.

Maria cannot force Camilla into a day program, and in some ways, unless her condition becomes severe and it is deemed that she does not have the mental capacity to make any decisions, there is not much that Maria can do. Medications cannot be forced upon her, and future visits to the doctor may be refused as well. If Camilla thinks that the doctor and Maria are in cahoots, she may refuse further visits and therefore decline any offers of treatment. Certainly she will not attend a day program for support if she denies there is a problem. Many people in such circumstances will leave a program for Alzheimer's disease patients when they sense that everyone is worse than they are and deny that they have any need for such a program.

In a case like this, when the parent refuses help and the dementia has not yet progressed to the point that a surrogate for decision-making can be appointed, sometimes the only thing a family can do is wait for some terrible crises to occur. The challenge for Maria, even if she does become Camilla's surrogate, is whether she is willing to force her mother to do something that she does not want to do. Their lifelong pattern of interaction was always based on her mother having very strong opinions and a very strong will and Maria usually backing down in times of conflict. She does not think she would be prepared to take the opposite position unless things were really terrible, which is not the case.

In fact, other than the bill payment issue, which can be dealt with, and the withdrawal of money, Camilla does manage. Work is an issue, and it looks like she will be let go as soon as she makes too many errors and misses days of work too often. Maria has spoken to the supervisor, who was very understanding and agreed to let Camilla go with a good excuse and send-off party to make her feel good. Camilla seems to shop for her personal items adequately, though Maria sometimes finds excess amounts of some products in the refrigerator, suggesting that Camilla may be forgetting what she has bought, but this is not a big problem so far. Maria does get calls from her mother from time to time about matters that have already been discussed or decided upon, but she has learned from her meetings with the Alzheimer's Society how to deal with those repeated calls. Maria also notes that Camilla reverts more often to Portuguese, and Maria struggles to respond, as her command of the language, which is not her mother tongue, but rather the one she heard spoken around the house, is marginal.

The real problems for Maria are long-term planning for Camilla and what to do with her own career. Getting her mother back to Portugal on face value sounds like a good idea, and with a large, accepting, and loving family that is willing to take this on, one might have jumped at the opportunity. However, if Camilla does not want to go, at least at this stage of her life, it would be very hard to force her to travel home. Maria might try to convince her to take a trip back to visit, with the hope that once there she will feel all the emotional and family ties to her native country and her family and agree to stay. But if that is not possible, sending her to Portugal for the time being does not seem to be a viable option. Maria must consider just how close Camilla is to these relatives in Portugal now that she has lived for so many years in Canada. If she has few contacts and a limited network in Toronto, and has kept some closeness with her family back home, this might turn out to be the ultimate answer to the problem, but it will have to unfold with time, as it cannot readily be forced.

Another option is to ask one or more of the Portuguese family to visit Toronto and stay with or close to Camilla so that she can relate to them and hopefully develop an attachment that might encourage her to consider the possibility of returning home, first for a visit and then maybe with the plan to remain there. If this were part of a plan, Maria would have to work closely with the relatives in Portugal to try to develop the supportive and caring environment that might lead Maria to think that a trip back would be a good thing, rather than something being forced on her by her "ungrateful" daughter.

As for Maria's career, she might have to discuss with her boss the realities of her life. It may not be possible for her to take on the overseas job until things have been settled with her mother. There are many sac-rifices that children can make in order to care for their parents. Children must accept that no one can plan for what will be; the real challenge in a caring relationship is how one deals with situations that one cannot control. It is hard to imagine that Maria would leave Camilla to fend for herself while she takes on an overseas portfolio. In all likelihood the plan would fail and she would have to return home as things deteriorated. Rather than undertaking such a move now, she might have to defer it, even at the risk of her career path for the time being, in order to be a dutiful and caring daughter. In an era in which many highly qualified workers face similar problems with aging parents, it is likely that if Maria explains the situation to her boss, some alternative career path can be worked out. She is clearly good at what she does, and most people in organizations value excellent people and invest in them long-term. So this may be a time for the company to support Maria so that she can be everything she might be for them in the future.

Being a single child of a parent with dementia is not easy. Not hav-ing other siblings to share the responsibilities and decision-making challenges is difficult. But there are ways to get help. On the advice of Camilla's doctor, Maria joined the Alzheimer's Society and finds the meetings and newsletters and other publications very useful. Speaking to other families who are struggling with similar issues really is a support for Maria. The doctor also arranged a few meetings with a social worker to assist Maria in figuring out what her options are, and she has found comfort in having someone to whom she can vent and express her inner-most concerns. The doctor suggested that if Maria needs more intensive support, she should consider getting herself to a psychologist or other counselor to help her work through her relationship with Camilla and to explore how her needs and those of her mother interconnect.

In situations such as this one, something usually happens that helps to resolve the issue. Sometimes, unfortunately, it is a crisis, such as an illness that makes things worse, that forces a certain direction of deci-sion-making. Maybe Camilla agrees to visit her family and decides that it would be best to stay, or a family member visits from Portugal and Camilla agrees to return for a visit and then remains there. Many things can happen. The important point is that Maria has to be supported in her quest to do the right thing personally. It is hoped that she gets the support she needs at her workplace so she realizes that ultimately she will be able to fulfill her career goals and dreams while at the same time being the caring and dutiful daughter that she is.

CASE STUDY 12
Finding the Middle Ground:
Engaging Mediation with Age-Related Issues

The dissolution of a long-standing marriage is never easy, for the couple or for any children, no matter what their ages. When all avenues of reconciliation appear futile the focus should be on diminishing the negative fallout from the breakup so that important emotional and filial relationships can continue, despite the situation.

Cynthia Woodhouse is 69 years old. Her common law partner, Barry Knight, is 65 years of age. They never "tied the knot" because they had a philosophical belief that the ritual of marriage was superfluous to their devotion and commitment to each other.

They live in Fort McMurray, Alberta, 270 miles northeast of the provincial capital of Edmonton. They've been there for almost 20 years, because Barry has been an oilfield worker since his early twenties and he followed the opportunities when oil sands started to be a viable option of oil extraction.

Cynthia and Barry are the biological parents of two children: Herman, 49, and Kent, 46. They also are adoptive parents of Dawn, who is 38 years old, and Katrina, who is 37 years old. After their second child, Cynthia had insisted that Barry 'get a vasectomy,' but later both regretted the decision and, agreeing they wanted more children, elected to adopt.

Barry has always been the main breadwinner in the family. An oil patch brat since childhood, Barry learned the ins and outs of the business by being totally hands on. His schooling was limited to the least amount he had to do to get by. He met Cynthia, the love of his life, in Calgary when they were in their teens and they were best friends for many years.

Barry is now about to retire. He has a very good pension plan. Cynthia, who worked part time on and off over the years, has always relied on Barry's salary to pay bills and keep them relatively comfortable, as well as support their children through community colleges, which is where all four of them went after high school.

Herman is a heating and cooling technician living and working in Calgary, currently in a relationship with a woman he's known since his second divorce six years ago. Kent, like his father, works in the oil patch for a large multinational. Currently, he's working on an oil rig in the Gulf of Mexico but when in Canada usually lives with his parents. He is a confirmed bachelor who loves his independence. Dawn is married to Evan and they live in Winnipeg, where she is a full time mother of three young children and homemaker; Evan works in a small plastics manufacturing company. Katrina and her partner Mandy live in Vancouver, where she works as a production assistant on movie and television sets.

The four siblings and their families have always gotten along reasonably well. There was a clear line of difference, though, between Herman and Kent and the two adopted children, Dawn and Katrina. It wasn't something anyone thought of as being serious, but there was an unspoken yet palpable "them" and "us" sense to the relationship.

Given that the family functioned fairly normally overall and the long standing good relationship and apparent devotion and commitment between Barry and Cynthia, it was with utter amazement that the four children read emails from their mother in which she said she wanted to leave Barry. The reasoning was somewhat fuzzy. It was essentially that Barry had always been a pretty good husband but that the past years made her realize that, having met Barry back in her teens, she'd never really explored the world outside of their relationship and family; that she'd had no life of her own and she was getting older and just needed to be free for once. She said she expected Barry to support her and someday she might want to come back.

Barry then started calling his four children daily (Barry was not big on technology; he had a cell phone he seldom used and never emailed, let alone texted). He was genuinely surprised, upset, and even afraid. He told them in separate calls that Cynthia was his everything; that he couldn't imagine life without her, even more so now that he was on the edge of retirement. He reported in his most recent calls that Cynthia had told him she was planning on moving out of the house and wanted to know how much monthly support he would guarantee her for the imme-diate future and, looking into the future, on an on-going basis. This, she said, should be decided based on whether or not she lived with him. Then she told him that she'd stopped feeling any strong emotional attach-ment or physical attraction to him some years ago. In reality Barry was painfully aware that their sexual life had petered out over the past few years but he attributed it to Cynthia's age and neither of them ever really discussed the issue, as once when he tried, her response was very curt and painful to him. Although he felt rejected, he was still hopeful that things would turn around, especially after he retired and they had more time together without the strains of work.

Herman and Kent seemed most affected by these developments. Each spoke with the other more frequently since the start of what appeared to be the unraveling of their parents' marriage. Herman won-dered if their mother had developed what he called "some kind of mental condition." Kent said he'd never noticed anything odd with their mother. Dawn and Katrina seemed less concerned. Dawn said they should just wait and see what happened; though she did talk with both of her parents several times and encouraged them to discuss things before making any decisions. Katrina basically had a live-and-let-live attitude, telling her siblings that they should abide by whatever their parents decided to do.

Kent spoke with his mother and urged her to go with his father to see a marriage counselor and work things out. His mother flatly rejected that. Cynthia is telling everyone she has made up her mind and it's now all about money, which, in essence, is her future security. She is tell-ing her children that the situation at home is getting to be unbearable because she is not speaking to Barry, but Barry won't stop speaking to her, asking her to work this out with him. She is trying to ignore him but this is very hard to do with them living under the same roof and Barry basically being responsible for all expenses.

Kent and Herman are increasingly worried for the wellbeing of their parents, and while Dawn seems concerned, Katrina clearly is not interested in helping out in any way. So the three of them determine something must be done to find some kind of resolution that will not have such a drastic consequence as their parents physically separating.

THE GERIATRICIAN'S POINT OF VIEW

This scenario is in fact not all that unusual although it does not always end up with the dissolution of long-term relationships, whether common-law or actual marriage. Many long-standing couples grow apart over the years but manage to find enough in their relationship to stay together, sometimes because in reality financially they can't afford to separate. For others there are major cultural and religious prohibitions and the fear of being severed from a family network might be too much to bear. If it were not for such common scenarios there would be little in the way of plots for novels, storylines for films, and the complex relationships of soap operas.

Infidelity and/or the desire to break free from a constricting, suffocating, and at the extreme, an abusive relationship, is in essence an old story. But each time it plays out, those involved experience the pain and conflict, despair, anger, hope, and sense of loss in a very personal and profound way. For the person leaving, it may invigorate a sense of new beginnings. For the one left behind it may provoke a sense of despondency that can be translated into a wide range of emotions and actions that can either be helpful or destructive to the individual or at the extremes to everyone around the couple in dissolution, almost as collateral damage. We must all know that at all ages falling out of love can be as emotionally powerful and all-consuming as falling in love, especially when the feelings are asymmetrical, which means that the feelings are not congruent but disparate or going in different directions.

What are the options for Barry and Cynthia and how may their worlds be salvaged as much as possible so that they can have a meaningful future either fully apart or with some semblance if not a full return to their previous state of coupledom? Anyone who works in the field of couple and family therapy knows that there is a wide range of outcomes to any couple dissolution ranging from the simple, "it's been great, but there is no future, goodbye," which is greeted with a "goodbye to you, nice knowing you," to passionate actions sometime resulting in tragic deaths, and everything in-between. The goal for those in this family network who really care what happens (which should be all of them) is what is often called "damage control" in the world of crises management.

Trying to get Cynthia back into marriage therapy may be a lost cause unless both of them are really interested in exploring what it may take to rekindle their relationship, and address whatever it is that is missing in their lives that they attribute to being with one another. Sometimes individual therapy may be helpful to each of the players to help them understand their own actions and feelings and come to a greater understanding of how such an outcome of their long-standing relationship could occur. Individual therapy can also help each of them in their perception of themselves and help prevent erroneous feelings of guilt or responsibility that may end up blocking their move into a useful, productive, and emotionally wholesome future whether alone or together.

If attempts at marriage counseling are clearly not going to occur, or do occur and are not helpful, then a mediator may be necessary. A professional mediator can help establish defined, agreeable goals so that Cynthia and Barry can not only move on in their lives, but the children (and even grandchildren) will not harbor deep-seated anger and lingering resentment toward them in the future, when Cynthia and Barry may need further assistance. Not everyone initially may feel that mediation is necessary and not every professional, whether social workers, psychologists, or lawyers, are aware of the potential long-term benefits of mediation. There has been a tendency to look at the dissolution of a marriage as an issue of asset allocation and arrangements regarding minor children. Since money is often the most contentious issue in a couple's relationship, the presence of love, sex, and *other relationships* frequently evokes profound feelings of betrayal and jealousy that often result in very destructive adversarial legal processes. It's common to read of cases in the media where couples are fighting over some aspect of a failed marriage and the focus becomes the children and custody (when they are underage), among other common issues like money, support, houses, and businesses. The black humor perspective of such situations is that of the lawyers happily milking the cow as the two farmers are fighting over who "owns the milk," when at the end of the process there is literally and figuratively no milk left.

More enlightened lawyers are turning more and more to the concept of mediation to avoid conflicts that are emotionally and financially very exhausting and expensive. The goal of mediation is ultimately to preserve the integrity and functionality of each of the parties and transform conflict and potentially destructive actions into a means by which all parties come out as "winners" in the end. We know that in the world of labor conflict and in the political arena the best outcomes often occur through the process of mediation.

Valerie Hazlett Parker, a well-known Ontario mediator, defines the process as follows:

> Elder mediation is a voluntary and co-operative process in which a professionally trained Elder Mediator facilitates discussions to assist people to address the myriad changes that occur throughout the family lifecycle. This process can involve a number of participants, including older people, family members, friends, and support persons. The focus is on addressing concerns while maintaining and promoting all of the relationships critical to the well-being of the older person(s). Numerous issues can be addressed, including: retirement; financial concerns; and family business succession; housing and living arrangements; relationship concerns, including intergenerational relationships, step-families and, for example, estate planning.

All the previous noted issues might be important to Barry and Cynthia as they try to plan in a responsible way for their future, either apart permanently, temporarily, or in some mutually-agreeable on-going relationship. Their children might also benefit from a non-adversarial approach to dealing with what is usually an emotional minefield. If these emotions are not approached in a calm, deliberative, and cooperative way it can lead to bad decisions and hard feelings that may carry on for years, negatively affecting everyone in the family.

Whatever it takes to get both Barry and Cynthia to agree to some sort of mediation should be attempted. Whether it comes from their children, individually or collectively; from mutual friends; from a trusted professional such as their doctor or lawyer; or from a combination of them, a good deal of benefit might be derived from the process. Failure to achieve some semblance of cooperation and acknowledgment that there are a number of sides to every human decision can lead to a situation in which no one is satisfied. Tragically, lingering hard feelings can carry over for years to come and the family itself could end up fragmenting — an unwanted outcome for all parties involved and one that should be avoided if at all possible.

CASE STUDY 13
The Stroke: Sudden Challenges and Changes

A self-sufficient parent suffers a series of strokes, creating an instant family crisis requiring careful co-ordination of care and attention.

THE CHALLENGE

Diane is 51 years old and married to Terry, who is 55. They have an 18-year-old daughter, Amanda. This is Terry's second marriage. He divorced his first wife after 15 years of an unhappy and acrimonious marriage that produced a daughter, Jill, who is 23 years old and lives on her own.

Diane's father left her mother, Wilma, more than a decade ago. A quick divorce followed, and he hasn't been heard from since. Diane, while never close to her father or approving of his lifestyle and treatment of her mother, still on occasion wonders about him.

Terry lost both of his parents in a fatal automobile accident six years ago while they were on their way to a vacation in Florida.

Because both Diane and Terry are the only children in their families, neither of them has any close family to speak of, other than a few distant cousins and an uncle out west. That's why they are so close to Diane's mother.

Until recently, Wilma lived on her own in a large, rambling house, an hour's drive in the country from Diane and Terry's home in Omaha. She'd lived there ever since her husband had left her. Wilma had never remarried, but for the past five or six years she has been casually seeing a widower who lived not far from her; they were just good friends (or so it seemed) who enjoyed being together.

Diane often drove out to visit her mother for an hour or so. Diane and Terry also regularly visited Wilma, with a protesting Amanda in tow. It is not that Amanda didn't like her grandmother; it was just that she was at an age where she would rather spend all of her time with her friends, music, and smartphone, and not her parents. However, despite not wanting to go — especially for weekend visits — Amanda usually had a reasonably good time once she got there. And Wilma, who at 72 years of age was full of energy, would take the bus to the city and visit for several days at a time a few times a year.

Wilma had always been in good health. The first time in her life that she was in the hospital was four years ago for a day surgery cataract procedure. She faithfully went to her annual medical check-ups, and she always fared well in the final assessments. Her one big problem was her weight. Wilma loved her food and loved to eat. She was about 50 pounds overweight, and no amount of frequent but loosely applied dieting got her weight down.

On one of her short visits to see her mother, Diane observed that Wilma was talking with a slight slur and that she leaned to one side in a way that she hadn't noticed before. But for all intents and purposes, Wilma seemed to be fine, just as full of energy as ever. Diane asked her mother if she was feeling all right, and Wilma assured her she couldn't be better. Yet something kept nagging at Diane, and she pressured her mother to make an appointment to see her doctor.

Two days later, Diane called her mother in the morning — a time she was always home — and there was no answer. Troubled, she called Wilma's friend, who said he hadn't seen her in a couple of days. After getting no answer a few more times, Diane called one of Wilma's neighbors and asked if she'd look to see if her mother was there. She wasn't.

Worried, Diane canceled her next two meetings and drove to her mother's house. Just as she arrived, there was Wilma getting out of the local taxi. Wilma explained that she'd been to see her doctor, who wondered if she might have suffered a very small stroke. But, Wilma said, everything seemed to be all right, although the doctor did suggest that she needed a good going over. And that's how Diane happened to be there when, an hour later, her mother toppled out of her chair, unable to speak or move. Diane managed to help Wilma to the car and drove her to the small local hospital.

Her doctor was summoned. He confirmed that she'd had another stroke and that this one was substantial. He arranged to transfer Wilma to a larger regional hospital.

The next two days were a terrible blur for Diane. She was told that her mother actually had suffered a massive stroke. Wilma's entire right side was immobile, and she initially lost all ability to speak. After the first day, she could communicate, but with only a few halting words. Terry was shaken, and Amanda was in tears. Even Jill, who didn't feel a great deal of closeness to Diane's mother, was moved to ask how she might help.

Diane arranged for her mother to be transported to a hospital in the city, where she could get more sophisticated care and diagnostic tests, and where she'd be closer to the family. A week later, Wilma was transferred again — this time to a rehabilitation hospital as a temporary measure. By now, although Wilma could utter a handful of words, it was clear from all the medical advice Diane had managed to collect that her mother probably would never walk again and certainly couldn't live on her own.

Wilma was on a regimen of daily therapy sessions, which seemed to help somewhat, but there was no significant improvement. Nor was there any further deterioration in her condition. All in all, Wilma was holding her own, and was trying to be as cooperative as possible.

Since entering the rehabilitation hospital, Wilma has had yet another stroke, albeit a much smaller one. She is now totally dependent on full-time care and assistance. She can't walk at all, and she has lost all use of her right arm. She is unable to move out of her bed or wheelchair without help. She has also developed some problems with swallowing and eating and occasionally chokes on her food. A nutritionist has made some recommendations about positioning her when she eats and setting the pace of feeding as well as modifying the consistency of foods.

Totally unprepared for this devastating event, Diane and Terry wonder what they should do next to help Wilma and make her as comfortable as possible. They aren't certain where Wilma could live. They recognize that, even though they have a small guest room in their house, Diane's mother needs a level of attention that they can't provide, and they have no room for a full-time caregiver. They also know they have limited time because of their job pressures, and limited resources because they paid for Amanda to go to a private school and now she attends Clarkson College, which is also a private institution. However, they do want to do the right thing for Wilma.

THE GERIATRICIAN'S POINT OF VIEW

Diane and her family must ask themselves, "What is the right thing to do?" The main focus should be deciding where Wilma will get the best care for her immediate and long-term needs and what the family can reasonably do with their present circumstances. While it might be the ideal situation for Wilma to move in with her family, it would be a monumental undertaking and also a very expensive one. They would have to renovate the house to accommodate Wilma's needs and arrange for full-time help. The cost of 24-hour care is prohibitive for most families, unless they are very well-off financially. This is not the situation with Diane and Terry, who are, in fact, struggling with their own financial situation now that their daughter is at a high-quality private college. Of course, selling Wilma's home and using the proceeds to help pay medical costs will help.

If keeping Wilma at home is not a viable option, the only other choice is to find a suitable long-term care facility. They can look for a facility either near where they live or near Wilma's own home. They need to weigh the importance of Wilma being near her social network of friends and neighbors against the convenience of being nearer to the family, who will be Wilma's main support.

Assuming that Wilma is not able to communicate, it may be necessary for her family to try to explore who among her friends might really be available to visit her. If the only important person is her male friend from her neighborhood, they might speak to him about how they can arrange for him to visit her from time to time. Perhaps they could either periodically pick him up or arrange for his transportation so that he could spend an afternoon at Wilma's long-term care facility and make a nice visit out of it. Wilma may or may not be able to recognize or fully interact with her friend, but if they could continue some kind of a meaningful relationship, it is worth pursuing this avenue for her benefit.

The rest of the visiting will be up to the family. Although it is not easy, they should try to develop plans that will make each visit a bit special. For example, they might bring some treats that are appropriate for Wilma. Of course, if they bring food, it is important to make sure that it is something that she can eat, especially since she has some swallowing difficulties. If Wilma likes flowers, it may be worth putting some plants in her room, as long as someone will take care of them. Taking pictures to share with Wilma would be a very nice way to keep her up-to-date with family events. Going for a walk around the premises is often a special event for nursing home residents and is generally something staff cannot do frequently. Some families hire private companions to take their loved ones on an outing or walk once in a while depending on the situation. If the staff thinks it is safe, going for a drive or some other kind of outing might also be a nice way to bring something new into Wilma's life. If music is something special for her, they should arrange for a CD player, tape machine, or mp3 player with headphones or small speakers for her room that she can listen to whenever she wants.

This would also be a very good time for Diane and Terry to explore with Wilma what she would like to happen should things take a turn for the worse. For example, if Wilma has strong views about end-of-life issues based on deep-seated personal or religious reasons, these should be confirmed. If it is thought that she would prefer not to have heroic treatments provided, this should be established as reasonably as possible.

The issue of feeding tubes might also be considered in view of the problems that Wilma is already experiencing with her eating. These issues should be presented in a way that does not frighten Wilma, as an assurance that nothing will be done for her or to her that she would not want if she could express her wishes herself.

If effective communication takes place, it may be possible for Diane and Terry to understand the limits and boundaries of care that Wilma would prefer if she were able to communicate at the time. So, for example, if she gets an infection, she would want to be treated if there were a good chance of full recovery. But she might prefer to not have cardiopulmonary resuscitation in the event of cardiac arrest, or she may not want a permanent feeding tube should she not be able to eat normally. Knowing Wilma's wishes now, when her condition is stable and non-threatening, would certainly make it much easier for Diane and Terry to live with what are often difficult decisions at a time of crisis.

These are not easy times. But with the goodwill and dedication that appear to be motivating Diane and her husband, and with a bit of luck,

Wilma should be able to manage reasonably well for some time in the nursing home, perhaps months to years. She might even improve in terms of function for a while, but inevitably something will occur from which she cannot recover. Diane and Terry should be ready for all eventualities and be thankful for any period of comfort and enjoyment that Wilma can experience during this very difficult period of her life.

CASE STUDY 14
Dementia and Depression: Reading the Signs

Discovering that a parent has significant health problems but is in total denial is a disturbing and often frightening experience for children. Such a stressful situation requires careful action to best help all involved.

THE CHALLENGE

Al and Denise Wilson have been married for 45 years. Al is 72 years old, and Denise is 68. They've both been in excellent health all their lives.

Al retired at age 65 on a full pension after working with the same company since completing university. At about the same time, Denise opted to take a downsizing severance package at the company where she'd been a secretary for more than 30 years, and this provided her with a good pension also.

Al, a structural engineer with a mid-sized consulting company, was actually relieved to retire when he did. He'd found the last couple of years at the office to be increasingly difficult. What bothered Al was that periodically, sometimes for a number of months at a time, he found he was having a hard time concentrating on his assignments, and the more complex a job was, the longer it took him to complete it. He never mentioned this to anyone, and he told himself it was because he was bored and tired after so many years of doing the same thing. He also had periods when he had problems sleeping, and so he attributed his lack of concentration to his periodic lack of sleep. Al also thought part of the problem may be that he was eagerly anticipating retirement.

After considering what they really wanted to do in their "golden years," Al and Denise sold their comfortable home in Toronto and moved into a retirement community on the shores of a lake north of the city.

The transition, which worried them a bit, went very smoothly. As they're still fond of telling people they meet, they both adjusted "like a duck to water"; they had no second thoughts and certainly no regrets.

They've thoroughly enjoyed their lifestyle in their new home. They culti-vated friendships with a number of other retired couples, played bridge weekly, and, best of all, golfed every other day. Last year, they splurged and bought a small sailboat and took some lessons. During the summer months they sailed most evenings for an hour on the lake.

For the past several years, Al and Denise have spent six weeks each winter in Florida at a condominium they co-own with another couple they've known for years. All in all, Al and Denise are very much enjoying their lives and feel that the years of work and careful savings are paying off handsomely.

Their only child, Mary, is 37 years old and lives in Toronto with her husband, Bob, and their two children, Amy, who is 17, and Tom, who is 14. Mary and her family are close to her parents and visit them about once every two weeks — sometimes staying for a weekend. Most holi-days are spent together.

Bob's parents live in North Bay and both are in good health. Twice a year his parents come to visit them in Toronto, and at least annually they trek to North Bay to visit for a few days. And, of course, they all talk to one another on the telephone regularly.

For all intents and purposes, all the family members honestly like one another and get along well.

About four months ago, Denise noticed for the first time that Al was "not his old self," as she described it to Mary at the time. He seemed to be more withdrawn, she told Mary, and sometimes indecisive about things like what to eat — something about which he'd always had very fixed views, with strong likes and dislikes.

Mary forgot about what her mother told her, and Denise herself put it somewhere on the back burner of her mind for the time.

As the weeks passed, Denise realized that her husband was spending less and less time in his small woodworking shop that he'd equipped in part of the garage. Finally, she asked him about it. Al said he'd just lost interest in woodworking, that it was too time-consuming and too hard.

Yet Denise knew Al truly enjoyed making small pieces of furniture and prided himself on the detailed work. That's why a few days later she asked about his woodworking again, this time to enquire when he'd finally build her the shelves above the washer and dryer. Al became very agitated. He said he didn't know when he might have the time to build the shelves. When Denise reminded him that he had all the time in the world, Al didn't respond. So the subject was dropped.

Then, just a few weeks later, Al changed his mind about going for their usual after-dinner sail, and he did so again a week later. This was definitely not like Al at all — he loved that little boat and the feel of the breeze on the lake. Denise asked him if something was wrong and Al said no, he just didn't feel like sailing these days, as he had some increased pain in his back, the result of an old athletic injury. He claimed that sailing seemed a bit risky for him and that he worried more about their safety out on the water. He seemed even more irritated when she asked again about the shelves. He told her that if she needed the shelves so badly, she should just go out and buy some.

Not long after that conversation, Mary, Bob, Amy, and Tom came for a one-day visit. It was a sunny, warm day and everyone wanted to go sailing, but Al said he didn't feel like it — and that was a first. Mary asked her father several times but got the same negative response every time.

During the course of the day, Denise pulled her daughter aside and told her about her father's recent change of behavior and how it was confusing to her. Mary was mystified. She watched her father very closely for the rest of the visit. She noticed that he sometimes appeared withdrawn, as if he were in his own world. He did not laugh in his usual way at her husband's wisecracks and puns, which was out of character. She mentioned this to her mother later on that evening, who said that this kind of behavior had been occurring quite often lately. Mary asked if there was anything else, and her mother admitted that Al was no longer interested in sex; whenever she approached him he found an excuse for not participating, usually complaining of fatigue or backache, a problem that he had had for years but that had never before interfered with what had been, up until a few months ago, a very satisfying sex life for the two of them.

Later Mary told her husband about her observations and her mother's comments, and he suggested that they should both see a doctor for a good assessment.

The next day, Mary called her mother and asked when her parents had last had a good medical check-up. Denise became alarmed and wanted to know why Mary was asking. Mary told her mother of her conversation with Bob the night before. She said there had been a lot written lately about depression, especially in older people, and it just seemed like a good idea for both of them to get thorough medical assessments from time to time, especially in light of the changes in her father's behavior. Denise replied that both she and Al had had a good check-up about two years ago but hadn't had any reason to see a doctor since, and that was a blessing.

Still, Mary urged her mother to arrange medical check-ups for both of them. She reminded her that just as she, Bob, and the kids get annual check-ups, so should her parents. And, Mary argued, it was a matter of something more than a regular routine examination, because it seemed clear that something was not right with her father, and the problem had to be identified and addressed.

Later that day Denise sat with Al on their deck, having a glass of wine before dinner. Al lately had started drinking more than a glass before dinner. He said it calmed him down, and Denise didn't think much about it. After all, they were retired, and he didn't have to worry about sleeping in if he had an extra drink or two.

She suggested that it was probably time for them both to go for a check-up; their doctor was still practicing in Toronto, so they could make a day of it — see the doctor, do some shopping, and then come home. Al shot back that he didn't need a medical check-up; he felt just fine, and if she needed one, he'd be pleased to take her. He wouldn't explain why he refused to go, even though Denise asked several times. Finally, Al stated emphatically that he felt just fine, that there was no use spending time on something that wasn't necessary, and that Denise was probably fine, too. He said they were having the best years of their lives, and that's the way it should be. End of discussion. No matter what approach she took, Denise couldn't get Al to agree to visit the doctor.

A couple of days later, when Mary called to talk with her mother, Denise told her of her father's firm decision and said she didn't want to provoke him or have an argument about it. So, for the time being, Denise said, they would skip the visit to the doctor and just see how things went,

because actually both of them felt well, other than the change in Al's interests and the fact that he seemed to sit around a lot more than usual. And
after all, Denise told her daughter, there was really nothing physically
wrong with them. Just because Al didn't want to build shelves or sail as
often and wasn't that interested in sex, it didn't really mean anything. These
things happen to people; she figured that it was a phase that would pass.

Mary didn't argue or push, feeling that she should respect her parents' wishes. For all her life, they'd been there for her as solid supporters
and sound parents, and she didn't think the current situation demanded
any kind of hard push on her part. She decided that if there were any further signs of a problem with her father, she'd personally arrange for and
take him to a doctor's appointment. And her mother seemed just fine.

THE GERIATRICIAN'S POINT OF VIEW

It is imperative that Al get medical advice. It appears from the description
that he is suffering from a depressive illness, which could be occurring
for several reasons. Depressive symptoms can be the earliest manifesta-
tions of dementia, such as Alzheimer's disease, and major depression can
occur for the first time in older individuals. Also, sometimes an earlier
bout of depression may not have been recognized for what it was, or
may have been attributed to nerves or stress or overwork, and therefore
ignored and not formally treated. A family history of depression sometimes helps with the diagnosis, and it would be useful to know if any of
Al's siblings or his parents ever had problems with mood disorders.

The main obstacle to Al's receiving help for depression is either that
he is not aware something is wrong or, more likely, that he feels ashamed
or guilty about admitting that things are not quite right. Many older
people, especially men who have always been in charge, have difficulty
admitting that things are happening to them that they cannot control.
Deep-seated feelings of inadequacy often occur and sexual problems are
not uncommon. This just makes things worse, especially if the person is
not used to expressing feelings and exploring problems with other people, even his or her spouse.

The danger of depression, especially when it occurs in older men, is that it sometimes leads to suicide. They may not give any real outward warning that things are that bad, but to the surprise of their loved ones, they kill themselves, often by some violent means. Other men respond by withdrawing into themselves, eating less, or consuming increasing amounts of alcohol and medications such as tranquilizers (which they may get from a doctor after complaining of sleep problems) that temporarily ease their feelings of despair.

A family in this situation needs to find a way to get their loved one to see a physician. Some depressed people will go on their own so that they don't have to involve their family in a problem they may consider to be shameful. Some people believe that depression is a sign of weakness and that they should be able to just pull themselves out of it. But that rarely happens. So what are Mary and Denise to do? Waiting for something to happen is not the answer.

In fact, if they do that and something terrible happens they would never forgive themselves. It would probably be worthwhile for Mary and Denise to arrange to be alone with Al and have a discussion in which they express their concern for him because of what they have been observing for the past few months. Al's response may be dismissive and he may be angry that they are intruding on his feelings. It might be helpful for Mary to bring some reading material for Al, suggesting that he read it when he is alone. She and her mother have to express their love and devotion to Al and tell him that they realize just how difficult it might be for him to admit to or express his true feelings.

They might suggest that perhaps he would prefer to visit the doctor alone rather than going with Denise. Of course, the hope would be that he declines that offer, because they want to be with him when he tells the doctor what has been happening. By himself, he might deny that anything is wrong with his sense of self and value.

Al may not respond immediately to such a conversation. However, reading the material provided by Mary and Denise might persuade him to agree to see his doctor. If this is the case, it would be worthwhile communicating with the doctor first by phone or whatever private means works best to explain the concerns of the family. Then, during the medical assessment, if Al does not admit to any problems, the physician can ask the necessary probing questions that may lead to a diagnosis of depression.

If a diagnosis of depression is made, the likely outcome will be an attempt at treatment with an antidepressant medication. There is a very good chance that the drug will be tolerated, especially if the physician begins with a small dose and gradually increases it, and will also be effective. If so, Al should become more sociable and less withdrawn and regain his interest in his hobbies and his wife. Many different antidepressant drugs and other components of treatment, including group therapy, may be offered, and usually one type of treatment or another will prove successful.

This is a time when a great deal of understanding and support is required, and Denise, Mary, and Bob will have to put all their efforts toward being supportive of Al and giving him the time and space to make his recovery.

One major concern, in addition to the high risk of suicide, is that the depression may be a symptom of dementia. For a substantial percentage of individuals, their depressive symptoms respond to treatment, but their mental powers and prowess continue to decline until it becomes clear that something beyond depression is taking place. The earliest signs of Alzheimer's disease are often revealed symptomatically with this kind of pattern. At present, there are no simple tests that can differentiate true late-onset depression from the type that will transform itself into dementia.

The positive news is that there are new drugs from which many people with Alzheimer's disease appear to benefit. Medical evidence suggests that even if there is no dramatic improvement in mental and cognitive function, the rate of progress of the disease appears to slow down, giving families and patients a bit more time to live life to its fullest and to make the necessary plans in anticipation of a progressive decline. (This includes taking steps such as appointing a power of attorney and making a will that will withstand external scrutiny or contest.) So, Mary and Denise need to lovingly get Al to the doctor, relate their observations, and explain their concerns. With a bit of luck, Al will be seen, a diagnosis of depression made, and proper treatment started. And maybe, with a little bit of extra luck, Al's condition will prove not to be the early stages of dementia and he can get back into his sailboat for many years to come.

CASE STUDY 15
Advancing Dementia: When Life Gets More Difficult

When parents are deteriorating, their children must make some hard decisions about how they might best help them to be as secure and comfortable as possible, while trying to maintain their own lives and meeting their family commitments.

THE CHALLENGE

Dorothy-May Miller is an 87-year-old widow whose husband, DeRoy, died three years ago of lung cancer. Dorothy-May never got over the shock of his death, although DeRoy had a long period of painful illness. After DeRoy's funeral, Dorothy-May remained completely devastated and was often unable to stop crying for several hours at a time.

She continued to live in the one-bedroom apartment in an Atlanta seniors' retirement community they'd moved to in the mid-1980s when DeRoy retired from his job with the railroad. They made the move partially to relieve the strain of caring for the house they had been living in and also because the seniors' facility offered increased levels of care. After DeRoy's death, Dorothy-May went out on her own less and less often and increasingly depended on her handful of friends who lived in the same complex, as well as the staff, for personal services.

Although Dorothy-May was in relatively good physical condition when DeRoy died, shortly afterwards she began to have a number of complaints about her health. The physician who provides on-site services to the community through its health center saw Dorothy-May with increasing frequency. To help her sleep and to calm her nerves, he prescribed a mild dose of lorazepam — a sedative often used for sleep. Then, six months ago, Dorothy-May slipped while walking on one of the many pathways in the community, fell backwards, pulling her walker with her, and fractured one of her vertebrae. She was in a lot of pain and couldn't get up on her own. One of her neighbors saw her fall and called for the nurse at the community's health center, who observed at once that Dorothy-May was suffering. The nurse called for an ambulance, and she was taken to the local hospital, where she required bed rest and fairly strong painkillers.

According to the doctor at the hospital, Dorothy-May became quite confused during the first night of her hospitalization, likely from a combination of taking pain medication containing codeine and being in an unfamiliar place.

They kept her a few days longer to make sure she settled down, which she did. She was discharged and provided with in-home care services, including a regimen of physiotherapy to help her get walking again.

Dorothy-May has one child, Owen, who lives in New Orleans. Owen is 67 years old and has suffered from a degenerative disk condition for more than 15 years; in fact, it's the reason he had to take early retirement from his job as a long-distance truck driver. His wife, Louise, is three years his senior and for several decades has suffered from schizophrenia. Her illness is reasonably controlled by medications, but even so, she still has some very difficult times.

Owen and Louise chose to live in New Orleans because Louise has supportive family there — two sisters and two brothers and their families, all of whom are very close to their sister. Also, Owen, who had always worked in the transportation industry, loves the tempo of the city, its very location, and the fact that it has so much history; as well, he is truly close to Louise's family. They have never had children.

While he has a deep sense of affection for his mother, he has never been terribly close to her, just as he hadn't been very close to his father. Owen has always respected his parents, but because he left home when he was 18 years old and has lived away from Atlanta since then, he simply never felt a pressing need to be physically close. In addition, neither parent had ever talked to Louise, nor could they ever accept that he'd married a "damaged woman," as his father had referred to her.

When Dorothy-May had her fall, the retirement community's director called Owen to tell him what had happened and that his mother appeared to be all right, even though she had been admitted to the hospital. Owen immediately traveled to Atlanta to see his mother and spent three days there — the first while she was still in the hospital, and the other two back at the retirement community, staying on an extra bed that was temporarily provided for him to put in her small apartment.

Owen had seen his mother only once since his father's funeral and he was surprised at how much she'd changed in three years. For one thing, Owen noticed how poorly his mother now moved; seldom would she even try to go from room to room without using at least a cane or, more often than not, her walker. He attributed this to her recent fall and painful back. Then he noticed that she often confused dates, times, and events. This alarmed him because he remembered that she had taken care of all her own banking since his father died, although there was never that much to do. When he asked his mother about her financial situation and if anyone was helping her with it, Dorothy-May told him that whenever she needs money, she calls someone at the bank who transfers the amount to her friend Wilma's account at the same bank, and then Wilma withdraws it and gives it to her. She also said that she writes only a few checks and that her rent to the senior's community was deducted automatically. Other than that, there wasn't much banking to be done.

During Owen's visit, he and his mother had dinner together in the dining room. Although Dorothy-May had some difficulty walking even with her walker as a result of the spinal compression fracture, she wanted to be among her neighbors and other residents of the community who took their meals at the center's dining room. During dinner Owen listened to his mother talk about some of the people she knew there. Even though she seemed to know something about most of them, she seemed to be vague about details. She also dropped veiled hints that perhaps some of the residents might be doing something wrong, or worse, illegal.

Owen spent most of his visit trying to arrange things for Dorothy-May so that she could maintain herself in the best possible way as she recovered from her injury. He requested some extra help in her apartment, including some bathing and dressing assistance. Dorothy-May initially declined this extra service, stating that she didn't need any help and that she didn't want anyone in her apartment for fear of having things stolen.

Over the course of his visit, Owen noted that he would have to repeat things he had told his mother over and over again because she kept forgetting what he'd said. But her memory for the "old days" was just fine, and he assumed that things could not be that bad if she could remember events from long ago in such detail. When he went home, other than the concern about his mother's memory problems, he was feeling that, all things considered, his mother was living safely and in relative comfort.

After his visit, Owen made sure he telephoned his mother once every two weeks for at least a few minutes. His conversations with her were relatively short, which didn't leave Dorothy-May much room to articulate in any detail any of her concerns or conditions. Owen didn't think he noticed any particular change in his mother, but he did sense that she acted as if he hadn't phoned before, and that she asked some of the same questions about himself and his life each time he called.

A few months after her accident, his mother did the totally unexpected — she called Owen. It was three o'clock in the morning and she wanted to know when his father was coming home, because she knew for a fact that he and Owen were at some party without her. Her voice was very tense, and when Owen said none of what she claimed was true, reminding her that DeRoy had been dead for years, Dorothy-May yelled at him to shut up and stop lying to her. Then she wanted to know how his "crazy wife" was, and Owen yelled back at his mother to stop talking like that and to listen. But she didn't. She just wanted to know over and over again when DeRoy would be back, and why Owen wouldn't help out and protect his aging, needy mother instead of going off to parties and living with some crazy woman.

By the time he got off the phone, Owen was devastated. First thing in the morning he called the community's director: what he heard floored Owen. The director said that ever since her fall Dorothy-May had been on a gradual slide in her state of health. She explained to Owen that there were a number of problems and that the doctor was concerned that his mother had signs of dementia, most likely Alzheimer's disease. She reported that Dorothy-May was still able to get to the dining room by herself and do her own grooming, and although sometimes the mix and match of clothes was a bit out of character for her, no one seemed to mind. And she was getting to the toilet on time, most of the time. But the director also told Owen that the staff was having someone help

Dorothy-May with bathing all the time now, since she feels unsteady in the shower even though it is a walk-in and has a chair in it to sit on.

The director suggested to Owen that he may want to try to visit more often and spend some time with his mother. She also reassured Owen that the seniors' community was equipped to care for people in Dorothy-May's situation, and that his mother might be moved to a unit where staff could help people like Dorothy-May with bathing, dressing, preparing snacks and any food not eaten in the dining room, and sometimes even feeding if it became necessary. There would be some extra costs involved, but that did not seem to be a big issue at the time.

Owen then called the physician who served the community's health center. The doctor discussed some possible issues that might come up with Dorothy-May and suggested that Owen talk about them with his mother "before it was too late." Owen has never really discussed deep issues with his mother, having left home as a young adult. He wishes, now that his mother is failing and he finds himself unable to communicate with her in a more profound and personal manner, that he'd done more to develop his relationship with her over the years. However, he does know that his mother is not a religious person and stopped attending church many years ago, saying to him that there was not much in it for her. She had always seemed to be a practical person with no deep-seated sense of mystery or symbolism.

To Owen's surprise, when he did speak to his mother again, Dorothy-May was able to state quite emphatically that she would never want to be left to live as a "vegetable," should she get seriously ill. She seemed able to articulate clearly her wish that if her condition couldn't be treated easily and the prognosis was that she couldn't return to her present state of physical or mental health, Owen should "let her go from this world." Owen was quite relieved to hear Dorothy-May state things so clearly. The doctor reassured Owen that should Dorothy-May fall ill, her wishes for minimal intervention of high-technology medicine would be respected. He had already noted those same wishes in her medical chart as Dorothy-May had stated them in the past — she had even written a letter to him stating her wishes — but the doctor felt it was still very important that Owen confirmed those wishes with her.

Owen told the doctor that he could be contacted in an emergency but that he trusted the physician's understanding of Dorothy-May's wishes should she be unable to express them at the time of a real medical crisis.

After these long-distance conversations, sitting in his small family room at the back of his frame house, Owen didn't know what else to do. He had his own personal challenges to face and suddenly he had an added responsibility to manage. He knows that Dorothy-May is safe for the time being, and he remains hopeful that he can provide sufficient support without having to leave home too often, because that is a physical, mental, and financial strain for him.

THE GERIATRICIAN'S POINT OF VIEW

The first thing Owen must do is figure out what has happened to Dorothy-May. It appears that she is suffering from some form of dementia, such as Alzheimer's disease, and perhaps something else as well. It is likely that she has been suffering from this condition for as long as a year prior to her fall. It does not seem likely that the fall itself caused her decline in mental function, but it is not uncommon for an acute medical event to lead to the recognition of dementia, which a person may have managed in his or her own environment for quite a while.

People with a moderate degree of dementia often succeed in managing their daily activities if they live in a reasonably supportive environment, such as a retirement home, seniors' building, or retirement community like the one in which Dorothy-May has been living. In Dorothy-May's case, for example, the staff at the bank has been very helpful, making sure that all of her financial transactions were conducted appropriately.

With a trauma like a fall, even if there is no head injury, which could potentially lead to a more rapid decline in mental function, the resultant hospitalization and need for analgesics containing codeine can increase the risk of a state of acute confusion, often referred to as delirium. This appears to be what happened to Dorothy-May. Although she made a reasonable recovery, the fact that the staff at the retirement community has recommended an increased level of personal care assistance is an indication that her mental abilities are deteriorating.

If Owen were able to arrange it, Dorothy-May might benefit from a referral to a specialist in geriatrics, geriatric psychiatry, or neurology — someone who has a lot of experience with older adults, especially those who have complex medical conditions and problems related to dementia. There are such services in most urban centers, and the There are Atlanta-based health services that have whole programs to assess seniors. One goal would be to differentiate the possible causes of her dementia in order to take the best available steps to deal with the condition and the possible consequences of it. Also, the specialist physician and health care team that often gets involved with the care of elders can act as one of the resources Owen could to turn to should his mother experience further decline.

By reviewing the events leading to the present state of affairs (the history), considering the physical findings, and running some tests (possibly a CT scan or other brain imaging techniques and some blood tests), a physician may be better able to define the kind of dementia that has affected Dorothy-May. This process is important because age alone is not considered a basis for a decline in mental function such as Dorothy-May is experiencing.

Although the likelihood of dementia increases substantially as one ages, it is still important to try to define all the possible confounding causes of the particular condition. For example, it is possible that the fall Dorothy-May experienced was caused by a small stroke that also accentuated her apparently rapid mental decline. It may be that she has blood pressure problems that were not noted previously or problems with her cholesterol. When all the findings are put together, the physician might be in a position to recommend treatments that could be useful in dealing with underlying risk factors that could cause further unwanted events.

If the physician believes that Dorothy-May is suffering from Alzheimer's disease, it may be worthwhile to try one of the special medications available for this condition. They have been in use for a few years now, and the evidence suggests that for a reasonable percentage of patients with Alzheimer's-type dementia (and those with some variants of that condition), these drugs can improve the level of mental awareness and interactions with people. In addition, it appears that the drugs decrease the rate of further decline of the condition, thereby keeping patients in a more stable condition for a longer period of time.

Dorothy-May may respond to the medication, which could improve the way she functions. But she may not respond, and decline may continue despite any medical treatments. Dorothy-May could potentially become more agitated, and the paranoia that Owen witnessed during that disturbing telephone call may become more apparent and interfere with her ability to function well in the social environment of the home in which she is presently living.

The next question Owen has to face is where his mother will live as her condition deteriorates. The retirement community claims it can provide a level of care called "assisted living," but should Dorothy need greater care than the facility and its staff can provide, she might need a nursing home. Some retirement communities include that level of care as part of their spectrum of services, but in some circumstances it might be necessary to move to another facility. It would be worthwhile for Owen to explore the options with the director and, if the retirement community does not have a nursing home level of care, to get some information about what facilities are available in the vicinity. He should visit them and also speak to the staff at Dorothy-May's retirement community to find out what their experiences have been with the nursing homes in the region. He should understand the process so he knows when to register her for transfer if this becomes necessary. Owen needs to set his mother up in a reasonably safe and secure environment that will be able to handle the likely decline in her condition, especially since he lives so far away.

To make the best choice, Owen should discuss with the director of the community as well as her family physician all aspects of Dorothy-May's physical needs and stress that he wants his mother's stated wishes to be respected as she declines.

Visiting his mother is difficult for Owen, but he could arrange to speak to the nurse at the retirement community's health center once a week, just to catch up on things. He should also continue to call his mother, of course, and could establish a routine of always phoning on the same day at the same time so that his mother is more likely to remember. It would help put Owen's mind at ease if he could also arrange for a friend or neighbor in the community to keep an eye on Dorothy-May and to call Owen if there were ever any worries.

Like so many children who live far away from ailing parents, Owen has to cope as well as he can. All he can do — all anyone can do — is try to do the best job possible.

CASE STUDY 16
Technology: Opening New Avenues of Care Management

Technology has been a game changer in eldercare. It's allowed myriad new applications to be mixed and matched, whether as in this case just monitoring in the home, or allowing for what used to be complex and invasive surgical procedures to become virtually outpatient experiences. The real beneficiaries are the elderly and their families.

THE CHALLENGE

Nelly Boduce is 91 years of age and until the past year has been sharp as a tack. She's lived in her own small two bedroom home in Sandusky, Ohio since 1949, when as a young couple, she and her husband Elmer secured a mortgage to buy the place for the grand sum of $3,050. The two of them lived in that home happily until his heart attack in 1997: the attack was severe and while he seemingly stabilized in the hospital, Elmer died in the intensive care unit three days after admission from a blood clot to his lungs.

Nelly and Elmer had eight children, six of whom lived into adulthood. The six live mostly around Ohio. Ellen and her husband Rex live in Toledo, not that far away. Kindra and her husband, Tim, and daughter, Emily, live in Shaker Heights, a suburb of Cleveland. Jan and her life partner Glenn live near Columbus with their four children. Adam and his wife, Agotta May, live in Ann Arbor, Michigan. Rick, three times divorced and with four children to still support, lives in Estero, Florida. Rita, who is the youngest sibling, lives on her own in Dayton.

The children did a very good job of staying in close contact with their mother after Elmer's death. They weren't a very close family, but they did strive to protect their mother by agreeing on who would call or visit when so there wouldn't be too much time without at least one of them being in touch. They often mailed greeting cards and short letters because Nelly wasn't Web savvy, let alone email accessible. The phone, for Nelly, represented high tech wizardry. It was relatively easy to do all that because Nelly was amazingly agile mentally and physically all throughout her eighties and so her children just came to assume that she would be able to carry on for some time.

Evidently, it was a rude surprise when Granny Nell fell and broke her hip and had to be hospitalized. She was on the orthopedic ward for almost ten days because of an episode of post-operative mental confusion that the doctors called "delirium," which gradually improved. Following the hospital stay she went to a rehabilitation program to improve her function and determine whether she could again manage safely on her own. But Nelly never got back to being her "old self" in mind and body; she seemed to be much frailer, and appeared to have aged since her fall, surgery, and hospitalization. The changes, although subtle, were real, and despite initial denial gradually were recognized by everyone in the family; now the challenge was what to do?

When Nelly finally got back home, the house suddenly seemed a lot bigger than it used to be. Getting around took a lot more effort, even though the place was pretty small compared to most of the homes built in the past 20 years. She worked hard to manage, but it wasn't as easy as she expected or wanted it to be. She became more and more uncertain as to what to do and how to do it best. She used the walker she'd been taught to depend on a lot more than she'd wanted to, but there was a sense of comfort and safety with using it that made a difference. And somehow, the home that was home for so long now seemed to her to be more distant and inhospitable; the level of comfort was lost to a kind of uncertainty that followed her from room to room.

Because of her own self-doubts and some degree of cognitive loss, Nelly started to call her children whenever she felt that she was or might be in harm's way. Both kinds of situations became real to her, and she'd call whichever child's name came to mind first. So they all, in effect, got a lot of calls. Sometimes she didn't recall that she had asked one of the children about a problem and then called the same child soon after and repeated the question. That's what got them started on exploring options that would help Nelly manage safely at home, which they knew was her preference, and how to do so with as little external intrusion into her privacy as possible. They concluded that perhaps there were technology-based solutions that could help their mother remain safely at home and also help each one of them ease the pressure of constant, unpredictable, desperate, and often repetitive phone calls. Nelly's children discussed this and discovered that there were a variety of technologies that promoted independence within a framework of increased safety.

Considering their options, they determined that using existing and emerging technology might be useful to supplement the time and care that they were prepared to provide, but that on its own was not enough.

As a first step, they got the Lifeline® (personal emergency alert system) necklace for their mother, which when activated automatically contacts the monitoring service to check on her needs at the moment. They picked the alert option that included the "sudden change in position" feature, sounding the alert if, for example, she fell and could not press the alert button. They decided against the two-way live audio option, because they also installed a home monitoring system that learns the behavior of those in the home and sends an alert if the pattern is changed in an unusual manner. So, if someone spends too much time in the bathroom, bedroom, or kitchen, beyond his or her normal practice, the alarm is sounded at the monitoring station, which first calls the person, and then, if there is a problem with the response or no response at all, contacts a family member. If the situation demands it, the system is capable of dispatching emergency services as well.

Once they believed they had Nelly securely monitored, her children felt much more relaxed. But it did take some time to convince Nelly that the devices actually worked. It took several overnight visits during the course of a couple of months and numerous practice sessions by Ellen, Kindra, and Jan to help her get comfortable with the devices. To her credit Nelly worked at it, practiced, fretted, and worried, but became much more confident wearing the Lifeline® monitor and knowing the house monitor worked.

A few months later, there were a rash of house break-ins and even two house invasions in Nelly's neighborhood and her stress level soared again. She called her children repeatedly for several weeks, noting that if she were sleeping soundly in the middle of the night or even napping deeply in the middle of the afternoon, she wouldn't be able to protect herself in the case of a break-in. Her angst got to be so deep that her children decided they should all chip in and get a security system installed at their mother's house. It wasn't that much more money and it brought their mother and themselves some peace of mind.

In the process of researching alarm systems, they discovered that if they got a more sophisticated system they could remotely check on her visually through their smartphones, laptops, and desktops; they could disarm the alarm system in case someone needed to enter; they even could check on and manage the heating and cooling system, the lights, and more. And if they got a few extra cameras mounted around the little house, they could take turns checking on her and eliminate the other monitoring service already in place and actually save money (even on home insurance costs). They explained all this to Nelly, who at first was against the idea as being too much, too expensive, and, she said, it was starting to feel like they were invading her privacy, they could watch her and hear her anywhere, anytime. However, after some good back-and-forth, Nelly agreed it was a good idea and the changes were made.

The past months all seems to be well with Nelly's life and her children are very pleased. But their experience is only at one level. Tele-medicine services for remote communities; portable monitoring of blood sugar and blood pressure, with results sent over the Internet; long-distance surgical procedures via robotics and digital commands; Medivac services to move people to more sophisticated medical facilities; and, the host of surgical procedures that have reduced the length, invasiveness, and recovery times are all vivid examples of how technology has transformed the practice of medicine and its monumental impact on the elderly and aging.

Nelly and her children are benefiting from only a few of the many modern and rapidly emerging technological services. Rather than interfering with human engagement and closeness, if utilized properly, many of the new technologies can enhance human engagement and family involvement.

THE GERIATRICIAN'S POINT OF VIEW

As a physician whose main role and goal in life is to enhance quality and quantity of life, it has been a personal struggle for me over the years to determine whether advances in technology promote or hinder these ideals. During the early days of the digital age, and distance learning and distance care, there were many like myself who felt a bit of skepticism and concern that technology might undermine the human factor in care giving and personal relationships.

However, over the years I have observed the meteoric advances in these technologies as they impact the actual practice of medicine, many of them to the benefit of patients and practitioners alike. The phenomenal advances in imaging technologies have virtually eliminated what were previously often very crude, inaccurate, and at times dangerous investigations to help unravel complex and often life-threatening medical conditions.

As a young medical resident training for a year in a nuclear medicine department, I recall witnessing the early nuclear medicine brain scans that allowed the fairly accurate and non-invasive diagnosis of "blood clots" on the outer surface of the linings of the brain (*subdural hematoma*) that might follow a relatively minor head injury in an older person. The previous methods of diagnosis were often cumbersome, inaccurate, and somewhat dangerous because the contrast material (that the x-ray could differentiate from normal brain and skull tissue) was injected through arteries going to the brain and multiple x-rays were taken to try and define the blood clot in order to eventually determine whether what might be life-saving surgery could be contemplated. When I saw the results of the first nuclear brain scan that clearly outlined the blood clot and the eminent neurosurgeon asked me, "Would you evacuate the clot on the basis of this scan?" I felt confident when I replied, "yes," to which he responded, "I will!"

This very minor example of the progress of medical technologies in diagnosis and treatment is clearly among the miracles of modern medicine that like any other component of medicine must be looked at through the lens of potential benefits versus risks. Sometimes with the introduction of a new medical technology, abnormalities are found for which a full understanding and explanation may not yet exist, and that may result in further investigations and treatments that may not be necessary and merely increase the risk of untoward effects. There is a tendency, especially in North America, to almost idealize the newest and most sophisticated technological advances with sometimes unexpected or untoward outcomes. Gradually, physicians learn to analyze the findings of the new technologies and the implications for potential benefit and risk, and sometimes can recommend a static approach instead. This approach seems counterintuitive in a world of technological advances and the quest for earlier and apparently better interventions. The development of what is known in the medical profession as *evidenced-based medicine* is our collective scientifically-based attempt to try to monitor and evaluate all medical advances, including new technologies, within the lens of proper study and assessment of true benefits and risks.

A powerful and entertaining demonstration of the impact of technology in arriving at a medical diagnosis, while at the same time establishing and confirming the deep human relationship between physicians (or nurses, or other health care professionals) and their patients is exemplified beautifully in the TedTalk® YouTube video (*http://www. youtube.com/watch?v=sxnlvwprf_c*) by the renowned physician-author Dr. Abraham Varghese (author of *Cutting for Stone)*. In it he discusses the importance of the physical examination and its historical and critical place in medical practice, not just for the purpose of helping to make a diagnosis, but of connecting the patient to the physician. Varghese contrasts the traditional method of touching and probing the patient with the current tendency to sit in front of a computer terminal and digest numbers and images, rather than relating to the patient on a personal, intimate level.

How does this relate to Nelly's family using technological advances to make sure she's safe and secure while still providing her the best quality of life possible? The important thing about this situation is that the family is using "technological fixes" with an eye to avoiding hype over new gizmos that may not necessarily be beneficial. In this way technology is being used to positively address some of the challenges facing Nelly and her family.

The first step in my evaluation of the whole picture is to make sure everyone in the family understands that Nelly's illness and surgery, her post-operative delirium, and her current tendency to be forgetful and repetitive, is likely evidence of cognitive impairment due to Alzheimer's disease. This condition is usually complicated by blood vessel disease as a consequence of the common conditions of high blood pressure, diabetes, and high lipid (cholesterol) levels. If this is indeed the case, the family must plan ahead, not just within the framework of technological solutions to Nelly's living situation, but with a plan in mind as to what to do when her clinical condition deteriorates. It seems to me that based on her illness it is only a matter of time, depending on good treatments for her underlying risk factors, before further decline and unexpected medical catastrophes occur.

An initial step is to get a proper geriatric (or comparable) assessment of Nelly's general medical condition and risk factors, as well as her mental status and function. Even though there are no "cures" for most causes of cognitive impairment, steps exist that might decrease the risks and maximize and stimulate brain function as much as possible. Some of these steps, depending on the circumstance, can be technology-based or enhanced. A simple example: blood pressure and glucose (blood sugar) control can now be administered and monitored at home cheaply and effectively, which is often preferred over the occasional and often anxiety-provoking visit to the doctor. If this is deemed a viable option, a plan has to be implemented that allows for home monitoring, as the technology that can accomplish this is readily and inexpensively available.

Once a full geriatric assessment is made, one can formulate a conceptual prognosis that will allow the family members to address some of the very necessary human, family, and personal value-reflecting decisions that should be known by family members of aging parents. It would be very useful for the family to explore with Nelly, in a way that is not threatening or negative, what her values and wishes are for the future, in the event that something untoward and unexpected happens. Although not high on the scale of truly complex technology, artificial nutrition and hydration can be achieved by a tube going directly into the stomach. It is, in essence, a reflection of modern technological medicine that did not really offer itself as an option a few decades ago; prior to inserting feeding tubes directly into the stomach, patients were subjected to the very uncomfortable method of inserting them through the nose into the stomach.

While exploring all the newest technological options, Nelly's family should not forget some of the simplest and oldest technologies that can promote safety and security. These include fire alarms and CO (carbon monoxide) detectors, with the provision that they are tested at least annually to make sure the batteries are working. Some detectors can be hooked into the monitoring systems that the family has installed in the apartment already, eliminating the need to constantly check the batteries. They should make sure that there is at least one land line that will continue to work even if the power goes off. There should be emergency lighting, of the type that goes on when the power goes off, and usually plugs into regular electrical outlets. An important reminder is to avoid or ban the use of candles, as these can be serious fire hazards. There should be night lights that either stay on through the night if Nelly has to get up and go to the washroom, or turn on when there is motion in their vicinity. Although relatively simple and low-cost, these technologies should not be overlooked.

Once the proper assessments, discussions, and long-term plans and options are considered and agreed to, the family can focus on the here and now and use whatever technologies there are that will help assure Nelly's safety, security, and independence. The risk, if any, is the assumption that these new technologies can replace the human touch and engagement. It might be seductive to conclude that a remote interaction with Nelly through a screen, like using Skype®, is a replacement for a personal visit with the hugging, touching, hand-holding, sharing of a meal, and looking at family photos as a way to connect.

As a complement to personal care, physical interaction, and love, technologies including the monitoring systems that Nelly's family has introduced can promote the important issues of safety and security, and therefore should be explored. The combination of personal attention and commitment, coupled with the best of non-intrusive and supportive technologies, holds a great deal of promise for the future of support for our aging parents and other loved ones.

CASE STUDY 17
Navigating the Health Care System: Knowing How to Get the Help You Need

Sometimes an elderly loved one whose health is failing can't be cared for by family members because either there are none, or they don't live in close enough proximity to be of constant assistance. In such instances, there is a need for someone who can take over the day-to-day care-giving roles that a family member might normally undertake, and, in essence, become the navigator of the health care system on behalf of the one in need and the family.

THE CHALLENGE

Ron is a retired pilot for Delta Airlines. After he retired, thanks to his initial education in commerce, he worked for an investment firm and ended up being an adjunct instructor in Wayne State University's business administration program. He had retired 13 years earlier at the then-mandatory age of 67. Now in his eighties, he is having many problems with his health and ability to function independently in his apartment in Woodbridge, one of the older communities just outside of downtown Detroit and close to the Wayne State campus where he continues to do some private tutoring.

Ron had some unfortunate experiences in his life. His wife of 38 years, Doreen, died five years ago after a long bout of pulmonary disease as a result of years of being a heavy smoker, despite the pleadings of Ron, who was a committed non-smoker. It was a bone of contention for them and eventually she agreed to not smoke in their old two-storey home, as Ron had developed severe allergies to cigarette smoke. Doreen maintained that his allergies were "psychological," but in the end she only smoked outside the house. As the non-smoking movement really took hold, finding a place where smoking was allowed became more difficult and she eventually found a way to stop. Nevertheless, the years of smoking resulted in chronic lung disease with lots of coughing, and in the later days, severe shortness of breath and frequent chest infections. She "in principle" refused influenza and pneumococcal vaccination, despite her physician's and Ron's urging (she did not "believe" in it), but instead took lots of supplemental vitamins to avoid infections. It was a severe episode of influenza with a secondary bout of pneumonia that resulted in her rather precipitous death that left Ron alone in Detroit.

Rosanne, their only daughter, lives in Toronto, as she, like Ron, has dual Canadian and American citizenship based on his having been born in Barrie, a small city north of Toronto. He moved to the U.S. after he started piloting for several American-based airlines. Rosanne was born in the United States but moved to Toronto to pursue her graduate studies in social work, married a Canadian architect, and has two children, both studying at Canadian universities. Gradually Rosanne has moved from clinical social work to a government-sponsored agency where she has a senior administrative role.

She tries to visit her father a few times a year and during the past year has noticed a significant decline in his daily functions and ability to look after himself. He has developed Parkinson's disease, and gradually his walking and self-care has deteriorated. He is very resistant to getting help even though Rosanne has tried her best to encourage him to do so if he wants to stay at home, about which he is adamant. "I do not want to move into one of those retirement or nursing homes. I would rather die in my own home, surrounded by my books and stamp collection."

Ron has been collecting worldwide stamps for more than 25 years. He started his collection when he was an active pilot and could explore and collect stamps from every destination he visited. Now he has people that he knows from his earlier years as a pilot continuing to send him stamps from all over the world. Ron carefully puts them in albums, categorized by country, and by whether the stamps are post-marked or in mint condition. Given the chance, he will sit down with any visitor and show off his stamp collection, relating stories associated with each stamp and the event or historical association connected to it.

Roseanne has noticed that during the past few visits, Ron's home is getting increasingly messy, a tendency he had all his life and was a cause of conflict with Doreen, who was constantly badgering him to "put things away." Also an inveterate "fixer," Ron would never call anyone to repair anything in his house, the result being many half-finished projects in the bathroom and the kitchen, and the perennial task of replacing ceiling tiles. The basement, where the washer and dryer were located, was an obstacle course he confronted every time he did the laundry: it required his going down a very narrow set of steps, which, with his Parkinson's disease, was becoming increasingly difficult and potentially dangerous. In fact, Ron had fallen a few times already, but fortunately those falls did not result in any serious permanent injury.

Ron did have occasional visitors, including Cecilia, a niece from Doreen's side of the family who lived in Dearborn, adjacent to Detroit. She came to visit twice a week for a cup of coffee at their favorite Biggby coffee shop on Woodward Avenue, and to "keep an eye" on how he was doing. She would report to Roseanne and lately was expressing concerns about his deterioration. She found that the fridge did not have a lot of food and Ron rejected any thoughts of Meals on Wheels, which was available in his neighborhood. He was able to walk a few blocks to a local diner that he liked, and since they'd known him for years he at least had a "proper" meal, but during the cold weather such outings were more difficult. He shopped for food at a local small market and Roseanne convinced him to pay with his credit card, which was shared and billed to her so she knew at least that he was shopping on a regular basis. But even then the details of what he purchased were not available.

Cecilia's report on the contents of the fridge was the only hint of a gradual decline in the range of products that Ron bought, although, there was at least some juice, a bit of yogurt, cottage cheese, and a few tomatoes, cucumber, and onions — favorites of Ron's, and something he included in almost everything he ate. But some of the expiry dates on the cheese indicated that he was not able to pay attention to such things, and maybe not getting what he needed to maintain a good nutritional status.

Roseanne visited during Ron's eighty-fifth birthday and arrangements were made for a dinner at one of his favorite restaurants. They were joined by Cecilia and one close neighbor and his wife. The neighbors took a kindly role with Ron and tried to keep an eye on him if they observed him leaving the house. They also saw him from time to time for a visit. After the meal, while Ron was waiting for people to return from the washroom, he turned to Roseanne and asked her, "How did I get here?" At first she was confused, and then realized that his recall of the earlier part of the evening was lost. It was then that she realized that she needed more help getting Ron the care he needed. The problem was, she was not in a position to pick up the slack herself.

When she brought up the subject of moving into a retirement home, he rejected it outright and wasn't convinced that he required help in the house or for any of his personal needs, not even acknowledging that bathing was increasingly difficult. He did not do it very often and failed to tell Roseanne that he had a fall in the bathroom a few weeks before, though she did notice a black and blue bruise on his arm and side of his face that he dismissed as "it's nothing, really" when she asked about it.

She was in a quandary and she wanted her father to be cared for but knew that she could not move him closer to her, or vice-versa, and there was no one she knew in the family or otherwise able to take on his care. She became quite fearful for his safety and security, and his ability to maintain himself in the little house that he loved.

THE GERIATRICIAN'S POINT OF VIEW

This is a common scenario that in the past was usually addressed by the family basically "taking control" and "forcing" the person they were concerned about to move into some sort of supportive housing or nursing home arrangement.

With the changes in many jurisdictions it has become less easy to make such a move without the consent of the person being moved. Even if she or he is not legally capable of refusing such a decision, many family members are loathe to make such a dramatic move against the wishes of the person they love and are trying to care for.

One option is to let things just move along as they are with all the inherent risks and wait for something to happen that forces the issue. This can be a fall, a fracture, or a serious illness that can cause circumstances to change. As a result, more difficult decisions have to be made because

some significant level of function or well-being has been lost that precipi-
tated the new opportunity to move in a more certain, safe direction.

Sometimes it's possible to persuade the person in need to attempt a
trial period at a retirement home with the agreement that it's temporary
and would only become permanent if the person agreed to staying after
the trial. I have used this tactic a few times with patients of mine, at the
request of the family, and it often worked out. This tactic worked with my
father, who initially was resistant to moving into a retirement home in
Chicago, close to where my sister lived, but agreed to it as a three-month
trial. He eventually agreed to stay.

If there is no way that the person is willing to try a facility-based
option, but might consider some help in the home and some services
from outside the home, it is usually a family member that takes on the
role of making those arrangements. What does one do when there is no
one to take on that role at all, or if the only family member(s) live far
away and would have to do everything from a distance?

There are a number of options that are worth exploring and vary
depending on the jurisdiction and what public and private services might
be available. Many cities and towns in the United States and Canada have
either publically funded or not-for-profit agencies that provide what are,
in essence, "case managers," who assist the elderly and their families navigate the many aspects of the health care system. Because of differences
in the funding structures of the two countries, and in the different states
and provinces, it is necessary for every family member to explore what
arrangements exist in the jurisdiction in which their loved one lives.
These case managers usually work within the framework of the agencies
they are connected to, usually know what the requirements are for getting various aspects of care, and will provide assistance in organizing the
care required.

A good case manager is essential to organizing complex combina-
tions of care that meet the changing needs of the person. They must have
good organizational skills and very good communications abilities so
that the patient and the family are included in the decision-making process. In fact, a good case manager will be acknowledged by all involved
as the person "on-the-ground" who knows the way around the system.

I know people who fulfill such roles, either with backgrounds in social work or nursing, who, in the United States in particular, are also very aware of the various funding challenges facing many recipients of home-based care with different levels of insurance beyond their basic government-sponsored Medicare and Medicaid benefits.

In Canada, though much of this sort of care falls under the umbrella of provincial health care, there are still varying levels of eligibility for public services, and, in some jurisdictions, additional charges that must be understood by the person receiving care and their family members. Although health care in Canada often involves less hassle and red-tape than in the United States, there are still substantial challenges to making sure all the pieces required for comprehensive care fall into place since services, regulations, and eligibility requirements vary from province to province and jurisdiction to jurisdiction.

The possibility of engaging what is often referred to as a health care *navigator* might become very attractive. If the public or not-for-profit systems were able to undertake and respond to the wide variety of needs that often occur in caring for an elderly and vulnerable person in a timely fashion there would be no need for a navigator. But as many of us know from other aspects of life, having someone to be one's "eyes and ears" can be very helpful, especially when many things happen simultaneously. Sometimes special expertise and a network of contacts within the health care system are required in order to achieve one's care-provision goals; a competent and experienced health care navigator has usually developed those necessary networks and connections.

Health care navigators are sometimes also called health care or patient *advocates*. If Roseanne were to Google "Health Care Navigator" or "Patient Navigator," or look at the many local and regional family eldercare support services listed online and in phone books, she would find a whole array of resources — some from organizations, and some from corporations who offer experienced professionals with specialized health care education and training.

If Roseanne is thinking of going that route, she must first do her homework and interview a number of potential candidates or a company representative to make sure what she is looking for is what she can expect. Remember, whatever arrangements are made, they do not remove Roseanne from a very responsible role. The main value to her is that she will not have to personally take on the many day-to-day issues that will arise in order to make sure the needs of Ron are being met in a humane, sensitive, and timely manner.

I personally witnessed a situation where a health care navigator was crucial in helping to get the right kind of support for a previously very fit and competent retired university professor (to be called Steve, for reasons of privacy), who suffered a complex medical and neurological condition that left him with severe walking and eating problems. The help of the navigator allowed him to avoid becoming a full-time resident of a nursing home, and instead return home to his Boston apartment with a sufficient array of home support services that would have been almost impossible to organize and supervise otherwise. Married and divorced once, with no children, the retired professor's only family lived out of state. Steve's two health care proxies were friends: one lived in Boston, and the other in Canada. The person chosen as navigator had the credentials and experience and knew her mandate and role — to get Steve the necessary medical assessments, and if these could not be arranged through the rehabilitation unit of the nursing home, to get him back to his apartment with whatever help he might require to be well cared for there. The navigator's team had relationships with an array of home care agencies, contractors, and physician groups, as well as legal and financial advisors. This allowed them to address almost any problem that might surface, and to assure everyone concerned that their client could comfortably and safely stay in his home.

Over the months prior to Steve's return to the apartment, arrangements were made to have a number of specialist medical appointments, and to organize a companion suitable to Steve's personality and interests, who would be able to provide social stimulation, and, weather permitting, to take him out in his wheelchair for long walks along the Charles River. Most important, however, was the arranging of a qualified contractor, who, with Steve's input, would modify the apartment so that it would suit his needs in terms of access, safety, and comfort. The navigator provided the family and close friends with frequent updates as to what was happening and was available whenever needed for meetings with Steve and his family to plan for the future.

The family was comforted by the knowledge that the navigator was not only there when needed and on short notice, but had the blessing of the client, and legal permission to make the necessary enquiries about health care and legal matters that had to be attended to when the family was unable or unavailable to do so. Without the navigator it is likely that Steve would have spent the last years of his life in a nursing home or other supportive housing facility.

Even when there is a navigator or case manager available to provide various levels of assistance to a client, there are still some things to keep in mind as a long-distance family member. Some of these are contained in an issue of *The Baycrest Breakthroughs* magazine (a publication from the organization with which co-author Dr. Michael Gordon is affiliated). This publication can be accessed at *www.baycrest.org*. In the winter 2012 issue there is an article entitled "Caregiving at a Distance: What do you do when you live miles away?" in which there are many fine tips about how to enhance your involvement as a long-distance family member. One of the most important of the 13 great tips in the article is the last one: "Take care of yourself! Caregivers living far away can feel guilty or anxious about not being there." It's important to consider joining a caregiver support group. This might allow you to express and share your concerns, fears, and successes in a supportive environment with others in similar situations.

CASE STUDY 18
We're On Our Own: How to Plan for the Future

A couple in their mid-sixties must consider how long and effectively they can care for an aging mother while planning for the day they will retire and eventually require care themselves.

THE CHALLENGE

Jean and Frank Scott have lived on the outskirts of Peterborough, Ontario, for more than 30 years, after having moved from Kingston where they were born, reared, and educated. Jean is 62 and Frank is 65. Jean is a schoolteacher and plans to work until she retires at 65 because she loves her job and the kids, and also because she wants to maximize her retirement pension. Frank runs the local hardware store. It has been a touch-and-go affair over the years, but it does have some value, and Frank hopes to keep the store going until the time is right to sell it and make some profit. Jean and Frank also have some RRSPs and have been making various modest investments to use for their retirement.

They have many friends and neighbors in the surrounding area but no children of their own. Jean has a sister who lives in Newfoundland with her family, and Frank has a brother and sister who still live in Kingston with their families. Jean's mother, Louise, aged 87, has lived with Jean and Frank since she lost her husband eight years ago. Her income is limited to little more than her small Canada Pension Plan payments, OAS (Old Age Security), and GIS (Guaranteed Income Supplement).

Louise managed well until about a year ago when she fell and broke her hip, resulting in complications — including a stroke that was either a result of the fall or happened just after it. She was found to have an irregular heartbeat and has since required Coumadin® (a blood thinner). She is also a long-standing diabetic and for the past few years has required insulin injections.

Although Louise has made a good recovery from the fracture and the stroke, she hasn't really been the same since and can't help much around the house. In fact, she now needs help with several normal personal activities. Because Jean and Frank both work, and there is no other family nearby, they've been dependent on the Ontario home care system to help provide in-home support for Louise, including bathing and meal assistance, helping her with insulin injections, and monitoring her blood sugar. Because Jean can get home from school by about four o'clock on the days she doesn't have after-school meetings, and Frank has some flexibility with the store when he has adequate help, they've managed with these limited care services provided through the local Community Care Access Centre (CCAC).

Early last fall, Frank and Jean received notice that the hours allotted to Louise's care were to be cut substantially because of funding restrictions to the CCAC by the provincial government. As a result, they've had to make some private arrangements with neighbors, friends, and a number of local teenagers to fill in the gaps left by the reductions. They are paying for the assistance, but their real concern is not the financial drain; it is the prospect of what will happen should Louise require more care. It will be a real challenge to make sure that she gets the services she needs without putting enormous pressure on Jean and Frank.

They worry that they won't be able to afford to keep Louise at home should she deteriorate to the point that she requires full-time help. Moreover, they've been thinking about what will happen to them during the next number of years should they fall ill themselves and need social services. Since they don't have any children or other family in the vicinity, they've expressed these concerns to their physician and the social worker from the CCAC, who worked with them in providing care for Louise. They're feeling very vulnerable in terms of their ability to cope with Louise's needs, physically and financially, and at risk in terms of their own future.

THE GERIATRICIAN'S POINT OF VIEW

There are two main issues involved here, the first being the very real and immediate anxiety about how to provide Louise with the best care possible while not putting Frank and Jean at emotional and financial risk. It is necessary for them both to continue working to maintain their income for as long as possible, as their retirement pensions and savings are not sufficient to ensure them a reasonably comfortable retirement for themselves, much less to ensure that Louise's needs will be met in the future.

They should have a very frank discussion with Louise about the issues and options and let her know that they will do whatever they can to continue to look after her. But they must also tell her that if circumstances change and they cannot continue with this plan, they will look for a nursing home that is close by and suitable for her. They should make it clear that this plan is not meant to abandon Louise, but rather to make sure that they can continue to participate in looking after her and still preserve their energy.

The financial implications may vary depending on Louise's income, but if she does not have anything beyond her government support, there should be no other funding expected from Frank and Jean for her nursing home care. They would clearly take all the necessary steps to make sure the facility is the one most suited to her needs, and it is obvious from their history and relationship that they would visit her frequently and take part in as many social activities as possible, including taking her home for weekends and holidays whenever they could.

The second issue, Jean and Frank's concern about their own future, is more difficult to address. The future is always impossible to predict. Government policies could change so that society may become more senior-friendly. Access to necessary health care and social services may not be a major problem. Or, of course, the opposite could become the case, and those without supportive families or friends may be in deep trouble should things go wrong in terms of health or independence. What Jean and Frank can do, at least, is discuss their concerns with the family that they do have — their siblings and nieces or nephews — so that should they fall ill and need some support, their preferences are known.

Preparing a living will, with the assistance of their physician, may help them feel comfortable with some of the difficult decisions that could arise in the future. Just naming a relative or close friend as a surrogate decision-maker and making clear their hopes and expectations for a time when they can't make decisions for themselves could lessen their worries. If family members or friends are not an option for this, Frank and Jean can turn to their lawyer and ask him or her to take on the role. In retirement homes or seniors' residences, should they eventually move into one, there is usually a way to get someone to agree to act as a support person or surrogate should the situation require it.

So, although it is understandable for them to feel some anxiety, especially as they face Louise's decline and the extra demands made on them, Frank and Jean can take many steps to assure themselves of safe and secure later years.

If the time comes when they are no longer able to look after Louise, Frank and Jean will have to examine the options for her long-term care, and there are many considerations. When looking for a long-term care facility, the options are often limited by geography. In some smaller communities there may be only one facility close by, and depending on the jurisdiction that facility may range from a retirement home with or without an assisted-living level of care to a regulated long-term care facility. Retirement homes usually fall under the category of unregulated homes because in most jurisdictions governments do not provide a regulatory framework or funding within which such facilities function.

Some of the better homes of this nature belong to voluntary organizations that try to ensure some reasonable level of quality of care — but staffing levels and services are not mandated by government. The facilities are usually privately run, sometimes as part of regional or national chains. In some, the quality of care is very high and the services personalized, but the cost, too, may be very high, and there is usually no subsidy offered by government. Many retirement homes, especially those with assisted-living levels of care, provide services that in other situations are usually carried out by long-term care facilities, often known as nursing homes or homes for the aged.

In some jurisdictions there is a range of options within a framework of special care housing structures that also provide important and supportive care. There are various kinds of group homes for those with physical and/or psycho-social problems. Many facilities of this sort provide excellent care for individuals with special kinds of problems, such as dementia of the Alzheimer's type.

When the option exists, many families try to get their loved one admitted to a regulated long-term care facility because the provincial government covers some of the costs and regulates the standard of care. The facilities themselves may be under the control of private for-profit corporations, government (usually municipal), or not-for-profit organizations.

The last category often includes community organizations, religious, cultural or ethnic organizations, or those related to some common heritage or historical link. (These facilities are sometimes referred to as "charitable homes for the aged.") Many large cities have long-term care facilities that reflect the ethnic and cultural bias of that community. For example, in Toronto there are Catholic, Muslim, and Jewish homes for the aged as well as those that cater to the Chinese, Italian, Greek, Finnish, and Polish communities — to name just a few.

The attraction of the not-for profit facilities is the assumption that there is a source of commitment to the care of the elderly beyond that of financial profit. The standards of care and dedication may be better than those run by private companies that may be accountable to shareholders and other corporate interests. That being said, there are many for-profit organizations, some of which belong to large chains, which provide excellent service and quality care.

Probably the two most important considerations when choosing a long-term care facility are location and quality of care. Ideally the facility should be convenient to family members to enable them to visit easily, so that frequent short visits can take place, which are preferable to infrequent but longer visits.

Of course, the quality of care is paramount but can be difficult to assess. One worthwhile exercise is to ask other people who have loved ones living in the facility what they think. You can also ask if there has been an accreditation process and whether the facility has received accreditation or if you can access recent inspection reports. Of course, a visit to the facility to watch how residents are treated and the sense of pride that the staff demonstrate in what they are doing can give a pretty good idea about the standards of care and caring. However, sometimes quality of care can only be assessed after the fact, so close observation during the acclimatization process is crucial. How is your loved one progressing? How often does the staff meet with families? How accessible are they? Answering these questions may indicate the quality of care that is being provided.

When you move a loved one into a long-term care facility, it is worth finding out who's who in the staff hierarchy and who should be contacted for information and progress. Providing the staff with health care expectations is very useful. For example, if a living will exists, the staff should be provided with a copy, or at least be told of the person's wishes for treatment and care. A meeting with the assigned or chosen physician (depending on the situation) is useful to make sure that both you and the doctor understand the general goals of care and the parameters around which medical care will be provided.

Some individuals are too frail and sick to be cared for in long-term care facilities. For example, individuals who require tube feeding, a respirator, complete bowel and bladder care, or who are bedridden or semi-conscious may need to be in a chronic-care hospital or a special level of nursing home that has a different framework of care than what is provided in long-term care (nursing home) facilities. Admission to such a hospital-type facility is usually based on a medical decision and may be the family's first choice or the result of a transfer from a long-term care facility should the person's condition deteriorate to the point that care can no longer be safely provided in the long-term care facility.

Choosing the right facility is very difficult for a family, and sometimes the bureaucratic process can be daunting to even the most informed. The decision-making process often seems very rushed to families struggling emotionally with the decisions. If possible, family members should seek the advice and assistance of a social worker who is knowledgeable in the field and familiar with the peculiar needs and preferences of the family. But the difficult decisions have to be made, and whatever those decisions are, the challenge is to make the best of it by being a loving and supportive family member and exploring ways to help the staff and the facility fulfill their goals to the best of their professional and organizational abilities.

You may have the chance to join a family council or advisory group, or volunteer to participate in recreational programs to augment the care and programs provided by the staff. Positive and engaged participation is usually far more productive and results in a better sense of dedication from the staff than constant complaining and finding fault, which unfortunately is the way that some families approach long-term care facilities. Constructive criticism is usually well received by a reputable organization, but more effective than criticism is a positive and participatory attitude from the loving family members who help those directly in the care giving role.

Caring is infectious, and staff usually recognizes family members who truly care for their loved ones, and they usually respond in a positive fashion that helps everyone.

CASE STUDY 19
The Difficulties of Decision-Making:
Deciding What Treatments Make Most Sense

One of the most difficult challenges faced by families is deciding what treatments might be appropriate to a parent in late-life and possible end-of-life situations. There are ways to ease the challenge and burden for children faced with such a daunting task.

THE CHALLENGE

Joyce, Brian, and Kenneth are very devoted to their father, David, who is an 87-year-old former engineer and a widower. They live in Oregon. David lives with his daughter, Joyce, her husband, Joe, and their two children, Ashley and Michael, in Salem, just south of Portland. Brian and his wife, Julia, and Kenneth and his life partner, Gloria, live in Dundee, just outside Portland, where they run a computer software business that they developed together. Brian and Julia have one child, Peter, and Kenneth and Gloria have twin girls, Elizabeth and Diane.

Clare, who was married to David for 42 years, died more than eight years ago. Everyone, including David, remembers the stress and emotional strain her failing health and death caused all the members of the family. She had metastatic cancer of the breast, and went through a great deal of stress and pain before she died. There were many difficult decisions to be made, and the three siblings found it hard to come to terms with the ambivalence often shown by David, who vacillated between being very aggressive in treatment decisions to just wanting comfort care administered. He was constantly scanning the Internet with the help of Brian and Kenneth to find out what new treatments were available and challenging the doctors, who did not always seem as keen as he was about some of the options. Through the process he created enormous friction with his children, who really thought their mother needed palliative care. She died suddenly of a complication as the cancer spread, which resolved the conflicts but did not leave anyone feeling particularly satisfied about the course of her illness. Since his mother's illness and death, Brian has become very interested in health-related issues and "natural" healing.

David, who was diagnosed three years ago with chronic myeloid leukemia, a malignancy of the blood system, has decided that he does not want to face any of the struggles that happened with Clare when it's his time to face life-ending issues and decisions. After careful research he decided that a living will would make things easier for his family.

He watched with great interest the unfolding media reports on the Terri Schiavo case and decided he would never want any controversy about his wishes should he not be able to communicate because of a serious, lingering illness. He realized that some of the problems he and his children had had with Clare was because no one had ever really spoken to her about her wishes; but then again, she was not the kind of person to talk about such personal things. If anything of that nature ever came up she would say, "Let's not dwell on negative things and just look at the positive. Things will always work out." Of course, because no one ever talked with her about her wishes, it was difficult to make some of the decisions that had to be made toward the end of her ordeal.

David is determined to not let that happen. He has even toyed with the idea of asking his doctor to assist him to die, if he should develop a terrible illness the likes of which affected Clare. And he has been reading a lot about Oregon's Death with Dignity Act and what the process would be should he ever decide to go that route. He has thought about it but hasn't communicated those ideas to his children, as he thinks that they'd oppose it vehemently — especially Brian, considering his preoccupation with health-related issues. He bases this on conversations that occurred when the law was in the process of being enacted in 1997. He thinks that Joyce, who works as a nurse on a surgical unit, might be less opposed to the concept because of some of the thoughts she's shared over the years about some of her very sick patients, for whom, like her mother, surgery did not cure a disease that was eventually terminal. But David has never discussed the option openly with her.

David mentioned his thoughts about physician-assisted suicide under the Death with Dignity Act to his doctor the last time he was there for the quarterly assessment of his blood disease, which was being held in check quite successfully with medications. His doctor suggested that rather than looking to that approach as the only option even if he were to develop a terminal illness (perhaps related to his chronic leukemia, which he knew could become acute), he should fill out a living will document so that his three children would really know what he would want should he not be able to participate in the decision. As the doctor said, "If you can make your own decisions, and you decide to go the route of physician assisted suicide under the Act, you can make that decision at that time, but in the meanwhile a living will might help your children make the right decision for you should you not be able to communicate because of your illness."

David listened to his doctor and managed to find on the Internet a number of living will forms that he felt would fulfill his needs. But none of them seemed to have all of the details he thought he wanted mentioned, so in addition to filling out the form he selected as the best, he wrote a letter of instruction he thought would make decisions easier for his children should they need to deal with a serious and terminal illness. He stated in the accompanying letter, "Should I have an illness from which it is unlikely that I am going to recover, such as a complication of my leukemia, and should I lose the ability to enjoy my life, I would like measures to be taken to assure my comfort and not allow me to suffer."

David mentioned to his children that he had filled out a living will and complementary explanatory letter; he told them where it was in the house and mentioned that he had given a copy to his family doctor as well as to his lawyer. He did not show it to them, but he said it was pretty clear in that it indicated the limits to treatments that he would want should he become seriously ill and not be able to communicate on his own behalf.

Eight months later, he was diagnosed with an acute transformation of his leukemia, which his doctor said had a very bad prognosis. He discussed his situation with his children and, based on their coaxing, agreed to a course of chemotherapy to try for a reprieve from the serious state that his leukemia had taken. He seemed to be moving into remission until suddenly one night he developed a very high temperature and chills; he just managed to call Brian, who rushed to the house and found him virtually comatose. Brian called 911, and David was admitted to hospital with severe sepsis related to the progress of his leukemia and the fact that the chemotherapy had caused a serious drop in the blood cells used to fight infection.

The next two days were a struggle for David. Everyone expected him to die, but by day three he seemed to stabilize; his fever dropped and he seemed better, although he remained semi-comatose. The doctor thought he would wake up, but by days four and five it became clear that something else was going on — especially since there seemed to be weakness of the right side of his body. A CT scan showed a stroke had affected the left side of his brain, and the doctors felt his long-term prognosis was very poor, even though the infection seemed to be under control. By day eight of his condition, he'd not improved and his blood count had dropped. The doctor said a blood transfusion would raise the blood count but the result would be temporary and the procedure had to be done that night to avoid severe immediate consequence. All the children agreed to the blood transfusion, but Joyce reminded her siblings about the living will.

Brian retrieved it from David's home and read it to his siblings. It seemed pretty clear, other than the issue of treatments to provide comfort. Joyce and Kenneth felt that no further treatments should be provided other than medication to control any pain or agitation that their father seemed to experience. They were against further transfusions, which they felt would just prolong David's suffering. However, after the initial transfusion, David seemed to calm down and appear more comfortable, although remaining semi-comatose.

Four days later his blood count dropped again, and everyone but Brian felt that no further transfusions should be given.

Brian disagreed strongly with his siblings. He said the blood transfusion provided comfort to his father, and that is what he wanted. The doctor agreed that some comfort did occur, but that it would be transient.

Brian convinced his siblings to a further set of transfusions — two units of blood — and another week went by of apparent benefit until the blood count dropped again. At this point, the doctor suggested to the children that further transfusions were of no real value and that their father should be allowed to die in as much comfort as could be provided.

Brian was the only person who disagreed with the doctor, and the three children appeared to be at an impasse — the kind that David had hoped to avoid by filling out a living will document and writing the explanatory letter provided to accompany it.

THE GERIATRICIAN'S POINT OF VIEW

After the Terri Schiavo case in Florida and all the intense media attention it generated, Internet sites that provided living wills appeared to get many more requests than previously. Apparently, people requesting the living will form were trying to assure themselves that should something terrible happen to them, their wishes would be clear and any controversy about their wishes would be avoided.

The tragic case of Terri Schiavo had less to do with living wills and intentions that Terri might have expressed at the young age of 27 (when she experienced her collapse that resulted in massive brain damage) than with the unfortunate difference of opinion and apparent animosity that existed between her parents and her husband. That was further exacerbated by the fact that the case became a lightning rod for political and religious groups that tried to use it to promote their particular views. It is unlikely that most adults in their younger years would contemplate a living will, and it is hard to imagine how one would capture all the possible events that could occur so that those who are left responsible for end-of-life decisions could adequately address them.

Despite all the media attention on this tragic case and all the discussions about whether a living will could have changed the outcome, most professionals in the fields of geriatrics and palliative care acknowledge that decisions about end-of-life care occur all the time in every hospital around the country without the kind of conflict that was seen in Terri's case. The tragic illnesses that affect loved ones, especially aging parents, and the difficult decisions that family members have to make usually occur within a framework of devotion and the desire by one's loved ones to do the right thing. (For more about the Schiavo case, see *http://en.wikipedia.org/wiki/Terri_Schiavo_case*)

The challenging question for those family members, and for health care professionals trying to give guidance and support to loving families, is: How does one decide what is the right thing? Within this often heart-wrenching process, does a living will help or hinder the final outcome so that all involved can feel comfortable with the decision that they have made? It is sometimes forgotten by families in the throes of making such difficult decisions that their focus should be trying to make the decision that they really believe is the one that the person who is ill would have made if his or her wishes were able to be expressed at the time of the illness.

How do family members know what their loved ones would have wanted? Sometimes they know from experiencing the person's lifelong history of religious beliefs. At other times, they may recall previous events that evoked observations such as, "I would never want to suffer like my brother did in his last weeks of life." A living will might be helpful for family members, but only if its contents are discussed with them. In fact, that is the key to a successful living will: making sure that the intent of any instructions are discussed with those who will have to follow and apply the intent of the instructions.

So David should have said to his children that should his disease change to become acute — which he knew it would —when it was clear that there wasn't any room for even a short-lived remission, he should be allowed to die with only symptomatic treatment. If those wishes were clearly expressed, it might have been easier for Brian to forgo the extra transfusions that he insisted upon and that added little to his father's well-being.

Since there wasn't any religiously based sanctity of life issue in question, the concept of quality of life likely would have been paramount in the final deliberations. The physician could have assured the children that David's symptoms could be addressed and treated in a humane and dignified manner to relieve suffering without resorting to blood transfusions, which provided a very temporary reprieve from death without any substantial improvement in his quality of life.

Some living will forms indicate the choice that those making the decisions should follow the medical advice being provided by the responsible physician. If this is the case, then it is very important to discuss with one's doctor what factors would be considered in the final decision-making process. It can be very helpful and soothing to a family for a physician to say that the issue was discussed and that what was meant was in fact being applied in terms of treatment.

Sometimes individuals do not articulate their wishes very well to their children, as was the case with David's wife, Clare. Although it might appear difficult, at the opportune time it is worth having a discussion with one's parent to explore the values and wishes that might form the basis of end-of-life decisions.

One method that often works well is for one of the children, such as Joyce in this case, to outline what she thinks the parent would want under the circumstances of a life-threatening illness: something along the lines of, "Dad, I have known you for 45 years. I watched you go through Mom's terrible illness when we could not decide what to do at the end. I think that in a similar situation you would want us to just make you comfortable. I suspect that you would not want to get into any treatments that wouldn't provide any substantial quality of life, but might extend it for a short period without out any real chance of permanent recovery. I don't think you would want a permanent tube feeding or dialysis, or resuscitation if there was very little chance of a full recovery — is that right?" If David had said to Joyce, "Right, you got it," the essence of the living will would have been communicated.

Such a conversation would have gone a long way to help Joyce and her brothers agree to give no further blood transfusions and to provide only treatments that would give their father a dignified, humane, and comfortable death. Any family that has not had that conversation should try it. Quite often the response is very positive, and an aging parent might feel relieved that the subject was discussed so that he or she does not have to worry about it in the future; it protects the loved one from unnecessary suffering and protects the family from avoidable anguish.

CASE STUDY 20
Finding a New Life: Corrections and Concerns

Many elderly people who have lost a spouse want to move forward and "get a life" at some point, yet often their children find themselves unable to understand or approve. This inevitably leads to confusion and potential conflict.

THE CHALLENGE

When Don Benson died after a lingering illness, his wife, Nora, understandably grieved for more than a year and a half. They'd been married for 51 years, and it had been a happy marriage throughout. They'd been extremely close — not just as husband and wife and parents, but also as the closest of friends and confidants. In fact, while they'd had many friends and a very active social life, they always told everyone that the best free time was the time they spent alone together.

Nora found much comfort and solace in the support she got from her son, Jeremy, and daughter, Lisa, at the time of Don's death. They stayed very close to her for the first few months and, even after, kept a close watch over her. They visited and phoned frequently and brought her to their homes.

Some six months after the funeral, Nora told her children that she appreciated their kindness, but she was feeling more stable and wanted some time to herself — to think about her life with Don, to sort things in the house, and to reflect. While Jeremy and Lisa at first worried that their mother was sliding into some kind of depression, they discovered, much to their relief that she seemed to be all right being more on her own.

At the time of Don's death, Nora was still a relatively young senior citizen of 72 years. She was in good health; the only significant medical procedure she'd had was cataract surgery three years earlier.

Jeremy was 44 years old and working long hours as a fairly successful stock broker when his father died. He was married to Miriam, a very happy woman who worked part-time at an upscale clothing boutique and spent as much time as possible with their 11-year-old daughter, Dawn.

His sister, Lisa, had just turned 40. She lived in a common-law relationship with Marvin. They had no children, and they always explained that they'd never intended to have a family because both were devoted to their careers and each other. Lisa was an actress who regularly landed supporting roles in local playhouse productions and appeared in television commercials and print ads. Marvin was a graphic artist by day and an aspiring painter by night, working on canvases that were displayed in some smaller galleries and in various restaurants.

The two families got along well, despite being very different. And both really wanted to help Nora in any way they could.

During the period Nora wanted to spend more time alone, her children and their families pulled back, respecting her wish. Of course, they still visited her and invited her to visit them, and they all spent time together during holidays and birthdays and other special events. Jeremy and Lisa also each spoke to their mother on the phone a couple of times a week.

As time passed, Nora seemed to regain her sense of confidence in herself and in life in general. She spoke less of the "good times with Don" and more about how she was going to move into a retirement home in the next year or so, about the canasta card club she'd joined, about her church activities, and about a local book club that she was thinking of joining. She also announced plans to become a volunteer at the local museum, a place that she had always enjoyed.

Her children were amazed and thrilled at what they considered to be a very healthy approach by their mother to the rest of her life. They were also delighted that Nora looked good; she dressed well, moved with comfort, and spoke clearly and lucidly about her life and day-to-day activities.

Six months ago, Nora told her children that she'd selected a retirement home and planned to sell the family home and move out within the year. She also surprised them with the news that she was going to take a seniors' bus tour across central and western Canada (which she had always wanted to see) that would last three weeks. She'd already signed up for the tour, which was departing from Toronto, a short bus ride from her home in Buffalo, New York. A week after her announcement, Jeremy and Lisa asked their mother if she thought that was wise. Nora assured them it was perfectly safe and told them with some pride that she'd had her annual medical check-up recently and had been given a clean bill of health. She also reminded them how much she and Don used to enjoy going on bus tours, train rides, and cruises.

And so Nora headed off, promising not to just send postcards but to call either Jeremy or Lisa every few days. She did just that, and she always sounded cheerful and contented. The three weeks seemed a long time to her children, who worried about her since she'd never been on any trip alone before.

But Nora returned unscathed and unharmed. If anything, at the "welcome back" dinner they arranged for her she seemed brighter and happier than they'd seen her in a long time. It was during the dinner that Nora told her children and their spouses that her life had changed. She explained that a few months earlier she'd met a very nice widower named Albert at the canasta club. He was 76 years old, tall, very considerate, and fun to be with. They'd had dinner together a few times. He was the one who suggested she go on the Canadian tour, for which he had already signed up, and they'd just spent a lot of time together and were very comfortable with each other. He, too, liked reading and had joined the book club, and he thought that the museum volunteer activity was great fun. And he lived at the retirement home where she planned to move.

Jeremy and Lisa were flabbergasted, as were Miriam and Marvin. They had not expected this at all. They didn't know what to say as they exchanged glances across the dinner table. It was only when Nora asked what they thought that they each said it was a surprise.

Jeremy immediately wanted to know more about Albert — about his health, about his financial situation, about his family. He had a lot of questions that just bubbled out of him. Lisa remained very quiet and listened to her mother patiently talk about her new friend.

After Jeremy had taken Nora home, he called Lisa. They talked for quite a while and agreed that this wasn't like their mother. They just couldn't imagine her finding someone else at this stage in her life. It simply didn't feel right to them, especially since their mother and father had been so close. Jeremy pointed out that he'd heard a lot of stories about widows and widowers who had hit on other elderly people in order to ensure their own comfort and financial security. He told her stories of stocks being transferred to such people in good faith, only to be cashed in by that trusted person, who then vanished. It was an unsettling phone conversation for them both.

Lisa had yet another nagging concern, and she called her mother the next day to raise it. Lisa asked her mother how she really felt about this man; Lisa wasn't comfortable calling him by his name. Her mother responded that she felt very comfortable and wanted to know why her daughter was asking. Lisa finally said what was bothering her: she loved her father and valued her memories of him and her mother together, and she just couldn't see how Nora could toss all that aside and select another man.

Nora was stunned and hurt. She told her daughter that one had nothing to do with the other. She said that tears still came to her eyes and she felt an ache in her heart when she thought about Don, but there was nothing she could do to bring him back; she could only cling to the good memories. But, she reminded Lisa, she still had a life and she wanted to live it. Besides, she and Albert were just friends, nothing more.

That didn't satisfy Lisa, and they ended the conversation on a tense note. Later, Lisa called Jeremy and reported what their mother had told her. Neither felt good about the developments, nor did they know what to do about it. The only decision they made was that together they must convince their mother to abandon her friendship with Albert.

A few days later Jeremy and Lisa went to see their mother to talk about their concerns. Nora became agitated and defensive and asked her children to let her have a life she could enjoy. They ended the session in a standoff — Nora determined to carry on with her plans, and Jeremy and Lisa equally determined to change her mind.

THE GERIATRICIAN'S POINT OF VIEW

The death of a spouse often leads children to assume that the surviving parent will remain single and that their role as children will be to care for and nurture the parent as a widow or widower.

In many cultures the idea of remarriage is quite alien, and widows especially bear the mark of their status quite openly. It is unusual for them to reconnect for many reasons, including societal standards and family expectations. But in still other cultures it is considered terrible for someone to be alone after the death of a spouse, and a lot of effort goes into trying to reconnect the person (especially in the case of widowers; the gender bias is clear).

In North America it is not uncommon for widows and widowers to remarry, although the likelihood for men is much greater than for women simply because there are more older women than older men. Also, our cultural bias finds it more acceptable for men to connect with much younger women than for women to take up with younger men.

So what's the problem with Nora's family? One would have thought they would be delighted that their mother is in a position to have a meaningful relationship at this time of her life. But it is not uncommon for children to react exactly as Jeremy and Lisa have. It would be useful for Jeremy and Lisa to explore the cause of their reaction so that they can come to understand it and prevent undermining their relationship with Nora or alienating her and her newfound friend, who may someday become more of a significant other.

Children often have emotional reactions to situations without looking at the situation from the perspective of the most important person affected, who in this case is Nora. Jeremy and Lisa seem to be forgetting that Nora's needs and wishes should be paramount, and as much as possible they should be supporting her to be a physically and emotionally independent person. If they really thought about it, they would probably come to the conclusion that if either of them were struck by the tragedy of losing a spouse, they too might one day want to reconnect. Emotional and physical relationships are so central to human happiness and fulfillment that to deny people such opportunities is to condemn them to a life of loneliness.

A lot of children think of a parent's desire to reconnect as somehow compromising their respect and love for the deceased spouse. Yet if you ask those in loving relationships what they would want for their spouses if they died, most would say that the most important thing would be that their loved ones not be left alone and that they try to find someone else with whom to share an emotional and physical relationship.

Some children are repelled by the thought that their parent might actually want to have a sexual relationship with another person, especially when they are older and after so many years with their other parent. Many younger people erroneously assume that human sexuality stops at a certain age. In fact, the main barrier to healthy and fulfilling sexual relationships in the older years is the lack of a partner rather than the lack of desire or physical ability.

Lastly, there may be other concerns that the children are not expressing that are financial in nature. Sometimes a surviving parent is left with a lot of money and assets that the children assume will pass to them after the parent's death. Therefore, a potential new spouse can be seen as a threat to an inheritance. It is also true that sometimes-dishonest individuals prey on unsuspecting widows and widowers to take advantage of their financial situations, using their emotional relationships as the basis for poor financial decision-making. I have seen very few of these cases in my practice of more than 35 years, but indeed this might be a valid concern of children who want to be sure not only of their future inheritance but also of the financial security of the surviving parent.

So what should the children do? Presumably they want to continue to have a loving relationship with their mother and at the same time ensure their mother's happiness and their collective financial security. If they keep acting the way they are, they are not going to achieve their goals.

The first step is for them to sit down with Nora and express to her their support and happiness that she is finding her own life again and that they respect and love her for it. They should also say that they understand why it is so important that she find a potential partner for an emotional and, possibly, physical relationship. They must emphasize their support for her happiness as a major priority in their lives.

With that said, they can then say that they just want to be sure that this new relationship does not put Nora at any risk emotionally, physically, or financially. They should offer to meet Albert and arrange a time when they can do so in a relaxed manner and welcome him as a special person in their mother's life The more they include him in family events, the more likely they will be able to figure out what kind of person he is and how he and Nora seem together.

With that kind of approach Jeremy and Lisa will be in a much better position to express other opinions and concerns. For example, they might suggest that should the relationship develop into something more serious or legally binding, Nora should seek the advice of a lawyer to make sure that her financial resources are protected. In addition, if Nora wants to protect her children's financial inheritance, there are legal ways of doing so. Taking such a step would probably go a long way toward soothing the suspicions and concerns that the children might rightfully have but may not be able to articulate to one another or to Nora as they contend with this new situation.

Many older people reconnect very successfully in their later years, especially after the loss of a long-time spouse. What more wonderful thing could happen to people who would otherwise spend their remaining years dependent on their children and friends? A new partner does not desecrate the honor of the previous spouse; if anything, many people who have been through such experiences find that they can share the importance of the previous relationship and use it as a basis for a new and fulfilling relationship. Children can play an important role in supporting and encouraging their parents' independence and need for emotional and physical fulfillment — an essential part of human existence.

CASE STUDY 21
Decision Time: Planning for the Inevitable

When one parent is ill and the other parent appears to be unable to make appropriate care-giving choices, the children must make some hard decisions about what steps to take to protect the dignity and well-being of both.

THE CHALLENGE

Margit and Tamas Ujhazy were childhood sweethearts. They were born in the same small village in Hungary, and they married when she was 16 and he was 19. A few years later, they immigrated to Saskatchewan when Canada was encouraging people to come to work there. Under the terms of the agreement with the government, for the first five years they had to work on a farm — which is what they did back in their native Hungary. After the five-year period expired, they moved to Esterhazy, where they rented a room in a private home and worked in the area — he as a farmhand, and she as a domestic.

They never prospered but lived frugally, and when Margit was expecting their first child they bought a tiny four-room bungalow that has been their home since the late-1950s.

Now, Margit is 70 and Tamas is 73. Margit had a serious stroke a year ago that has left her totally incapacitated and in need of round-the-clock care in a nursing home. She is able to speak, but not easily, and often mixes English with Hungarian. Meanwhile, Tamas continues to live in their home and work part-time at a local hardware store.

They have two children — Elizabeth, 40, and Arpad, 37. Elizabeth, a radiologist, lives in Vancouver with her second husband, Bob, a software programmer. Arpad, a chartered accountant with an accounting firm, lives in Edmonton with his wife, Nancy, and their three children. Since leaving home, neither Elizabeth nor Arpad have been very close to each other or to their parents, until their mother's stroke prompted both siblings to become more actively involved.

When their mother suffered her stroke, Tamas called his children — something he hadn't done in more than a decade — to tell them what had happened. Both Elizabeth and Arpad went to Esterhazy to see their mother and visit with their father. It was Elizabeth's first visit home in more than five years and Arpad's first time back home in four years. Elizabeth and Arpad now call their father every Sunday and stay in touch with each other through weekly emails to compare notes about what Tamas has told them.

Recently, their mother was diagnosed with bone cancer. Tamas told them about the diagnosis in one of their weekly telephone calls but said that everything was under control. In a subsequent telephone conversation he told Elizabeth that nursing home staff had complained that Margit yells a lot and said that they think that she's in extreme pain. But Tamas says she's not really in much pain at all; rather, all the noise she's making and the claims of pain are her way to get more attention.

Elizabeth asks her father who their family doctor is and decides to call her. When they eventually connect, the doctor tells Elizabeth that Margit is indeed in extreme pain, which is why she's often yelling out.

The doctor wants to place her on morphine patches but explains that Tamas refuses to agree and, at most, allows only Tylenol 3 to be administered. The doctor also tells Elizabeth that Tamas, who's been diagnosed with early signs of Alzheimer's, proudly points out that his wife has a history of bearing pain very well. Tamas has said that while everything possible should be done to keep Margit alive, morphine patches are unacceptable. It's not clear to the doctor why Tamas feels that way.

Now Elizabeth and Arpad face a dilemma. The doctor has explained Tamas's wishes and suggested that their father may not be making choices in a sound frame of mind. Elizabeth and Arpad agree that Arpad should see their father to talk about what needs to be done for both their parents. Uncertain of what they should do about either parent, the two siblings decide that their father's views should be sought and, if they make sense, applied.

When Arpad meets his father in Esterhazy, Tamas tells him that his mother often took to yelling out loud when she felt she was in pain but that this was a natural overreaction that shouldn't be taken seriously. He reminds Arpad how much and how loud Margit used to yell even if she just bumped an elbow into a door or got a slight cut on a finger. Arpad can't remember any yelling at all by his mother, so while he wants to believe his father, he's very conscious that his mother is suffering terribly from her bone cancer while incapacitated by her stroke.

No matter how much he talks to his father during his weekend visit, Arpad can't convince him to approve the morphine patches or any other pain management assistance for his mother. And the more they talk, the more Arpad realizes that at times his father is very logical and lucid, but at other times he is seemingly confused and uncertain of past events. Arpad wants to believe his father, yet he's torn by nagging doubts and a growing concern for his mother's condition. By the end of the weekend, Arpad feels the visit was an exercise in futility and that even if his mother has a low pain threshold, that has nothing to do with the fact that she's got bone cancer, which he recalls is one of the most painful types of cancer there is.

When Arpad returns home, he calls his sister and they have a long discussion about what they can and should do for both their parents. Both realize that there is little they can do long-distance and that neither really wants to take on the responsibility of becoming a dedicated family caregiver. They exchange stories of their childhood and teenage years that demonstrate that their parents didn't do as much as they should have for either of them — and then they realize that they are groping for a justification to do little or nothing.

Ashamed, agitated, and confused, Elizabeth and Arpad finally decide that they must try to help make their mother's suffering as manageable as possible and that they need to try to deal with their father and find a way to get him the help he'll need when their mother dies, and as his Alzheimer's continues to develop.

THE GERIATRICIAN'S POINT OF VIEW

Elizabeth and Arpad face a situation in which there really isn't a right answer. Here they have one parent who appears to be suffering unnecessarily from pain due to cancer and another whose dignity they are trying to respect, even as he shows evidence of cognitive decline. The respect for one parent's needs appears to be in direct conflict with the needs of the other parent. As both children try to show respect for their parents, they must struggle with the impact of whatever decision they make.

To ignore the need for proper pain management in a parent suffering from malignant bone pain seems cruel and unacceptable to them. However, since their father is the person making decisions, they are trying to respect him even though the consequences for their mother are not acceptable emotionally, nor are they acceptable as part of a standard of medical practice for palliative care.

For most health care professionals, withholding pain control in the palliative stage of malignant disease is considered an abrogation of one's professional responsibility. Therefore, in order to care for their mother and try to maintain respect for their father, Elizabeth and Arpad are going to require enormous sympathy and assistance from the health care professionals caring for both of their parents.

If, indeed, Tamas is showing early evidence of Alzheimer's, this should be formally addressed by his physician. It might be that the diagnosis is incorrect and that there is another explanation for the change in his personality and decision-making process. For example, depression can appear to cause memory lapses and other cognitive changes that may be misdiagnosed as dementia of the Alzheimer's type. Some medications (such as sleeping pills and sedatives) can also cause lapses in cognition, memory, and judgment, and Tamas's doctor should evaluate this possibility in an objective fashion.

If, after appropriate review, assuming that Tamas agrees to the evaluation (which can be facilitated by his physician if the children explain the situation), no clear clinical explanation for his views and no disorder that might compromise his ability to be a surrogate decision-maker is found, the children are faced with a serious problem. They will have to get as much assistance as possible from physicians and nurses whom their father trusts to try to help him understand the importance of proper pain management for their mother. It would be worth exploring why he is opposed to morphine patches. If he is concerned about her becoming addicted or overly somnolent, perhaps alternative methods of pain management might be suggested that he will not perceive as risky or that might "end Margit's life." This might include a less potent analgesic given on a round-the-clock basis coupled with drugs such as tricyclic antidepressants that can accentuate the effects of analgesics.

If Tamas still refuses some appropriate regimen of pain management, the children will have to decide whether they should apply to replace their father as surrogate decision-maker because of his failure to fulfill this role according to most legal frameworks (i.e., acting in the best interests of the person on whose behalf you are acting). This will not be an easy decision and could potentially cause a rift, temporary or otherwise, in the relationship between Elizabeth and Arpad and their father.

If, on the other hand, it is found clinically that their father is cognitively impaired and incapable of making proper surrogate decisions, he can be replaced by the children. This may also result in a negative response from him, the only difference being that the children can perhaps get some help from the physician in explaining why the surrogacy has to be changed. In that way, the doctor can bear some of the responsibility for the decision, and then proper decisions concerning Margit's palliative needs can be made without the children appearing to be going against the wishes of their father.

The children must be prepared for the likelihood that after their mother dies their father is going to require an extra measure of help. If he is, indeed, manifesting evidence of dementia and early Alzheimer's, he may feel the loss of his wife profoundly and his symptoms may be exaggerated. It is likely that he will need help in his home. Or perhaps he will eventually need to live elsewhere. Such a decision should not be taken precipitously, but rather in a measured manner, as the mourning period may be prolonged.

The hope is that their father's dignity can be maintained as much as possible while they still meet the first imperative — ensuring that their mother has a peaceful and pain-free death.

CASE STUDY 22
When Love and the Law Conflict: Who's Right, Who Has the Right?

The conflicts that emerge when family wishes and the law clash can create barriers that often leave the aging and vulnerable loved one in limbo for way too long, and their families bitter and divided.

THE CHALLENGE

Sometimes even the seemingly most sensible laws made with the best of intentions and ethical and legal principles falter when they come into conflict with family devotion and a sense of "protecting" those we love most. For those whose role is to unravel such challenges, the results are often disquieting and tug at one's heart while at the same time causing one to consider the ideas of "right and wrong" in an ethical and legal sense.

Leonard was 87 when he had a terrible near-asphyxiation event while in Florida, where he'd been going for many years to avoid Winnipeg, Manitoba's winters. He had been living with dementia of the mixed vascular (blood vessel disease) and Alzheimer type for about five years and was already in need of constant care from Janette, a personal support worker (PSW) who lived with him round-the-clock, with some relief on weekends. The winter move to the condominium owned in Hallandale was arranged and assisted by his two older children: Rebecca the oldest and Martin in the middle, with the usual plan of each of them, as well as his youngest daughter, Lisa, visiting for a one-week period during his three-month stay, at the end of which one of them would accompany him and Janette back to his Winnipeg home.

Leonard needed help with most of his daily living activities (eating, bathing, and toileting), but if food were prepared for him and cut into small pieces he could usually eat by himself and there had not been any apparent problems thus far with his swallowing. It was therefore a shocking event that with the personal support worker turned from the table for a few moments to put something into the refrigerator, Leonard inhaled something into his airway and started choking. The attempt by Janette to expel the food with a forcible abdominal thrust failed twice so she called 911; paramedics arrived about 10 minutes later and managed to dislodge the food from his airway, but Leonard had by this time lost consciousness.

In the Florida hospital it became evident that he had suffered significant brain damage, which when added to his underlying dementia, as explained by the doctors, meant that it was unlikely that he was going to regain even a small amount of his previous function. And that meant, in essence, no speaking, interaction, and perhaps even an inability to have any significant appreciation of what was going on around him. Arrangements were made to have Leonard returned by paramedic-accompanied flight to Winnipeg to be directly admitted to an appropriate health care facility, which required some complex discussions and applications sent from Florida with all the salient information.

The issue of palliative care was raised by Rebecca, his eldest daughter. Martin, his son, rejected that option although apparently there seemed to be some dissension by Lisa, the youngest daughter. When they were told that in order to keep him alive they would have to insert a feeding tube the two eldest children, who in fact shared the formal decision-making role, agreed without hesitation. An application was made and he was eventually transferred to a skilled nursing home (known as a Complex Continuing Care facility) in the Winnipeg area. Once he was admitted and settled and all the information was being acquired about him from the team social worker, Rebecca, almost as an after-thought, mentioned that Leonard had a living will (advance directive). She said they had only found it after the feeding tube had been inserted, when they went to Leonard's apartment in Winnipeg, and that they were not aware of its contents prior to the choking event.

The document was presented; it was dated 10 years previously, when presumably Leonard was still able to express his wishes in what is legally called a *capable* manner. The document was signed by him in the presence of a lawyer. In it was stated quite clearly that he would not have wanted a feeding tube under the present circumstances, as he had indicated explicitly that he would not want artificial life maintenance in the event that he would not recover from a condition that would leave him without the ability to participate in life. He used the term *heroic* measures as well, as a way of indicating that he would not want cardio-pulmonary resuscitation (CPR), but did not give any details about what else he would have meant by the use of that term.

After the document was produced, the social worker asked Rebecca why they didn't know about this before Leonard became ill with dementia and certainly why it wasn't discovered after his acute asphyxiation. She said they "just found it" when he was in the hospital as they were looking through some of Leonard's papers and assured the social worker that she and her brother and younger sister were never apprised of its content by their father. The siblings indicated that they assumed that should something happen the lawyer involved might be contacted and she would have the document on file. They only knew about that lawyer because when their mother was ill the lawyer was involved in advising Leonard what the law allowed him to do when he opted to discontinue life-maintaining therapy, which for his wife included not just a feeding tube but a respirator. That experience seemed to provoke the idea of the living will, surmised Rebecca as she spoke to the social worker.

The social worker relayed this information to the head nurse and the attending physician, who expressed concerns and recommended that the ethicist working for the institution, as well as the facility's lawyer, should be consulted for advice. They all knew that in Manitoba a living will was supposed to be respected by substitute decision makers but were not sure what to do if, after the fact, a living will came to the attention of those responsible for making the decisions on behalf of the person who made the living will.

After conferring with the ethics consultant and the lawyer, it was deemed that according to the law the advance directive, which was quite clear to all who read it, meant that the feeding tube would have to be removed or its use discontinued and that a DNR order would have to be put in place, since that is what was indicated quite clearly in the living will document.

A family meeting with Rebecca and her younger brother and sister took place with the social worker, head nurse, family physician, and ethicist, and the law was explained to them. In addition, articles were produced outlining the dismal results of Cardio-Pulmonary Resuscitation for people in Leonard's state and it was reiterated that Leonard had indicated that he would not want CPR. Following this meeting, with some reluctance, Rebecca and Martin agreed to the DNR order in their capacity as the substitute decision makers. The real disagreement came when they said they could not agree to withhold potentially life-saving treatments such as antibiotics in the face of an infection, and most certainly could not agree to discontinue the artificial nutrition and hydration despite a clear indication of that wish by Leonard. Rebecca said she did not believe her father "really understood" what he was signing and that it was probably a template living will made by a lawyer which he just signed without knowing in totality what it meant.

Martin was clearer in his reasoning when he said, "As his son, I just cannot bring myself to take a step that I know will lead to his death. I could not live with myself to think I was responsible for allowing him to *starve* to death." He continued, "I suspect he wrote this after our mother died because he was mourning his loss and of course experienced her long and drawn-out death, but I do not believe he would want to do this to us, having to take such steps to allow him to die. The lawyer should never have allowed him to sign this document and we won't agree even if you have to take us to court; in fact, we will fight it tooth and nail."

Lisa, who did not speak much during the meeting, seemed to indicate by the few words she did say that she believed that her father should be allowed to have his wishes fulfilled, but both Rebecca and Martin, by their words and body language, indicated that her views mattered little as she "did not really understand, and in any event she wasn't a formal Substitute Decision-Maker" (also referred to as proxy for health care).

The staff met after the family left and the lawyer indicated that they were duty-bound to challenge the family's position as they were in violation of the law, which in Manitoba is embodied in the Care Consent Act that with a range of variations is mirrored in many jurisdictions in the United States and Canada. The idea of patient autonomy is so ingrained in the culture and in the law that it is very hard to ignore what would be defined as *capable* wishes of a person about medical treatment. The other issue often raised is whether artificial nutrition and hydration is a *medical treatment* or just a human obligation to feed and provide fluids to an ill person, outside the realm of medical treatments. In most jurisdictions, the legality of artificial nutrition and hydration as a medical treatment has been established. However, there are many people with strong religious beliefs who maintain that it is outside the realm of medical treatments and so is not just obligatory, but that discontinuing it would be the terrible offense rather than the other way around.

The consensus of the legal and ethics consultants, even in the face of the social worker's reminder of the strong personal feelings on the part of the family and the "lack of malice" in their wishes, was that as an institution they were obligated to respect the law and that they, too, in their roles of substitute decision-makers/proxies was to respect the expressed wishes of their father. The institution informed the family of its obligation to pursue the legal channels to challenge their decision and that meant taking the case to a tribunal that adjudicates such cases. In most jurisdictions it's called the Consent and Capacity Board, although in the United States cases such as this one often go into the general court system rather than a specific health care-related tribunal.

The family members were informed and indicated that they would be willing to present their case before the tribunal, and were counseled by the social worker to get a lawyer to represent them; likewise, the legal department of the facility requested the advice of a lawyer whose expertise was in this field.

Meanwhile, Leonard's condition did not improve. In fact, he had an episode of pneumonia which was treated with intravenous antibiotics from which he recovered, but there was no improvement in his level of consciousness that at this point was hardly existent even though the family maintained he "recognized" them when they visited and remarked on movements of his eyes as "proof," even though there were never any verbal utterances of recognition.

The case was brought before the tribunal, and despite supposed evidence brought to bear by Rebecca and Martin (who were the main witnesses during the hearing, with Lisa playing almost no role) about Leonard's Judaism and its importance in his life, and the testimony of a rabbi about how nutrition and hydration were not considered *medical treatments* in Judaism per se, their arguments were not persuasive. Their contention that Leonard could not have known the implications of what he was signing were clearly refuted by the lawyer under whose guidance he made his living will. The lawyer clearly indicated the standards and process by which she undertook what she deemed to be this very important task and indicated that from all of her notes it was clear Leonard fully understood and appreciated (the standard of *capacity*) what the lawyer wrote and what he signed. At the end of the hearing the Board's opinion was that Rebecca and Martin had to abide by the instructions in the living will within a timeframe outlined in the decision. A few days later they launched an appeal of the decision. Throughout this exercise, Leonard was being maintained in a state that seemed to be in conflict with his living will instructions and his children were taking on the adversarial role that it was them "protecting" their father against the system and believing that it was only they who cared about Leonard.

THE GERIATRICIAN'S POINT OF VIEW

It is very sad when a situation arises where the loving instincts of family members end up coming into conflict with the person in whose best interests they believe they are acting. Laws such as the Health Care Consent Act and other laws like it in other jurisdictions were created in order to protect the wishes of people who can no longer speak for themselves. There has been a profound evolution in the legal system during recent years regarding the importance of respecting such expressed or strongly implied wishes. The introduction of the concept of a living will or, more formally, advance directive, has only come into being in the past few decades. Prior, it was always the family acting as substitute decision-maker or proxy that decided what would be done for family members with no formal legal framework for determining the basis of how decisions were to be made.

Now there is a legal framework in place in most jurisdictions to assure individuals that they can elect how they might wish to spend the last period of their life if they take the right steps. Not every family is comfortable discussing thoughts such as this, which means that in many situations like that of Leonard, when there is no shared documentation as to wishes and no apparent open discussions with family members or those who will take on the decision-making role, the substitute decision-maker must struggle with the often heart-wrenching decision-making process. Some of the decisions are vital, especially when one of the options is to refuse what may be deemed to be life-maintaining therapy, such as respirator care, tube feeding, treatment of very late-life infections, and cardiac arrest. The decisions are clearly dramatic and emotionally laden as the person making them may feel that he or she, and not the disease itself, is responsible for the death.

I usually try to counsel family members to "have the conversation" with those to whom they have entrusted their decision-making in such a way that the family members (or friend, or third party — sometimes the case when no close family or friends exists) has a reasonable understanding of the person's preferences or wishes. This is not easy for many people. The question I am asked is: "When do I bring this up? It seems so morbid and negative?" I tell people who ask this that most of the research on the subject suggests that most often older people want to talk about these things to be sure that their wishes will be heard and respected. Sometimes a good opportunity comes when something happens to a close family member or friend and discussions occur as a family where a parent may say something like, "I hope that such a situation will not happen to me — such a tragedy." As it turns out in the case of Leonard, that seemed to be part of the motivation of his undertaking a living will after his wife died, in order to avoid some of the things that happened to her.

When I am meeting with a patient and any of the family, usually children, by the nature of my geriatric practice, I actually ask if the subject of artificial nutrition and hydration (or "feeding tube," which everyone seems to understand) has ever been discussed. Sometimes the patient (many of mine have some degree of dementia) and family say, "we have discussed that already and there is no issue — it has been decided, no feeding tubes no matter what." More often than not, there is a silence as the family member indicates that there has never been a "conversation" about that issue and so I press on with the subject. My approach is to make the discussion as free of tension and dread as possible.

My usual scenario goes something like this: "Ruth, I want to ask you something." (I am usually on a first name basis with my patient by this time; if not I would use the Mr. or Mrs. designation). "Do you like ice cream?" To this question there is almost always as affirmative answer, although at times the person may add (depending on their degree of cognitive abilities), "I haven't been able to eat it as much during the past few years because of my diabetes, but you can get the low sugar kind, you know, and some of that is pretty good." I then go on: "How would you feel if you could never ever taste ice cream again. What if, in fact, you could not only never taste ice cream again but never taste anything again. That your food would be put into you through a tube into your stomach and you would not even know you were eating. How would you feel about that?" By this time the patient is usually intently staring at me and listening. I then stop and say again, "So Ruth, how do you feel about that possibility?" At this point the vast majority of patients with whom I have had this little conversation have looked at me and said, "Are you crazy (or something like that), who would ever want anything like that? I do not think that is something I would want."

Then I turn to the family members and say, "You have just heard it loud and clear. You may have this conversation again. But you have to keep it in your mind and heart because if, *God or Nature forbid* (I always include the whole spectrum of beliefs as one never knows what drives people's belief systems), Ruth has a stroke or a serious infection you may find that someone on the "care team" will come to you and tell you she is not eating and that they have to put in a feeding tube to keep her alive. You have to be steeled against that decision because once made it is very hard to reverse, so you must be prepared because it can easily happen."

What steps can an older person take, beyond discussing and writing their wishes in as clear terms as possible? Sometimes going to a good lawyer is not sufficient for a lay person to understand the implications and meaning of their instructions in medical terms. For example, using the term "heroic" in a written advance directive no longer has a lot of consensus as to its real meaning in contemporary medical practice. If the person means respiratory life support, they should say just that. If they mean no artificial nutrition and hydration on an ongoing or anticipated permanent basis (sometimes after acute surgery there may be the need for a short period of artificial nutrition and hydration in contrast to a permanent feeding tube), dialysis, and no antibiotics for an infection, which if left untreated is likely to result in death, then they should make those specific wishes clear. Cardio-pulmonary resuscitation (CPR) is another dramatic topic, but in reality in the frail elderly it rarely if ever works and often results in what some might construe as an assault on a dying body rather than a beneficial clinical intervention. A response to each of those possible scenarios should be discussed so that there is no opportunity for someone acting as the proxy, who may have differing personal belief systems or guilt, to not abide by the instructions.

The next issue that comes up that can be very sensitive in terms of family dynamics and avoidance of, or production of, conflict is who an older person should choose as her or his substitute decision-maker or proxy. The usual and understandably natural tendency is to look to one's children, if one has any, on the assumption that they "know you best" and will always act in a way that you would want them to or that is "best for you." The next tendency, if there is more than one child, is to make them proxies together, meaning that they all have to agree in order for a decision to be made. The latter decision is often fraught with problems, as it is not always easy to get all concurrent proxies to agree, sometimes for geographical reasons, but often because of conflicting philosophical and personal values. Experience shows that many children in the role of proxy somehow believe that once they are in that role (which of course is predicated on the parent not being capable of making decisions on his or her own, which sometimes needs a special medical and legal evaluation to be determined), it is in essence "their call"; that is to say, *their* decision based on *their* personal views or preferences.

In fact, that is a very common error in the understanding of the role and legal mechanism of being a substitute decision-maker or proxy. You are supposed to act based on what you believe your loved one would have wanted had he or she been able to give an opinion, and that should be based on sound evidence, which in some cases is in a written living will. The next standard, if true wishes cannot be determined, is called "best interests," which takes into account the scope of implications for a treatment or decision and whether or not that treatment or decision is in line with commonly agreed-to principles of health care and humanity, or associated with unnecessary hardship or suffering: a much harder standard to interpret.

In the case of Leonard, the proxies are not following the legal parameters of how they should act. They have a capable wish available and verified by the lawyer who made the advance directive with Leonard but have chosen to ignore that wish because of their own values and feelings, including Martin's statement of "I could not live with myself if I decided to let him starve to death." But the issue is not about what Martin feels; it is about what Leonard has entrusted him and Rebecca to do to fulfill their obligations to him. Rebecca, by invoking her Jewish religious values, is projecting those on to Leonard, who by all accounts, although a lover of his Judaism, did not exclusively allow Jewish values, rituals, and law to govern his life.

The youngest daughter, Lisa, who had no formal legal designation, seems to be the only one who expressed at any time, and primarily in confidence to the social worker and doctor, that she believed that Leonard would be upset that his two children were not abiding by his instructions. However, not having any legal role and not wanting to create serious family strife, which she knew would be the case from her history with her two older siblings, Lisa opted to just leave it to the tribunal to decide. She expressed quiet satisfaction with the tribunal's decision and seemed stunned that her siblings decided to appeal it, further delaying Leonard being left to die in peace as Lisa felt would have been his wish. The appeal reversed the judgement of the tribunal, leaving the decision in the hands of Leonard's two older children. This left many people, including the institution's lawyer and ethicist involved in the case, disappointed that the whole concept of autonomy and the meaning of an advance directive had been negated.

This case study opens up the question of how and to whom one should entrust end-of-life care, and if it's possible to ever be absolutely certain that one's children will be able to bring themselves emotionally to make such difficult decisions. I have heard people say that they have asked a non-family member, such as a very close friend, to act in that role in the hope that the emotional bond is such that the person will not balk at fulfilling the proxy role. I also know of people who have asked their lawyer to act in concert with a family member to assure themselves that their advance directive will be followed. If you are thinking of doing this you must check within your jurisdiction to make sure that it can be done legally, without any concern about conflicts of interest or professional standards — the laws associated with this can vary quite drastically from region to region. You may be worried that your family could perceive this decision as a slight against them, but a good way to avoid such a reaction is to explain to them that you know how difficult these decisions can be for family members, so you removed them from the central role — and the guilt associated with it — and transferred that "burden" to someone else.

In this case the result is not nearly as important to highlight as the process and the challenges that arose for the family and for Leonard. Each case eventually resolves itself one way or another. But one can hope that at the end, those involved will be able to live with their decisions and believe in their deepest of hearts that they did *the right thing* for their parent.

CASE STUDY 23
End of Life: Caring and Sharing

It's natural for children to become intensely concerned and involved when a parent is in the process of dying, and even more so when the other parent isn't well. The real challenge is to know how to become constructively involved rather than intrusive.

THE CHALLENGE

Simon Beauchamp is 73 years old and dying of lung cancer. His wife, Emma, is the same age. Because she's a severe diabetic and more than 40 pounds overweight, as well as physically and mentally exhausted from trying to care for her husband over the past two years, Emma is no longer able to care for Simon with the level of intensity required.

They live in the outskirts of Baltimore, Maryland, in their three-bedroom suburban home. They have regular help with lawn and snow care. As Simon's condition continues to deteriorate and Emma is increasingly less capable of caring for him in their home, they've turned to the local community home care provider for additional support. With budgetary constraints, that support is nominal — a homemaker who comes to help bathe Simon and do some light housecleaning twice a week for two hours each visit.

Simon and Emma have one child, Allison, who is 46 years old. She lives in Hagerstown — a bit less than a two-hour drive away — with her husband, Daryl, and their two children, Melissa and Mary. Allison works as a bank teller, and Daryl is a program director with the city's parks and recreation department. Allison has tried to help her parents as best she can, but Simon and Emma have been stubborn all along, consistently rejecting her repeated pleas to have her father put in a nursing home so he can get the attention and services he needs and to reduce the pressure on her mother.

Simon, Emma, Allison, and Daryl are fully cognizant that, according to their family doctor and the oncologist who's been examining him,

Simon will probably die within the next four to six months. However, the family is having a very difficult — nearly impossible — time talking about it in any constructive fashion. They're frozen in inaction.

Simon is in a state of denial. He rationalizes his terminal condition and most days proclaims, "This is the first day of the rest of my life, and I'm going to improve." While this may seem a positive mental attitude, with Simon it's actually a deep longing to regain his health while wishing away the reality of the situation.

Emma, meanwhile, is angry that Simon didn't stop smoking years ago when she did. She blames him for being on the verge of a premature death, and while trying to make him as comfortable as possible, she too often verbally attacks him for his selfishness and lack of self-control. Emma is emotionally distraught, and she is also worried about her own health, placing the blame directly on her husband for the state of their lives.

And instead of appreciating Allison's concerns and expressions of support, both parents blame their daughter for meddling in what they believe is their own problem. They can't see her as the adult she is. Allison, in their minds, is still a child who should listen to their words and wisdom and show respect for their wishes, which are entrenched in a paradigm of parent-child control.

Allison is totally frustrated and angry with her parents. She's determined to help her father die with dignity and with the most support possible. Yet, whenever she calls (daily) or visits (weekly), her father argues that he's in stable condition and on the road to recovery.

Meanwhile, Allison's mother continues to complain that her father is his own worst enemy, rejecting all the positive things she's doing to help him. Emma often tells Allison that her father actually deserves to suffer because he's so long ignored all the good advice that she, their doctor, and even their friends have given him.

From Allison's perspective, her father is ignoring reality and not planning for his own death. Her mother is hurting as a result of her husband's inevitable impending death and her own anger. And no one is doing any planning that will reduce the amount of pain and uncertainty that's about to happen in their family.

Allison doesn't have power of attorney for either parent, although she's talked about it with both of them a number of times over the past few years. Nor does she have any other legally binding rights to make decisions on behalf of either parent. In short, legally, Allison has no say in what happens with either parent, and that probably won't change.

She's also spoken several times to her parents' family doctor. In his seventies, the doctor treats her the same way her parents do — with a level of disdain and distance, talking down at her rather than with her.

He always concludes conversations with assurances that everything is under control and that he knows what's best for her parents. Meanwhile, in conversations with the case manager at the home care agency, Allison gets the distinct impression that she's talking to a stressed, overworked, well-intentioned, but overwhelmed professional who is trying to provide whatever services she can while meeting her many other obligations within the constraints she must face every day.

THE GERIATRICIAN'S POINT OF VIEW

The challenge for children of aging parents is to try to provide care and concern while respecting their parents' wishes to do it their way. In essence, it's the same challenge that parents face when their children are growing up: to allow them to make decisions and do things that may seem to fly in the face of their own best interests and that may not reflect the opinions and advice of their parents.

In some child-parent relationships, the conflict in values and opinions is so great that the relationship is disrupted for many years, if not for life. Usually, as children mature, they begin to better understand and accept their parents, and usually, but not always, parents understand their adult children. Some parents can never get out of the mould of treating their children as children, rather than as adults who happen to be their offspring.

So what can Allison do? First she must accept that the most she can achieve is to give her best care and advice to her parents and then let them make their own decisions, even if she thinks they are not the best ones possible.

In terms of getting that message across to her parents, it would probably be worthwhile to try to meet with them to tell them that, as part
of her love and devotion to them, she wants to do whatever she can to
help. She can say that her perspective on what is going on may be different from theirs, but that she is willing to accept their views. She should
say that while she wants to help, she will not interfere with their decision-making but will be available if necessary when they need her.

Allison might suggest to her mother that blaming her father for what
has happened does nothing to help the situation and may in fact make
things worse. However, if it is her mother's nature to need to assign blame,
then Allison is not going to get very far with that approach. Nevertheless,
she must try to focus her mother's efforts on doing what is necessary to
make her father as comfortable as possible.

As for the physician, Allison is unlikely to be able to build a constructive two-way relationship with him. But it may be worthwhile writing to
him and thanking him for all the years of support that he has provided
to her family. She should express her concerns about her father's present
and future needs and at the same time acknowledge that the doctor may
understand her father well and that she will trust that he will make the
right decisions if and when they are necessary.

Allison also may want to ask the home care agency what kind of
home care might be available should her father decide that he does not
want to enter a palliative care or hospice unit — or for that matter, any
other kind of facility — no matter how bad things are.

It is not uncommon for people suffering from cancer to deny the
reality of their disease, and trying to convince them of the truth may be
counterproductive. Most terminal cancers progress to a point where the
symptoms force the person suffering to face the illness.

But the element of hope should never be taken away from someone
who realizes that he or she has a terrible disease. For the family that may
mean focusing on relieving symptoms, rather than on trying to cure the
disease. Sometimes something urgent or acute happens that shakes the
person suffering from the disease into reality. For example, with lung
cancer it could be bleeding from the lung. Or it could be evidence that
the cancer has spread to the bone, causing great pain, or to the brain,

causing seizures or headaches. Whatever it is, the shift in symptoms that cannot be ignored may help everyone focus on the reality of the illness and on the future.

At this point, Allison has to find ways to avoid getting angry with her mother for being angry and frustrated herself. She can be supportive of her mother without taking on the responsibility of trying to ensure a particular plan of approach. By removing the sense of responsibility for the outcome, Allison may be able to participate in the care of both her father and her mother without feeling that she has failed just because things do not go the way she would want them to go.

Unless there is a sudden turn for the worse, a time will likely come when Allison will be able to provide support and care for her parents. It may be necessary to take a more passive approach right now so that her parents can work out their issues as a couple, however abnormally she may think they are doing it. She should continue to visit on a regular basis but avoid being judgmental when she does. She should call on a periodic basis and, again, listen a lot but not give advice unless it is asked for, as difficult as that may be.

When her parents are ready for her help, she can then be there without resentment. It is crucial for her not to blame them for what has happened and for not allowing her to be involved when she thinks it is necessary. The timing, within reason, has to be their timing, and she has to accept that she can only do what she can do and, of course, what she wants to do, which is to provide the best love and support she can in this very difficult situation.

Meanwhile, Alison should prepare herself for her father's death. One of the difficult tasks that children are likely to face when a parent is nearing the end of life is dealing with the reality and the anticipation of loss while trying to maintain their relationship with the still-living parent. Some children, other family members, and even friends withdraw from a loved one as a way of dealing with the coming loss. One often hears people say, "I couldn't face the experience. I would have nothing to say and I was afraid of breaking down." Some individuals find ways to relate and communicate in the deepest and most profound and loving way to their family and friends when they are dying, while others project anger and sorrow and repel those who try to express their love.

Children and other family members must recognize that the knowledge of impending death is not easy, even for the most exceptionally balanced and emotionally secure individuals. It is important to overcome whatever hesitation may exist in visiting and being with the person as he or she nears the end. This time is not about the feelings of the person doing the visiting, but about those of the person who is being visited.

Most people do not want to be alone when they are dying, even though some act in a way that appears to push away even those they love. It is usually valuable to make a point of visiting, and if possible to do so in a predictable fashion so that the person can count on the visit and have something to look forward to. It is not necessary to do anything elaborate when visiting, but a small gift, especially something the visitor knows the one they are visiting might value, is often very much appreciated.

But what does one do during the visit? Just be there. Talk about anything, big or small, but usually personal and on a positive note — what is happening to friends and children that the visitor believes their loved one would enjoy hearing about. Bring pictures that reflect good experiences with the intention of helping the person continue to participate in the positive aspects of life. When asked by family members if they should be emotional, I usually tell them if that is the way they feel, then it is okay, but always to remember that it is the person who is ill that is the center of the exercise, not them. I usually encourage families to let their loved one know just how wonderful a person they are and how meaningful they are and always will be to those who love them.

Lastly, I recommend to families to do as much touching as possible: hold a hand, give a kiss, and provide a soothing massage if that seems to be welcome and helpful. Do not expect the person to respond in kind, which is not important. This is a time for giving on the part of family and friends and not expecting anything in return from the person who is ill and coming to terms with his or her own impending death. After it is over, those who were able to give of themselves, to be patient with impatience, and to express affection and devotion will reap the benefits for many years after the event. They can usually find comfort in the way they behaved at the end, even when the loss is great and the loved one is no longer with them.

CASE STUDY 24
Moving On: Living Life without a Loved One

It's not easy learning how to cope with the grieving, how to live on when a spouse or a parent dies, and how to deal with the trauma, guilt, and pain that's involved.

THE CHALLENGE

Marilyn O'Connor is a recent widow. Her husband, Conrad, died six months ago. Although everyone knew that Conrad's death was inevitable and that it was just a matter of how long he could hold out against the pancreatic cancer, his actual passing still came as a shock.

Marilyn, her son, Wes, stepdaughter, Wendy, and their families and several dozen friends attended a graveside service for Conrad on a dreary, overcast fall day with on-and-off-again rain showers that matched their own feelings.

For two months before his death, Conrad had been a patient at a palliative care unit at their local hospital. Marilyn, 68 years old, spent hours with her 72-year-old husband every day. And while many nights she had a series of friends spend time visiting with her and offering support, Marilyn was deeply troubled and very afraid of life without Conrad.

For both, this was their second marriage. Marilyn had left her first husband some three decades ago because of his alcohol problem and her concerns about herself and her son's well-being. She managed to get herself back into the stream of things as a single mother and did well with her new job at an advertising agency.

Conrad's wife died when her car hit black ice on December 24, 1968. She was killed instantly in the crash, but their two-year-old daughter, Wendy, survived with just a few bruises and a long-lasting confusion about what happened to her mother.

Marilyn and Conrad met at a wedding in 1972: she attending as a friend of the bride and he as a relative of the groom, who was at the last moment pressed into serving as best man. It seems the groom and his intended best man had a major disagreement just days before the wedding, and so Conrad was recruited.

A few weeks after meeting at the wedding, Conrad called Marilyn to see if she and her young son would like to join Wendy and him at an Easter egg hunt. So the relationship began, growing into a warm, comfortable friendship, and then into a strong emotional attachment. Two years after meeting — and over time finding that their children got along amazingly well — Conrad proposed. Three months later, they were married at a simple ceremony attended by a handful of friends.

In the years since the marriage, Marilyn and Conrad grew very close to each other and their children. During the summer months, the family often went camping together, and each winter Marilyn and Conrad would go on what they used to call a "just us" holiday for at least a week to a Caribbean island or some other warm vacation spot.

They were not rich, but they were comfortable. Conrad was a partner in a small law firm, and Marilyn continued to work part-time in the creative department of the same advertising agency where she had started after leaving her first husband. Meanwhile, Wes and Wendy emerged as good kids who grew into serious college students and responsible adults. Conrad often told his friends that he and Marilyn were extremely fortunate to have two such wonderful kids.

Wes was married at age 30 to Amy, the daughter of Vietnamese refugees; they have two daughters and live in Edmonton. Wendy was married when she was 27 to Mark, who was just establishing his dentistry practice in Toronto, and four years later she gave birth to their only child, Damian.

Conrad retired precisely on his sixty-fifth birthday; Marilyn had stopped working ten years earlier, instead spending time in volunteer work. Until Conrad was diagnosed with cancer, they traveled as much as possible, played golf together, spent a lot of time hiking in forests, and had a quiet but satisfying social life.

When they retired, Conrad and Marilyn decided to live in Orillia, an hour's drive north of Toronto but within short driving distance of many golf courses and large parks for hiking. The retirement years were good to them, and for them. Conrad, always an animal lover, became involved in the local humane society as a volunteer and fundraiser, but because they wanted to be free to travel they decided not to have an animal of their own.

The pancreatic cancer was a real blow to them all. It was totally unexpected, and right from the outset their family doctor and the oncologist who was seeing Conrad made it clear that the prognosis was very poor. In fact, the oncologist strongly recommended not operating and suggested that any form of treatment was not going to be beneficial in any way. For the first few months, Conrad and Marilyn decided not to tell Wes or Wendy about the cancer, but then thought better of it and explained to them and their spouses, Amy and Mark, exactly what the situation was.

The family rallied in support of Conrad. Amy's and Mark's own parents — with whom they'd always been on very good terms — would call often to see how Conrad was doing, and they stayed in touch with regular emails. Wendy, who lived in Toronto, visited her father every other day and helped her stepmother with housework, and Wes called him at least two or three times a week just for a few minutes.

However, it was clear that Conrad was in a rapid state of decline, with ever-increasing pain that was being treated with increasingly stronger doses of morphine and other pain relievers, given by mouth, injection, or patches. It was also clear that caring for him at home was becoming more and more difficult for Marilyn.

Watching Conrad in his pain and seeing him shrink before their eyes was painful for Marilyn and Wendy. The oncologist finally suggested that they consider placing him in the palliative care unit. This was devastating for Marilyn to hear, but after talking it over with Wendy and Wes, she agreed that it seemed like the best thing to do. Although the admission process was painful to them, the assistance of the unit's social worker, Cynthia, did make some of the decision-making easier.

Near the end, Marilyn was allowed to stay over in the special family room at the palliative care unit. Emotionally she was exhausted, and by the time Conrad died she hardly had any tears left to shed. Cynthia was very supportive of Marilyn, and a few times during the final days she gave Marilyn the opportunity to talk out her feelings about the loss she knew she was going to experience. Wendy had resigned herself to the inevitable but still wanted to find some element of hope to cling to.

Wes flew to Toronto the day his stepfather died, arriving at the palliative care unit just hours before the end. Neither Wendy nor Wes had much contact with Cynthia, although she did offer to meet with them if they wanted to. They declined.

After the funeral, Marilyn found there was a huge empty space in her life. She became withdrawn and very quiet. She rejected her friends' offers of company, choosing instead to spend hours looking at old photos and videos of her holidays with Conrad.

Wendy spent weeks in a very depressed state and kept questioning why her father's condition hadn't been diagnosed sooner and why more couldn't have been done for him. She called her stepmother every day, emailed back and forth with Wes, and found that she was having a difficult time concentrating on her work. Mark offered as much support as possible, but his practice kept him busy six days a week, so he was limited to doing the best he could to console her and try to spend more time with Damian.

Three months after the funeral Mark found his wife was still incapable of getting back to what he thought should be their normal life, and he saw that Marilyn was also still in a deep state of grieving. Mark suggested to Wendy that some counseling would be helpful. This caused a huge outburst of anger from Wendy, who lashed out at Mark for not understanding — his parents were still well and together, while her father had died just when he was beginning to enjoy his life.

Wes, meanwhile, seemed more collected, but in their weekly telephone conversations, Mark felt that he, too, was still in pain but just burying it.

THE GERIATRICIAN'S POINT OF VIEW

Dealing with death is not easy. It doesn't matter what a person's background and experience might have been, the death of a loved one is a major challenge to a person's equilibrium. However, since death is intrinsic to life, everyone eventually has to come to terms with the realities of someone they love dying.

What can family and friends do to help with the process of bereavement and grief? This is not an easy question to answer, but there are people with a lot of experience in the field and processes that have proven helpful to those going through the experience.

Many religions and cultures have traditions that promote the re-establishment of social networks in order to work towards reintegrating grieving family members back into relationships that are crucial for a fulfilling, joyful life. In other cultures, the role of the bereaved spouse is almost institutionalized so that there are barriers to reintegration back into the social fabric of the community.

Before anything can be done for Marilyn and her family, someone has to recognize that something is not right and probe possible avenues to improve the situation. The idea is not to try to forget the pain of death and loss, but rather to turn it into something positive that provides a reason to participate in life's activities once again. Many palliative care units, because of their recognition of the difficult path that family members often take after the loss of a loved one, offer bereavement services and counseling to assist family members.

It would have been nice if the palliative care unit where Conrad was a patient had such a program. It may be that it does, but for some reason no contact has been made by the appropriate person to Marilyn or Wendy, as the two of them seemingly are suffering the worst part of the grieving experience. If Wes is the most likely person to get Marilyn and Wendy to accept assistance, it might be worth having him speak to a member of the palliative care unit's staff to explore what options exist.

Most palliative care programs have social workers involved in the care and support of family members. It is this person, especially if the family has had a good relationship with them during the dying process, who can become a valuable asset in the process of working through the grieving period. Since there was a social worker involved in Conrad's hospitalization, and because Marilyn had the most contact with her, the logical place to start might be to approach Cynthia about the possibility of calling Marilyn. She could ask how things are going and invite Marilyn for a chat as part of the hospital's bereavement program. Wes could call Cynthia and explain what is going on and ask what might be done to further help Marilyn and Wendy.

Cynthia's overtures might be rebuffed and thought to be intrusive, but most social workers and counselors who deal with bereavement are pretty good at managing initial rejection of offers of assistance. On the other hand, most people experiencing grief understand that life has to go on and usually respond to gentle and caring overtures of help. Counseling can help to normalize the psychological and physical symptoms often associated with grieving and create a safe environment in which one can explore painful feelings. Even when death is expected and family members are prepared for the final event, the grief reaction may not be any less intense or prolonged than when a death is sudden.

Loving and caring family members can be instrumental in such assistance, although the kind of response that Mark experienced from Wendy is not unusual. The timing of the next attempt to discuss the issue has to be carefully considered and prepared for, and could be couched in the desire to help deal with the next stages of life. Mark has to be sensitive to Wendy's sensibilities, but he can build on being able to help her stepmother, while they both remain available for each other and their child.

Each situation is different, but the goal has to be to regain meaning in life, which does not imply forgetting the person who has died and who was loved. Sometimes a way can be found to commemorate the person who died that will have extra meaning to survivors. That is often why endowment funds for students, projects, or donations to charitable societies are suggested as a way of remembering the life of a loved one.

The wife of one of my patients decided to set up an endowment fund in her husband's name for the psychiatry unit that was so helpful in his overcoming severe depression. He spoke about it very highly after he recovered from his mental illness, prior to his death from another cause. In addition, she decided to become a volunteer at the hospital in which the psychiatry unit was located so that she could help other people.

In this case, Marilyn might want to consider setting up a fund for the palliative care unit to provide a better place for families to stay during the final days of their loved one's life. Or she might offer to work for the Cancer Society as a canvasser or in its office. This kind of work often allows for relationships to develop with other people who have lost loved ones to cancer; this common bond against the enemy of cancer often leads to social involvement.

Another option might be for Marilyn to get involved with the humane society as Conrad had, and continue with an activity that was dear to his heart. Similar options might be attractive to Wendy, although the main focus appears to be to meet Marilyn's needs. It is possible that if her needs are met, Wendy will refocus her energies on the future rather than on the past.

Whatever is done, the family has to be sensitive to the needs of Marilyn and Wendy, especially as they seem to be having the greatest difficulty. It is not that Wes would not benefit from bereavement counseling, it is just that he may have to get involved after the pattern and process is already established with his mother and sister.

The goal, of course, is to get on with life, because that is what life is all about. The people that do not accomplish that goal often become embittered and lose the ability to enjoy and share life with others.

If Conrad knew what was happening, it seems likely that he would tell his family to remember him as someone who enjoyed life and that he would want them to continue to live in a loving and expansive way. His death should be a catalyst for them to remember the wonderful things in life and to strive to enjoy them, rather than a reason to dwell on the past and the sadness that it contains.

OUR OWN EXPERIENCES

MORE THAN THE BIRDS AND THE BEES:
Having "the Conversation" with Your Parent

by Michael Gordon

Those of us who are parents will probably recall the discomfort, embarrassment, and anxiety that surrounded the experience of the "birds and the bees" conversation with our children, usually when they were budding adolescents.

Many of us tried to time the discussion during the early pubescent period so as to make sure our children knew the important messages and were not pulled into sexual activity as a response to their surging hormones. For many families a decision was made as to who would have the conversation, often mothers to daughters and fathers to sons. Even if that gender split was decided, the actual discussion was often not an easy one and lots of blushing and blustering might precede the actual content of the talk. Some parents supplied books to supplement their discussions, some to replace their discussions, and some just decided to let their children figure it out since there was so much opportunity from peers. At the time my children were going through this stage of life, the school system was attempting to provide proper instruction, but what parents often heard was that it was very physiological in nature, with a modicum of "fear" thrown in related to venereal disease, and that there was little focus on the emotional and social components that surrounded this very charged subject.

I recall the evening I had decided to discuss this sensitive issue with my then-adolescent daughter while we were on a "just dad and daughter" weekend in New York City, the place of my birth. It was a very exciting weekend that we had planned for many weeks. We were staying at my best friend's (from university days) apartment, with me sleeping on a futon on the floor and my daughter Neta sleeping on the sofa in the living room: sort of camping out in his apartment, which was in a wonderful area on the upper west side of Manhattan. The two of us had tickets to a show but the plan was to go to a Chinese restaurant near the theatre first, as we both loved Chinese food.

As the large and very tasty egg rolls were served I started my "speech" that I had prepared in my head; "Neta, I know that you may know a lot about what I am going to speak to you about, but when you were little I vowed that when the time came I would talk to you about sex, which is a conversation that never happened to me." She blushed and started to say something. "Let me finish. Grandma and Grandpa are great people and very intelligent and liberal, but I think during my adolescence it was not common for parents to speak to their children about such personal issues. So I learned, as most of my generation did, from friends, from books, often hidden from view, and some of what I think I learned was very incorrect and inaccurate."

Neta started again, "But dad I really know about this — we get it at school and I do read a lot." I knew what she was telling me was right, but I continued: "I know that you do probably know, but let me have my say so that at the end of our conversation I can feel comfortable that I did what I had always vowed to do, and if there are any questions you can ask me and then at least I can feel assured that you really do know the essence of what it is I think you should know factually and emotionally." The egg rolls were sitting on our plates getting cold. I said, "Take a bite and I will continue while you eat." I then went on to discuss the basic anatomy and physiology of sexuality (after all I was not just a father, but a doctor father).

While I was doing it I was reminded of lectures I gave while I was teaching anatomy and physiology at a newly opened nursing school in Ramallah on the West Bank during my years of training at the Shaare Zedek Hospital in Jerusalem. The students (all girls) were from small villages in the West Bank. There was an agreement between the Israel Ministry of Health and the administrative authority in the West Bank to develop a nursing school that would train local girls. When I was offered the position by the hospital's chief of staff he told me that the request was that the lectures be given by someone whose mother tongue was English as that would be the language of instruction. I was skeptical but he was persuasive, and after my initial meeting with the director of the school, who was an American University of Beirut-educated nurse, I was convinced.

Before each two-and-a-half-hour session (which included a 15 minute break) I was given a couple of cups of Turkish coffee, which of course was very energizing. It was the 15 or 20 minutes of chatting with the school director that was the most enlivening, as she had a great vision for this new facility. I had no books so all my illustrations were hand-drawn on an old blackboard with various colors of chalk, which I was told was in itself a rare luxury. At the beginning of the school session, the girls, about 25 in number, appeared very shy, had difficulty looking straight at me, and much of the time kept their eyes averted. Over time they became more engaged and eventually quite lively as I invited them to speak, comment, and ask questions, which I was told was unusual as a teaching method when doctors were teaching nursing students. The director told me that the girls found the lessons very exciting.

When the time came to do the anatomy and physiology of the genital system, including sexuality, I was concerned that for most of these girls it was a subject spoken about only between women. The director said to me when I expressed my concerns: "You are the teacher, so teach them what you think they should know in their studies as future nurses — just be very matter of fact." As I started the lesson, having written in large letters on the blackboard, "Anatomy of the male and female genital systems," I could hear the twitter among the girls. First I started drawing the female genital system, and I could see the girls looking at each other furtively and writing feverishly in their notebooks with attempts at copying my very simple blackboard illustration. After a few hesitant questions we took our break and I told them, "Now we will do the male genital system," and started drawing the basic outline of a male penis. I could almost feel the heat in the room go up as I saw the blushing on the faces as the girls looked at their notebooks and cautiously raised their eyes to look at the simple illustration I had done with three colors of chalk. As I proceeded, in the director's words, very "matter of factually," the heat in the room lowered and the girls stared at the board and copied the illustrations. I wondered if they would show these pages of their notebooks to their parents, especially their fathers.

When it came time to address the physiology of these systems I could see their keen interest and realized that no one had really discussed this with them before, even though some said their mothers had discussed some aspects of female sexuality, but mostly related to menstruation and not with any detail to sexual activity. So their interest was naturally high and, although there was some discomfort initially, this passed as the lesson progressed.

This was the association I had while speaking to Neta, who in fact was born in Israel, and left with me and my first wife when she was two years old. She had never visited Ramallah with me but it was during her infancy and toddler stage that I was engaged with the nursing school teaching, eventually moving on to medicine and surgery with the same cohort of students, who by second year were becoming quite mature and secure in their knowledge and new roles as soon-to-be practicing nurses. After the discussion with Neta was finished we ate our meal, me with a sense of relief and I suspect Neta with a sense of amusement. We then went to the show.

With this recollection stored way in the back of my mind as I developed my interest in dementia, I also became involved in palliative care. It became apparent to me that for many individuals with late stage dementia, there was unlikely to ever be any discussion with those who would ultimately make decisions on their behalf surrounding what they would want to happen if there were a conflict in treatment choices. The concept of "what to do if?" was the kind of idea that many families and their loved ones had never broached for a variety of reasons. The main reasons expressed to me by family members are their discomfort with the subject, the fear of causing anxiety in their parent's lives, the concern about seeming "morbid," and the belief that what might happen would not happen to those they loved. This last element of denial is a common characteristic of many people. By not facing the subject and dealing with it, the results and outcomes may later on be filled with many regrets and misgivings. Sometimes even when the discussion of these issues does take place, the actual process is not always easy for those involved.

Two of the case studies in this book, numbers 19 and 22, focus on some of the issues and concerns surrounding this challenge often faced by family members. To expand on the cases and discussion from those scenarios, I use as an example a situation I had to deal with some years ago. A patient was admitted to the complex continuing care unit at the institution where I work. She had had a devastating stroke, which followed a number of previous smaller strokes, from which she had made a reasonable if not complete recovery. At that time of the latest stroke she was still able to live at home with help and seemed to be functioning at a level that was acceptable to her and her family, one son being a doctor and one daughter a social worker.

After a week of virtually no recovery following the stroke the family was approached about the insertion of a feeding tube for the purposes of artificial nutrition and hydration, as by this time it became clear that she was not going to recover in any significant way and certainly not soon enough to sufficiently maintain her nutrition. The family agreed and more than a week later she was transferred to our facility. For the first few weeks she seemed quite stable and the family desperately hoped she would rouse and begin to recognize them and become more alert. This, however, did not happen. As the weeks passed it became clear that although she appeared "comfortable," the likelihood of recovery became dimmer and dimmer. One day I met the son in the hall. I had known him from work I did with him at the general hospital, at which he and I were on staff. He said, "Michael, we have to speak. I think we made the wrong decision and now want to change it. What should we do?" I suggested that he ask the social worker to arrange a family meeting with me in attendance in my formal role as the ethicist for the facility.

At the meeting both he (who was formally the substitute decision-maker) and his sister (the third sibling, a son was out of town, but we were told he concurred with his two siblings) indicated that when they agreed to have the feeding tube inserted they did so out of a feeling of desperation and hope. Now that they had witnessed for many weeks her state and the expected prognosis, they realized that as they knew her, even though such a situation was never actually discussed, she would not have wanted to be maintained in her current state: semi-comatose, being fed through a feeding tube, not recognizing her family in any meaningful way, and not being able to express the dignified aspect of her person, which they both emphasized. When the son showed us a picture of her during her active days as a volunteer at the hospital where we both worked, I realized that I actually knew her in that role and agreed that she was a very vivacious person and very proud of the way she dressed and looked. They requested in their role of substitute decision-makers that the tube feeding be stopped and that their mother be allowed to die peacefully with no further interventions other than for comfort care.

Their request at the time fulfilled the regulatory requirements of the province of Ontario, that allow for the refusal of and discontinuation of therapy either based on a person's wishes or that of the substitute, if it is based on their best knowledge of the person they are acting for or is in that person's "best interests." All these criteria appeared to have been met. But some of the staff, including the medical and some nursing staff on the unit, found the decision "objectionable." They felt that she was stable and not really "suffering," so why should her feeding be stopped? It became a very contentious issue, and even though the regulations in existence, and the ethical principles espoused as part of their underlying knowledge and practice of the facility were understood and acknowledged, the "gut" feeling of the staff was very strong. On top of that, the physician actually said that she "could not write the order, for 'religious reasons,'" which raised a whole separate issue of the role of personal belief systems when they might be in conflict with secular regulations and law.

The resolution only came when the family, in concurrence with me and other senior staff, including those on the palliative care unit, agreed to transfer her to the palliative care unit in the same facility. As part of their philosophy of care, what was requested by the family was allowed as part of their program parameters for patients and/or substitute decision-makers to refuse further treatments other than for comfort care and symptom management. That was clearly the case in this situation.

The transfer took place, the patient was comfortable, and the tube feeding was discontinued. After 10 days with a degree of gradual decline and a bout of terminal pneumonia, the parent of her devoted children died as peacefully as one could hope for. After a period of debriefing with the staff it became clear that had the discussions taken place earlier on in the course of her hospitalization, had it been clearer that this would have been the wishes of the patient, and had the family indicated this during the early part of her hospital course, the staff might have been more prepared and been less resistant and upset by their decision.

This was for me one of many cases that I have dealt with that has convinced me that "having the conversation" like the ones we often have with our children about the "birds and bees" is absolutely essential when it comes to end-of-life decisions. The main subjects, as alluded to in some of the previous scenarios, include the use of artificial nutrition and hydration, cardio-pulmonary resuscitation, and treatments for acute inter-current illnesses that often precede the final days of life such as pneumonia and urinary tract infections — these being partially due to the failing body's inability to ward off such infections and the inability to mount an effective immune response.

Therefore, one of the many recommendations that have become part of the discussions I have with patients, either those in my geriatric clinic or when I am lecturing to family and professionals, is to "have the conversation" and discuss these important issues. It is important to be prepared for all the possibilities that may occur when acute illness strikes, since in a general hospital the recommendations, for example, for artificial nutrition and hydration often do not take a long time. Once agreed to, even when there is a modicum of doubt and hesitation, it can be very heart-wrenching to reverse. In the same way that the "birds and the bees" was a crucial conversation for our budding pre-pubescent and adolescent children, end-of-life discussions are critical as well for all who will end up being part of whatever decisions have to be made.

ROZ AND MAX

by Michael Gordon

My father's voice was shaky. "Mommy had a little stroke and is in the hospital. They called it a 'transient attack.'" My 82-year-old father, Max, was calling me in Toronto from Brooklyn, where he and my mother, Roslyn (Roz), also 82, lived together in the cottage-like home they had owned for almost 40 years. He explained that my mother had suddenly had trouble speaking and her face had gone crooked. By the time she arrived at the hospital by ambulance she had recovered, but she was admitted for testing.

As a geriatrician practicing in Toronto I knew that my mother, a diabetic, had atrial fibrillation and was at risk for a so-called embolic stroke (blood clot to the brain). The cardiologist explained that her CT scan was normal and that he had anti-coagulated (thinned) her blood. He was trying to convince her to go on a long-acting anticoagulant called Coumadin® (Warfarin), but she was adamant that she didn't want that drug because of the risks of bleeding and the need for frequent blood tests. I was not surprised that my mother, a very active and spry person, would not want to be encumbered by frequent tests and doctors' visits.

When I called her, she said she was fine and wanted to go home. "The food is lousy and they keep sending me for tests," she complained. The cardiologist recommended putting her on Aspirin (ASA), which is also used to decrease the risk of blood clots. It isn't the ideal drug treatment, but at the time, the more recent studies showing the benefits of Coumadin® were not yet in the mainstream medical literature. I reluctantly agreed to his decision and felt that I should not influence my mother against her wishes to take a treatment that had substantial side effects.

Immediately upon exiting the hospital parking lot, my mother, eager to leap back into the stream of her activities, insisted on dropping in to visit an ailing relative. "Can you imagine," she recounted to me, "that I caught my foot in the car door and fell and banged my knee! I look like a school kid — all black and blue." What relief I felt that she was not on Coumadin®— she might have bled and bruised herself even more from the fall. It seemed so incongruent that my mother, such a graceful and fluid dancer, had a propensity to fall! This tendency, and her level of activity at her local seniors' center, meant that anticoagulant therapy would be highly risky for her. Her cardiologist's decision appeared at the time to be the right one.

During the next few weeks, each time I spoke to my mother, who said she was fine and active and dancing away at the seniors' center, I felt relieved at the decision that had been made. Then came the distraught call from my father: "Mommy collapsed and I called 911. I couldn't move her from the bathroom — she is in the hospital." She was at a local city hospital, not the HMO (Health Maintenance Organization) hospital where she had previously been a patient.

I called my sister, Diti (a nickname for Diane), in Chicago and we coordinated our flights to New York. The taxi ride from LaGuardia to the house in Brighton Beach was filled with scenes remembered from childhood as we passed familiar landmarks. We got closer to our house, and I recognized the bicycle path where my father took Diti and me for long bike rides when we were youngsters.

The news at the emergency department was shattering. My mother had had a massive left CVA (stroke), leaving her paralyzed down the right side of her body and requiring ventilator-assisted breathing. It was the kind of event that one uses the Coumadin® that she had adamantly refused in order to prevent. It was the beginning of the Memorial Day weekend in May, with the hospital short-staffed and frenzied and the emergency room a holding pen until beds on wards became available. And there lay my mother amidst beds and stretchers of bodies, on a ventilator, suddenly so frail and helpless. I took my father's hand as we approached her bedside. It was impossible to reconcile this scene with the images of my gregarious mother, twirling across the dance floor with vibrancy and joy. I gazed at her, and in that instant I realized that our lives with my mother would never again be the same. I clung to echoes of her laughter as she would tell a story or watch the antics of my children. I knew that my beloved mother had a tough and uncertain road ahead.

At home my father explained the events again: "She was in the bathroom, all dressed up getting ready to go to the center, when I heard a scream and a bang, like something falling. I had trouble pulling her out of the bathroom and used the bathroom rug under her to help move her. I dragged her out of the bathroom but I couldn't get her up. I called 911, and they rushed her to the hospital. She hadn't been feeling that well but insisted on going to the center. I told her she shouldn't go because she might collapse on the way — and then it happened in the house."

In a way it was comforting to know that, up to the very moment she was felled by the stroke, my mother was enjoying her active life.

My mother was moved to a six-bed hospital room, and the nurse reported that she had opened her eyes for a moment a bit earlier but had not responded to her name. The CT scan confirmed the stroke, and a program to anti-coagulate her was started. I was a bit shocked that she was on a ventilator on a regular medical floor, rather than in the intensive care unit (ICU). But the medical resident explained that there were no ICU beds and they thought it was best to move her out of the emergency room. We arranged for private duty nursing to supplement the regular nursing staff, which we could see was inadequate for the task at hand.

I noticed that my mother was on a regular mattress and asked about moving her to a pressure-reducing one. The nurse said, "This is the Memorial Day weekend, and we can't get a pressure-reducing mattress until Tuesday." I was really worried about her developing a pressure ulcer from being immobilized for three days, but the nurse reiterated that there was nothing she could do. She promised that the nurses would shift her position as frequently as they could. The problem seemed to reflect the condition of the whole hospital, which was rundown, having been built sometime when I was a youngster in the 1950s. Now, like many of New York's public city hospitals, it was understaffed and dilapidated.

We all sat around the bed and took turns going out, walking around the hospital floor and going down to the coffee shop, not knowing if Roz was going to survive and, if so, what kind of recovery she would make. On Sunday morning my mother opened her eyes and, with apparent recognition, tried to talk but could not because of the tube in her throat. Her right side was completely paralyzed and her face was drooping, but at least her eyes were open and she seemed to be able to focus on us and follow our conversation. She indicated that the tube was bothering her. The doctor said he was going to try to remove it and hoped that she could breathe on her own. When the tube came out it was wonderful to see her whole face. She tried to speak, but couldn't because of the stroke. My father left the room and started crying in the corridor. Diti and I held him and told him that we would do whatever it would take to get her better.

The next few months were full of both hope and despair, with endless physical and emotional stress, as Diti and I alternated or overlapped our visits to Brooklyn. Supporting my father on the phone was not easy; he was despondent. With every small improvement he was hopeful, and with every small setback he was devastated. There were moments of humor and pathos, deep drama, and the sharing of basic human emotion with other families whose loved ones shared the various hospital rooms with my mother. One time, soon after the ventilator was removed, my mother indicated by scrawling with her left hand that she wanted a cup of coffee, or as she would have said in her Brooklynese, a "cuppa cawfee." My mother loved coffee, and it was a joy to provide her with a cup, even if it went through the feeding tube. It was only after that tube was finally removed that she was able to drink some coffee very slowly through a straw and enjoy its taste.

My mother played the piano and was an accomplished ballet dancer in her youth and as an adult. She was a devotee of dance and music. When Diti and I were children, even though we did not have a lot of money, my mother made sure we had music lessons and often took us to concerts, shows, and ballet performances, which we enjoyed even though we always had the least expensive seats. Those times were special experiences in my life and set the stage for my own lifelong appreciation of music and dance.

I thought that bringing music to her would be therapeutic. We bought a portable tape recorder with earphones and put on Tchaikovsky's *Nutcracker Suite*. Her face lit up and she started moving her good hand and her head rhythmically to the music. Most poignant was that she started pointing the toe of her left foot the way a dancer does. We went through tape after tape, my mother responding to music that I knew she loved: Gershwin, Mozart,

Beethoven, and one of my favorites, Rachmaninov, whose *Piano Concerto No. 2* was one of the first records our family ever owned. She kept the earphones on throughout most of the day, and we instructed the privately hired caregivers to keep the music going. It added meaning to my mother's day, and without it she had little to look forward to.

She had some major setbacks: a week after she was admitted a blood clot lodged in her left leg, and Diti struggled to get urgent medical help. Emergency surgery successfully removed the clot and appeared to salvage the leg. It was during that time of post-operative intensive care admission that the most terrible outcome of her hospitalization fully developed: a deep and painful pressure ulcer on the lower part of her backside. During this period, we became very close as a family, dealing with fears and hopes and sleeping again in the very small home that we grew up in. Diti and I strengthened an already great and affectionate respect for each other. It was an unfortunately painful way of enriching our close and loving relationship.

We optimistically welcomed my mother's transfer to the hospital's rehabilitation unit. We began to fantasize that she would go home, and we began to explore what it would take to modify the little house to accommodate her. How would my father, who had significant angina, be able to care for her? We explored how much outside help would be required in the home but also looked at nursing homes in Brooklyn. Diti investigated nursing homes in her neighborhood of Oak Park, Illinois, thinking that both my parents could move there. We even inquired into how she could be moved by an air ambulance. At one point my father almost accusingly asked me why I could not get her into the geriatric center where I worked in Canada. I explained the immigration issues, but because he persisted I looked into it and was told that we could not take an ill person into the country, even with monetary guarantees, because of the high financial risk to the publicly funded health care system. It was when I was in the process of exploring this option further that my mother's condition suddenly got worse with the development of gangrene in her left, non-paralyzed leg.

When the gangrene was diagnosed the surgeon told us she would need a leg amputation at least above the knee, if not at the hip, depending on what transpired. This would mean she would be left with a completely paralyzed right leg and little or no left leg. It was hard for us to imagine that Roz, a person who loved to dance and move to music, would have agreed to such a state of affairs if she had been able to discuss such a choice with us. Since she'd had her stroke, we could not really communicate effectively with her, but we did the best we could as a loving family who felt we understood her values.

We had arranged for Jessica, a wonderful woman who had looked after another family member for years, to assist in her care and feeding, as our HMO would no longer approve private duty nursing. We observed that the unit nurses were too busy to provide adequate care. That a loving and caring person was with her for many hours during the evening and night, especially when Diti and I were not in New York, was very comforting to everyone in the family.

Then came the ultimate choice. My mother required morphine to quell the pain from her gangrenous leg and from the very deep pressure ulcer on her backside. Her level of consciousness was variable, but through moaning and grimacing when she was awake she indicated that she had terrible pain. Diti, my father, and I struggled with the decision. It was impossible to imagine her living with the expected state of leg paralysis and the amputation. With heart-wrenching effort we decided to decline surgery but rather to treat her with painkillers and let nature take its course.

The physician suggested putting in a feeding tube, but we decided that it would prolong her agony and we rejected that as well. The doctor, who had palliative care experience, sympathetically agreed with us, but some of the nurses accepted the decision only reluctantly. One nursing supervisor had the audacity and insensitivity to ask me why I was "starving my mother to death" by not putting in a feeding tube. I had to control my rage when I explained that our family wanted my mother to have as peaceful a death as possible under the circumstances.

I spoke to the doctor, who concurred with our request to treat my mother palliatively, using morphine round-the-clock as is done with patients dying from cancer. Despite the medical order, it soon became apparent that the nurses kept waiting for my mother to express pain before giving her the injection. Diti or I had to persistently ask, sometimes almost beg, the nurses to give her the morphine at the appointed time and reiterate that the order read "every four hours round-the-clock," not "as required," the latter being the usual non-palliative morphine order.

The vigil began. My father had the greatest difficulty watching her suffer, and we generally did not leave him alone in her room. Diti or I sat with our mother for hours on end, listening to her rhythmic breathing, with the rasping sound from secretions gathering in her chest. She was not awake and did not seem to hear what we said even though we spoke to her of our love for her. I put the earphones from the tape recorder on my head and turned on Rachmaninov's *Piano Concerto No. 2*. That piece has had a profound effect on me since the first time I heard it in our one-bedroom apartment in Brighton Beach when I was about seven years old. It sustained me through medical school, and now I listened to it over and over again as it wove itself into my mother's labored breathing.

Exhausted, we decided to go home for the night. Jessica was to stay there to be with Roz. Early in the morning, Jessica called with the news: "Come to the hospital now; it's over." Sadly, my mother died with Jessica, rather than with any of her family, by her side. Diti and I went to the hospital. Our mother was lying in the bed, uncovered, with an ECG machine connected to her, a last rites ritual of a medical system that seemed to forget dignity but was enthralled with technology. I started pulling out the intravenous line, and the nurse began to object. I firmly told her I was a physician and her son and could not bear seeing her in this undignified condition, uncovered and with tubes connected to her. Neither the on-call physician nor any of the nurses uttered a word of condolence. It was just business as usual. We covered her with the sheet and collected the few items from her side table and went to the office to sign the papers. Her ordeal was over. The ten weeks of coming and going as the long-distance son and daughter was over. Now there was only my father, in the small bungalow that had been our home and now was his alone.

After the funeral and the mourning period, we tried to help my father organize and clean the house. He said he wanted to stay there and assured us that he would be fine. One of us called almost every day. The few friends and neighbors and his sister who lived in Queens tried to lend a hand, but mostly he wanted to be left alone. We knew he was shopping for groceries because the supermarket debits showed up on the credit card, which he shared with Diti. He rejected the idea of rejoining the seniors' center and claimed he had gone there only to please Roz. We figured the real reason he refused to go was that he was afraid that he would break down and start crying, something he did whenever he talked about our mother.

Our periodic visits revealed that he was managing, but the state of the house was deteriorating. He rejected any outside help in cleaning or cooking. We thought he might be depressed, but with time he seemed to express his normal interest in reading his papers, especially the financial sections, and he watched television. He continued to visit some friends from the seniors' center but refused to attend any activities despite urging from everyone. He rejected most invitations to join his sister in a meal, but when Diti or I visited he would agree to eat out with us and his sister and her husband and seemed to enjoy himself.

We struggled with his future, even though he said he was fine. I decided to try to get him resident status in Canada. My father agreed to apply, acknowledging how much he and Roz enjoyed their frequent visits to Toronto. After the certificate allowing him entry arrived, he said, "I'm not sure I am going to move. Will I have to take a new driving test?" I could not answer for sure but was pretty certain that he would eventually have to qualify for an Ontario license. He expressed reluctance to submit to reapplying for a license, as he was concerned that he might fail the test.

During a visit to Toronto he expressed other doubts. "You know I will probably have to pay more income tax in Canada," he commented.

"But you get more in the way of services here," I replied.

"What kind of services do I need?" he asked.

I reminded him of the cost of the long-term care facility that we visited when Roz was sick, and he nodded in agreement. But after the week-long visit, he was eager to go home, and once there he said he wasn't ready to move. I tried to cajole him, reminding him how hard it was to look after Roz with us being so far away.

"I understand, but I can't make the move yet," he replied. His certificate of immigration expired. He was staying at the bungalow in Brooklyn. Diti and I reluctantly agreed that he had to do it his way.

He occasionally visited me in Toronto or Diti in Chicago. During each visit he seemed a little frailer, but he was still independent in all of his activities. He became increasingly sloppy, but that had always been part of his character. We enjoyed his visits, and he took pride in seeing his grandchildren and experiencing some of their activities like hockey games and playing their musical instruments. But he was always eager to return; sometimes he suggested he would cut his usual week-long visit short, agreeing to stay the full week only when I told him the cost of changing his flight.

The house in Brooklyn was looking worse and worse. He tried to fix the bathroom shower faucets but succeeded only in breaking the wall in the process. The float in the toilet broke, and being the engineer, do-it-yourself expert, he fixed it by rigging a primitive combination of clips that could be pulled in order to flush. He became embroiled in a lawsuit with a neighbor whose new medical building compromised his ability to use the house's side entrance. That five-year legal case became the focus of all of his psychological energies, and most telephone conversations centered on the topic. The case was finally settled out of court, although my father was never satisfied and complained he never had his "day in court."

We visited to celebrate his eighty-ninth birthday. Diti arranged a dinner with his sister and her husband. On the way to the restaurant we stopped to buy him a new television as a birthday gift. At dinner, he ate well, but slowly and very tentatively. Afterwards, when he was alone with Diti as the rest of us went to get the car, he turned to her and asked, "How did I get here?" Diti and I took him home and noticed some over-the-counter sleeping medications on his bedside table. Because of a recent episode of low back pain, his physician had given him some strong analgesics.

During this visit, Diti and I noted the dramatic deterioration in my father's functioning. The house was a complete disaster. There were mouse droppings everywhere. We found multiple checks written for the same bill, each addressed but not sent out. And we found monthly checks made out to a charity, but not one that had ever been special to him. It seemed he had forgotten to whom he had sent money. He admitted to falling a couple of times and had recently hit his head and cut his forehead. He blamed it on tripping because of the clutter in the house.

Diti and I agreed that the decision could no longer be left to him. Diti said, "We are moving you to Chicago." We waited for his standard adamant refusal. Instead, he nodded in agreement. Diti told him she would go back to Chicago and see what was available that would provide independence and privacy. He agreed again.

It was now Diti's turn to go through the process of thinking about how and where to move my father. With great luck she found availability in a retirement home five minutes from where she lived. Three weeks later, we both returned to Brooklyn to help him move. The plan was for Diti to drive to Chicago with our father in his small car. We spent a weekend trying to clean up the house but mainly identifying the papers and personal effects that he would want to take with him. We lined the streets with green garbage bags filled with things we had decided could be tossed.

It wasn't easy to identify essential papers, income tax forms that had not been filed, and bills that hadn't been paid. But gradually things fell into place, and Diti and my father were ready to leave. At first, he climbed into the driver's seat, saying he would drive because he knew the route better than Diti. I was concerned that he would actually insist on driving, but Diti managed the scene by gently saying, "You can't drive, I need you to navigate." And with that she held his hand to help him out of the driver's side of the car, put him in the other side, and gave him the maps. He seemed satisfied in this role.

That night I received a call from Diti. "What a trip," my sister laughingly said. "First of all it took two hours to get out of New York because although Daddy thinks he can navigate and I assumed he could, we got lost a few times before we got on the highway." She continued, "Then the fun began. It was like traveling with a two-year-old just recently potty trained. I drove into every rest stop and insisted that he go to the bathroom. It made for a very long trip. His back was hurting and he really was slow, so I had to pull him out of the car, hold his hand to go to the bathroom, and help him back. He kept asking if I was tired, offering to drive." I was relieved that they had made it to the halfway mark only a little later than expected. Diti went on, "Daddy thinks this is a pretty swanky motel because it's a cut above the Motel 6 he's used to, although it's not really that fancy. But he thinks it's great. He even asked if it has a casino and said if I want some money to gamble he would give it to me." We both roared with laughter.

The next night I spoke to Diti again. "We made it, but it was a trip that was so exhausting I cannot believe I did it." I asked if he recognized the neighborhood when they drove through it even though he had not been there for some years. "Oh yes. He named the streets and started giving me directions on how to get to the house. He asked about the shops and was surprised when I told him that some of them were no longer in business."

His apartment at the retirement community had been newly painted and carpeted. It was nicely furnished and even had paintings on the walls, and it had a lovely modern kitchen. Diti and I assured him that we would not sell the house unless he wanted to, but reminded him that he had to make a minimum five-month commitment to the apartment. Diti asked the home to furnish an extra bed so that she could stay over on a moment's notice, if necessary, which my father liked.

After two weeks, in keeping with my father's independent, stubborn nature, he declared he was ready to go back home to Brooklyn. Diti reminded him that he had agreed to stay five months and that he would be obligated to pay for the apartment whether or not he stayed, which helped clinch his agreement to stay on a bit longer.

Diti visited him several times a day during those first weeks to help him acclimatize, often staying with him during the daily luncheon program on his floor. She sat with him and engaged others in conversation to break the ice and help him meet people. She placed his medications in a pillbox to prevent the kinds of mix-ups we suspected had been happening in Brooklyn. When she couldn't visit, she called to do everything to encourage the success of his move.

The township offered a program of discounted meals at local restaurants for seniors. Max loved this program and especially enjoyed one restaurant that offered good food and ample neighborhood action. The waitresses began to know him, remembering that he preferred soup, not salad, along with his French fries, chocolate ice cream, and tea. Diti thanked the restaurant owner for helping our father to adjust and see what a wonderful place Oak Park was. Max, a true product of the Depression, appreciated being served a $10 meal for $3. He began to say what a nice neighborhood he now lived in.

One evening he called Diti saying he was feeling really bad. He was having a terrible bout with constipation — something that had plagued him for many years in Brooklyn — and said he needed to go to the hospital.

Thinking a trip to the hospital wasn't necessary, Diti instead gave him water, stool softeners, prunes, and watermelon as he sat on the toilet. He used glycerine suppositories and finally was successful. Diti stayed overnight on the bed set up for just such a situation. The next day, she was able to challenge his thought that maybe he could go back to Brooklyn. She asked him, "What would you have done last night if I hadn't been five minutes away?" He conceded. This was the turning point to his agreeing to the permanency of the move.

Diti knew that he was making a very positive adjustment when he began to relay details of conversations he was having on his own with people in the lunchroom. Sometimes he would read his *New York Times* (he was the only resident getting this paper delivered) in the lounge rather than going back to his apartment. He always wore a baseball cap that had "Indiana" written on it, and he found that it provided a nice icebreaker, as people would ask him if he was from Indiana. In his most engaging way he'd say, "No, but I passed through it on my way from New York." Diti was able to lessen her visits to once a day and then occasionally miss a day here or there. He would tell people that Diti had "shanghaied" him, and she would retort, "No, I kidnapped him." After three months in the apartment, he announced he wanted to visit Brooklyn. His decision to move had happened so fast that there were people to whom he hadn't said goodbye. He worried they would wonder why he never answered his telephone.

Diti took him home and they visited the few really special friends he had left behind. He repeatedly described his new living arrangement in Oak Park very positively. At the end of the Brooklyn visit he said, "I am ready to sell the house." We were ecstatic! Fortunately, the next-door neighbor was a realtor, and before they returned to Chicago a contract was signed. My father conceded that life in Oak Park was a much easier and nicer life than he had had in Brooklyn during the previous few years.

One month after the move, his new medical insurance was in place. He had a complete medical examination by a colleague of mine and his medications were modified so that many of the problems that had plagued him in Brooklyn, like his back pain, were brought under control.

To our delight, with these changes and some additional medications that he needed, his mental state improved remarkably, as did his mood and interactions. A few more months passed, including the Chicago winter, and my father settled in nicely at the retirement home. He gradually began to participate in the various social activities. Each phone call seemed more positive, and Diti said he admitted that he had been doing very poorly in Brooklyn and expressed gratitude that we had "forced" him to move. He even said, "You saved my life." I found our phone conversations to be like those from years ago. I could discuss world events and politics. One Sunday evening, which is when I usually called him, I asked him about what was in the *Times* and he said, "I don't get the *Times* anymore." I asked with concern, "Why not, are you having trouble reading it?" (This was a man who had read the *New York Times* every day of his adult life.) "No," he replied, "I started getting the *Chicago Tribune* instead because it has local news. I thought it was worth knowing what's going on here." To me that was the best indicator that he was staying in Chicago and that his mental function was probably as good as anyone could possibly hope for.

The issue of his driving came up from time to time. We had made a decision not to allow him to drive, and Diti kept his car in her driveway. In reality he had no reason to drive, but as is often the case, he considered not driving a serious blow to his independence. We understood the impact that the loss of his license might have for him, so we agreed to look into the Chicago regulations, hoping that with time it would become less and less of an issue. His insurance was changed from New York to Illinois, and he saved thousands of dollars with that alone.

We got him new Illinois plates — handicapped ones because of his bad back and angina — but put off applying for a new driver's license. A couple of times Diti took him for his favorite drive to the country and found a secluded place to let him drive. Each time, after no more than 15 minutes, he was tired and willing to give up the wheel.

Things were progressing very well, with most of the details of my father's health gradually being addressed. One of the outstanding issues was his hearing. He had been resistant to wearing a hearing aid even though it was clear to everyone around him that he had hearing problems. We modified his phone and encouraged him to seek advice, which he refused. On one of his visits to Toronto I arranged for him to have an excellent hearing evaluation at the Baycrest Geriatric Centre, where I work. The audiologist was very perceptive when she responded to his statement, "My hearing is fine, you know." She showed him the audiogram, appealing to his engineering expertise, and said, "Mr. Gordon, you are correct that your hearing is okay, but you have major problems with discrimination of sound. Although you might hear the sound, you cannot figure out its meaning." He accepted the explanation but later on again declined a hearing aid, saying that it was not necessary. Meanwhile Diti and I struggled with telephone conversations, repeating ourselves many times and speaking slowly when it was clear that my father had failed to understand what we had told him.

Then, in March 2001, on a Friday just prior to my family's winter ski vacation, I received a call from Diti: "Daddy fell this morning in the bathroom, but he seems okay and I am taking him for his scheduled hearing aid assessment." That appointment turned out to be fortuitous. While registering at the local hospital for the assessment, Max had a momentary seizure-like episode. His face grimaced, his left arm went up involuntarily, and Diti screamed for help. He was immediately transferred to the hospital's next-door emergency room.

The nurse picked up the phone as my father was being hooked up to the cardiac monitor and said to me, "The tracing looks to me like he is in some kind of heart block." The next day, the cardiologist confirmed that he might need a pacemaker but wanted to observe him further over the weekend to make sure the problem was not related to any of his medications. I assured Diti and my father that should he need a pacemaker the procedure was very safe and effective. By this time my family and I were in Quebec on our holiday. While my wife and children were out skiing, I stayed at the condo and did my writing and reading, staying close to the phone.

The day after the pacemaker was inserted; my father had an episode of vague chest pain, which turned out to be a small heart attack. The medical team at first thought that he could be treated with an angioplasty (a balloon widening of the heart's blood vessels), but it soon became clear that he would require urgent bypass surgery.

I explained the urgency and poor prognosis without surgery to my father over the phone. He said, "Let me think about it." I replied, "You have about five minutes to think because if it's not done you probably won't be around for very long." He said, with hardly a moment's hesitation, "Okay, if that's the case." Surgery was booked for the day we were driving back to Toronto. There was no way I could get to Chicago to be with him, but I spoke to him the night before and I arranged a flight for the morning after my expected arrival back in Toronto. Diti kept me posted during the drive home. I arrived the day after surgery, while he was still in the state of recovery but already quite awake.

Max had indicated to Diti, prior to the operation, what outcome he would accept from his surgery and what limits he would want on care should it not be successful. I was very concerned about the possible deleterious effects of major surgery on his mental function, but other than a short period of confusion related to the pain medications, his mind was quite clear. He even started making humorous remarks to the nurses, who appeared to thoroughly enjoy him. They were all very impressed with his rapid mental and physical recovery. Within the week he was on the cardiac rehabilitation unit. Two more weeks and he was sent back to his retirement home. He now knew, for sure, that his move to Oak Park had literally saved his life.

With his ninetieth birthday coming up, I planned a visit to help celebrate. It coincided with a conference on aging in Chicago, so I took advantage of the opportunity to work and celebrate at the same time. The three of us went out for dinner, and after the meal my father said, "I want to see if after I eat and walk I get chest pain the way I used to." I remember those years when my father would stop before he went for a walk to "catch his breath" and usually take a nitroglycerine pill to try to ward off or relieve his angina. We walked up the street and then down and my father said, "I don't feel anything; the surgery really worked." Of course he had not had the surgery because of angina but rather because of the small heart attack, but a side effect of the surgery was improvement of his angina.

Soon after, an offer came through on selling the house, which we accepted, and Diti and I were confronted with the prospect of actually cleaning the place. We knew that my parents had saved almost everything, so the unpleasant task of making it ready for possession loomed over us. We had planned to bring my father down to see the house again before we emptied it, but because of his heart surgery we had to cancel that plan. It was, therefore, left to Diti and me to do the job. I suggested that we just hire a dumpster and have the house emptied. Diti, rightfully as I soon learned, disagreed vehemently.

It was late Friday night when I arrived. Diti had already packed many bags with clothes and an equal number with garbage, gradually emptying overfilled cupboards and dressers, of which my parents had many. At one point she stopped and asked, "So you want to just throw everything out?" as she handed me my original birth certificate, which she had plucked from between some old papers stuffed in one of the dresser drawers. Although I had long ago obtained a copy of it, I held the original in my hand and wondered what other treasures we might find in the little three-bedroom bungalow.

Each item resulted in a comment or observation, and some past association was evoked. There was no rhyme or reason to where things had been stored. A box of childhood and family pictures was in one drawer; Diti's Grade 5 school essay was in another; my high school yearbook was in yet another. We found the bill of sale for the Sohmer baby grand piano that our grandmother had purchased for our mother in 1935, the one on which I learned to play. We found the receipts of the mother's milk our parents had to purchase after I was born prematurely because I could not tolerate anything else.

We found a letter from our bubby (grandmother) to our mother, then pregnant with Diti and still in Dearborn, Michigan. It assured her that we could live with her in her Brighton Beach apartment and that my mother needn't wait until my father's transfer from Dearborn, where he worked for the U.S. Department of Defense. The letter brought back memories of the apartment we lived in before we moved into our house many years later: the large single bedroom where Diti and I and our bubby slept, our parents sleeping in the living room with a bookcase separating their "bedroom" area from the rest of the living room, which contained the baby grand piano, a sofa, and some chairs.

The most poignant discovery was a typewritten letter from our mother to her father, who had unfortunately abandoned the family to pursue another relationship. The letter pleaded with him to be the father she remembered — when her mother sang opera and he played the English concertina. The letter brought us to tears as we read of the pain she struggled with in trying to come to terms with the problematic relationship she had with her father. It also left us puzzled because our mother had never typed. We wondered who might have helped her write this letter. We couldn't know if it was ever actually sent and we were looking at a copy, or if she had never mailed it to him. It reminded us painfully of the absence of our mother and the many struggles of her life. We could not ask her questions about the letter.

As we found other things, we were grateful that we were doing this job while our father was still alive. Later we could ask him who people were in old photographs or named in documents. I asked about a hospital record we found showing that I had required a blood transfusion as a premature baby. He confirmed that the blood for the transfusion came directly from him to me — the way all transfusions were done in 1941. The scar at the elbow crease of my left arm from that transfusion has often been the subject of conversation when I donated blood.

We found a document required by Max for work that listed all the personal details of immediate relatives, including dates of birth and city and country of origin. It was a wonderful record of our family history, confirming our Jewish Lithuanian heritage and showing that our name, Gordon, had never been changed as so many other immigrant names had. As well, this document confirmed the Scottish link to our name, something I had discovered years before while studying in Scotland.

We were very happy to find pictures of our mother in her youth in artistic poses from her ballet and interpretative dancing days. Other pictures much later in her life showed her dancing at the local senior citizens' center, which was such an important focal point of her life. Although she gave up professional dancing aspirations when she got married, throughout her lifetime she and my father were the subject of much admiration whenever they danced together in public. I recall at my wedding in Winnipeg to my wife, Gilda, at which guests remarked to me how wonderfully they danced and especially how expressively and beautifully my mother moved. At the retirement home, my father is still able to take part in the social dances, and Diti danced with him when he was 93. She recognizes that being able to dance with him is a great gift and part of the legacy from his life with our mother.

We slogged along filling green garbage bags and showing each other nostalgic finds, always making sure that anything my father might want or need was kept. We called him occasionally to ask if we could throw out some item or other. He asked us to keep some old *New York Times* clippings, of which there were many, as he wanted to read them again. On the second day of our clean-up, Diti yelled from the basement that she had found something special and chided me again for having suggested that we just call in a hauling company to take everything. It was two huge boxes of personal letters. It seemed like every letter ever exchanged among us was in these boxes. There were hundreds, including those from my six-month trip to Europe when I was 19 years old and many more from my six years of medical studies in Scotland, my one year as a draft-dodging landed immigrant in Montreal, and my four years living in Israel. There were letters from the two years that Diti spent in the Peace Corps in Tunisia. There were letters from old friends. We started reading them, some to each other when we shared the person or the experience, and some on our own, because they were very personal.

The letter that caused both Diti and I to laugh most together was one she wrote from summer camp when she was 14 years old. In it, the essence of her intelligence, sensitivity, and maturity came out loud and clear, and within its commentaries and questions was evidence that our relationship was built on and continues to flourish because of the strong values and trust that our parents had in the two of us. Cleaning the house increased the bonds that tie the two of us and made us realize even more that the legacy of our parents is imprinted indelibly upon us.

Finally, we finished the job (after a few more visits to get the house ready and to put everything left over into the dumpster that was eventually required) and closed the deal. The home of our youth was no longer ours. My father no longer had a place to return to in Brooklyn. Chicago was now his home, and at least he had Diti (whom I had renamed "Deity" in honor of her divine devotion to our father) close to him to help him care for himself. I was still the distant son, trying to be of assistance by phone and the occasional visit and through very close communication with Diti.

She had assumed the major part of caregiving. She had done it all with the greatest love and devotion that anyone could ever expect from a child. We have concluded that it is all part of being a caring and loving family and that there really could and should not be any other way, although we know that many times things do not work out so well in families.

My father came through a lot. We recognized that we had to just take things one day at a time and enjoy the fact that he still had a life with a lot of interests and satisfactions and that we were still able to enjoy his presence, his humor, and his sweet and engaging personality. Since his heart surgery, my father had done quite well, with the first three years following it being ones of relative stability and enjoyment. He accommodated himself to the retirement home, and the staff had clearly developed a special fondness for him. I knew that he was comfortable in his new home when, on one of my visits, I arrived early enough on a Friday that I had a chance to join him for the community member lunch program. This program, sponsored by a grant from the city council, allowed people from the community to dine at bargain prices in a dining area rented from the retirement home. The convenience (it was located on the floor my father lived on), discounted costs, and outside company all made this program very attractive to my father.

As we walked into the room filled with tables and diners, with my father wearing his ubiquitous baseball hat, many called over, "Hey, Max, sit here. Is that your son?" We eventually picked a table with a few other lunch program participants, and I found that they all knew almost everything about me. Clearly my father was a favorite among the diners, and he must have spoken often about me, as they were right up-to-date with my personal and professional life. I must admit, it was a very warm feeling to know that they knew of me through him, since he, unlike my mother, who loved to talk about me to anyone, anywhere, had always been more reserved when it came to referring to his children. The fact that everyone knew Diti because of her frequent visits clearly was an entrance point to their knowing more about me, the "famous" doctor son from Toronto.

Another year had passed, and I watched my father gradually physically slowing down. Although he could still manage most things, and he attended the retirement home's social events often with Diti, his gait was slower and more deliberate. On one of my visits, I told Diti that I wanted to have a talk with him again with her in attendance about his future wishes should he become ill. Even though there was nothing pressing at the moment, I wanted us all to be clear as to what his wishes might be for future care if there were a crisis or terrible affliction. So after lunch we went back to Diti's home. We were sitting on the sofa and easy chair, my almost 94-year-old father, my sister, and me, and we started to speak.

I reminded him that we had actually talked about his wishes some years ago while walking on the boardwalk in Brighton Beach, where he was still living at the time. I had reminded him of our painful experience with the terrible way Mommy had died during her final illness and said how much I would like to avoid anything like that with him should something just as terrible happen. I asked my father on that quite balmy spring day what he would want in a comparable circumstance. After a few moments of silence, I outlined to him what I thought his values were based on my knowledge of him and through observing him as the suffering husband of our ailing mother. I told him I thought he would not want "heroics" if he could not make a good recovery. He answered, "Exactly." That was how things stood in terms of communication until this Saturday afternoon in Chicago when Diti and I were going to speak to him on the subject again with both of us present.

My sister and I had decided that we should have an open heart-to-heart talk with him so we could be sure about his wishes and desires for the future, even though he had recovered wonderfully from his bypass surgery and was managing very well in his new environment, being sociable and involved. We also decided that we had to straighten out his burial wishes; our mother was buried in New York, where the adjacent plot was reserved for him, but he had mentioned cremation a while back, which appeared to be out of character.

"Dad, we are both very happy with how well things are going with you here in Chicago," I started as we comfortably sat next to him. "But you know that something sudden and terrible could happen, like it happened to Mommy and could have happened to you when you had your surgery." He nodded with the slight welling of tears as often happened when we talked about our late mother's illness, even though almost eight years had passed. "We want to know what it is you would like us to do should you become ill in a way that you cannot make decisions for yourself and it is unlikely that you will improve."

"I trust you to decide for me," he responded. "You have been very good to me and your decisions have been good, even the one to move to Chicago." Although that was nice to hear again, it was not what we needed at this time. There was no question for any of us that he never could have managed by himself in our family home in Brooklyn. It had become rundown for lack of maintenance — he had refused any outside help, a phenomenon that I often see in my own clinical geriatric practice in older people who fiercely protect their privacy and independence.

"Yes, we know that you have designated us as your power of attorney, but we want to know that if we have to make decisions, they will be the ones that we think you would want us to make," we replied.

I continued, "If, for example, you have a stroke or develop Alzheimer's and can no longer communicate reasonably well, enjoy ordinary things like food, be able to get up and about, listen to the radio, read the newspaper — even if it is only the *Chicago Tribune* — and things are likely to get only worse, what would you want us to do?"

"Leave me alone," he replied.

"Do you mean not do anything to keep you alive, for example, if you got pneumonia?"

"Yes, that's what I mean. Nothing heroic — just let me go in peace." We looked at each other and felt we were clear about what he meant.

"Now what about *when* you die, where do you want to be buried and why did you once say to Diti you wanted to be cremated?"

He smiled and said, "I don't want to be a burden to anyone and cremation is easy."

"But it really isn't what we would normally do because of our Jewish heritage and culture, so don't worry about being a bother to us," Diti answered.

We then looked at the pros and cons of his being buried in Chicago while my mother's grave was in New York. "The cemetery in New York is the one from our community, Eyshoshuk, in Lithuania, and it is befitting that you and Mommy be buried there as part of our historical heritage," I said.

"But who will come and visit us and pay tribute?" he asked.

This was clearly an important issue for him, which was interesting, as he generally was not one for symbolism or ritual. He was usually very empirical, having been a respected engineer in the United States Department of Defense. Now he was talking about a strong symbolic value.

My sister replied, "We'll just make it our business to come and visit as part of a weekend in New York."

And I followed up with a quip: "And then, after the cemetery visit, we'll celebrate the two of you as our most wonderful parents and your legacy to us and your grandchildren by going out to eat Chinese food, which has always been a way we celebrated important family events."

We all had a good laugh, and it was agreed.

There was a sense of relief among all of us, now that those important issues were addressed. We agreed that the talk had been very helpful and had settled some important questions that we might have to struggle with at some time in the future.

This personal experience was partially the result of my repeated professional involvement with situations in which families have not adequately discussed or explored the values and wishes of those for whom they will be responsible. They often struggle with the decisions and feel guilty when a difficult choice is made. It is often very painful for families to make difficult decisions, even with the help of health care staff.

Diti and I, both health care professionals, struggled with the decisions as they related to our mother, so we know that open discussions when there is no crisis help to clear the air. The goal for us was to achieve a comfort level so that when there is a difficult challenge it can be addressed with warmth, love, and the security that our choices reflect previously expressed values and wishes. Discussions like the one we had with our father do not make such difficult decisions easy, but it makes them easier to live with after the fact.

Sometimes there is a need for a sense of closure as one moves forward on life's journey. I had such an opportunity sometime after I had the discussion with my father and Diti. It was March 2004. I had not had a chance to visit my best friend, who lived in Manhattan, since my father had moved to Chicago from New York. He had helped us pack up the house after my father moved and had been a very close part of our family during my university days and thereafter. The March school break was coming up, and I decided to make a short visit to New York and take my 14-year-old son, Eytan, with me, as he had a camp friend in New York and had expressed an interest in visiting her. Now we were in New York for a long weekend.

We were staying at my best friend's upper west side apartment in Manhattan, a great place from which to undertake our daily activities. In addition to walking the streets and doing some shopping, with the main focus on my son's love of rock music, we had short visits with two cousins, one the daughter of my father's youngest sibling (his sister, with whom I had been very close as a child). It was she who had taken me to many of the shows and outings that entranced me as a child, and she has always been very dear to me. The other was the daughter of one of my father's brothers, who was famous for his sense of humor, with an endless array of stories and jokes that he used to entertain me and my cousins during family gatherings.

On the last day of our trip we agreed to combine a visit with Ellis Island, the entry point of my grandparents from their native Lithuania and Russia at the beginning of the twentieth century, with a visit to Brighton Beach in Brooklyn, where I spent my childhood and from where my father had been moved to Chicago. The museum on Ellis

Island is tasteful and moving and resonated strongly with me as I recognized the street scenes of the immigrant neighborhoods of lower east side New York and the garment district sweatshops that I had heard about in great detail from my seamstress maternal grandmother. Eytan and his sister, Talia, had heard many stories from me about their maternal great-grandmother (my bubby) and had seen some old pictures of her that I retrieved from my parents' home when we emptied it after my father moved to Chicago. As we sailed past the Statue of Liberty on the way back to the dock, I imagined what it must have been like to enter New York's harbor for those millions of immigrants and refugees who had to pass through Ellis Island before entering the country.

We got on the subway and took it to Atlantic Avenue to change to the train to Brighton Beach. At the station I explained to Eytan that this was the place I had arrived each day for three years while I attended Brooklyn Technical High School, one of the special schools in New York that prepared students for entry into science and engineering, which had been my career plan prior to my decision to study medicine. The small blue and white tiles on the station walls looked exactly the same as they had in the mid-1950s when I waited with my arms full of books to return to Brighton Beach, which was the last stop on that subway line. From the train windows I pointed to Cunningham Junior High School, where the new curriculum at the time had required boys and girls to learn typing, performing the repetitive exercises on heavy Underwood typewriters. It was probably the single most useful course I ever took in my educational career, one that prepared me for my university years, where I was one of the few students who did not have to hire a typist for term papers.

We descended the stairs to Brighton Beach Avenue, for much of its length in the shadows of the elevated subway line, which periodically roared above the street. Immediately, it was clear that we had entered another world, one in which mostly Russian immigrants lived and worked and whose stores and restaurants all sported signs written in Russian and sometimes also in English. If this were like Quebec, the language police would be having a field day giving out summonses to shop owners for not highlighting English as the primary language for commerce. As the faces passed, gold crowns on the teeth, a common approach to dental prosthetics in the former Soviet Union, were everywhere to be seen. As I pointed sights of note to Eytan, he reminded me that he had actually been in Brighton Beach some years ago to visit his grandfather with me and recognized the neighborhood, a fact I had forgotten in my plans to show him the place of my roots.

We walked along the boardwalk, away from the famous Coney Island and toward my childhood home. The level of the sand along the celebrated Brighton Beach had for some reason gradually been elevated until it was almost even with the boardwalk, a sharp contrast to the six- to eight-foot drops from the walkway to the beach that had existed during my childhood years. It was strange to look straight across the sand rather than down at it as we walked along on this crisp, sunny March day. We returned to Brighton Beach Avenue, and I had to stop as I saw the sign: "Mrs. Stahl's Knishes and Pizza" in bright green and gold letters. The venerable home of the best knishes in the world had been turned into just another fast food eatery, with some attempt to attract those who remembered the delicious aroma and taste of those luscious knishes that could be eaten in the small cramped space in the previous restaurant, taken out to eat on the street, ordered for home celebrations, or shipped (as the old sign said) "To anywhere in the world" — which they sometimes were. Knishes and pizza are a reflection of the melding of cultures and cuisine in the transformed world of my youth and that of my parents, Roz and Max — today's Brighton Beach.

We walked toward West End Avenue, from where we had moved my father to Chicago. From the time of my last visit about a year ago with my daughter, also to show her for the first time in her life my old neighborhood, the whole structure of our small, attached bungalow had undergone a dramatic transformation. Parallel to a small medical center, which had already been built during my father's tenure as a widower, was another similar medical clinic, and together the two buildings framed the entrance to our little home on both sides so that it appeared to sit back between them, small and insignificant. I pointed out the door to the house, tucked back, having been changed since my father had left it. It was at that moment, while taking a picture to send to my father and Diti of the house and the two medical buildings with my son sitting on the curb, that I realized this visit was likely to be the last time I would ever return to the neighborhood of my childhood. The era was over; my life and the lives of my parents and sister in this small bungalow where I had studied for high school and college were over. I would tell my father of the transformation during our next phone call and send him the picture. As Eytan and I walked back to the subway, I knew that the memories I shared with my parents and Diti of Brighton Beach would be forever in my soul, and that these memories I shared with my youngest son would be the last additions to the narrative of this chapter of my family's life.

When my father agreed to sell our little house, after he settled in Chicago, both Diti and I were delighted that he had agreed to leave the place of memories with my mother, Roz, and all we had shared during those formative years of our childhood. Saying goodbye now had little emotional impact but did leave a bittersweet sense of the history and sharing that I had just done with Eytan and that allowed him to have a small glimpse into the continuity of the history that he shares with his immigrant great-grandparents, whom he did not know, with his grandparents, whom he did know but mostly as a very young child and only intermittently, and with his father, for whom Brighton Beach was the place that helped to mould who we are.

How and if Eytan and Talia will find the connections to all of us as they form their own lives is of course not certain. The distances make it difficult to maintain a sense of intimacy with my father. Eytan and Talia and my older children from my first wife, who knew their grandparents better, will hopefully carry some of their legacy into their own lives in one way or another. I can only hope that the legacy and continuity that I bring to them of my heritage will become part of theirs, and that when the time comes they will be able to understand me and my needs and desires in the same way that I have struggled to understand those of my own parents.

A number of years passed since this visit with Eytan to the Brooklyn home. Things in Chicago seemed to be going on pretty well with my father more settled in the retirement home and Diti entering a routine of visiting and providing small supplements of care beyond what he received from the retirement home, which was quite sufficient for his needs. He had gradually accommodated to his new living arrangement and was becoming part of that community, which he seemed to enjoy to the level of his comfort. He continued to get his lunch at the community program housed on his floor and I would enjoy seeing him interact with mainly seniors from the neighborhood who came for the highly subsidized and quite nutritious lunch — they even had a "deal" on bagels and bread from a local bakery, which one could buy for personal after-meal use — he loved to get a few bagels — a throw-back to his childhood and adult years in Brooklyn. I must say from my years of exposure I had become in essence a "bageloholic," meaning that I could never eat just one and when I lived in places that did not have good bagels, I felt deprived. Toronto eventually started having good bagel bakeries that had either the New York style bagels or the Montreal-style which were quite different and although good were not my favorite.

Things were going along when one evening I received the type of phone call one hates to receive. It was from Diti, "Daddy fell and I think he may have broken his hip. He is in the emergency room." As I arranged for an urgent flight to Chicago the back and forth phone calls revealed that he was getting up at night to go to the bathroom when he "missed" his walker, which he had become used to as an extra support for his walking. Despite his original resistance to using such a walker as he, like many seniors, did not want to "appear old," once he started using it he marveled at its design (being an engineer at heart) and used it to its fullest potential. He was instructed on how to use it properly and safely and despite a mild degree of cognitive impairment he was able to grasp the understanding of most things. He still watched television and could give a reasonable account of current events and still looked at the stock pages and knew which stocks he owned. There were some problems with recall and he tended at times to be repetitive and needed help taking his medications on time and accurately, but he still managed pretty well with no need for extra amounts of personal care beyond what the retirement home provided for accurate taking of his medications.

The fall was by the side of the bed and because he could not get to the phone he lay there until the morning when the nurse came to give his morning medications and found him on the floor, conscious but in pain. By the time I arrived in Chicago and got to the hospital he had been admitted and investigated and it was clear he had a hip fracture that required surgery. He was booked for first thing the following morning and I reviewed the details with the admitting physician and was at the hospital with Diti early enough to be there for when he went into surgery.

The next day he went for his surgery which according to everyone went well and he came back to the ward with the intention of transferring him to a rehabilitation unit in the same hospital soon after his return to the surgical floor. As an unexpected and unfortunate event, soon after surgery, before he was transferred to the rehabilitation floor, he fell from his bed and fortunately did not incur any serious damage — but that highlighted the need for all of the special scrutiny and monitoring that he required to avoid a second and what could be a devastating fall.

I had to return to Toronto and was kept informed by Diti. He finally was transferred to the rehabilitation unit and according to the first reports from Diti the plan of action seemed to be good with their goal of getting him to his previous level of function so that he could return to the retirement home and his own unit. I was receiving reports from Diti as to progress on the rehabilitation unit and although the original assessment and plans seemed fine, over time she began to express some concerns about his progress, his mental status, and the response of some members of the team who seemed to interpret his status as due to an underlying inability to participate in any of the rehabilitation activities to a significant extent.

I had planned a visit for a couple of weeks after his surgery and made it coincide with what was to be a team meeting with the rehabilitation staff. When I arrived on the morning of the planned team meeting, having taken an early morning flight and benefiting from the one hour time difference between Chicago and Toronto, I was shocked to see my father. He was confused, I would say delirious, picking on the bed clothes in the typical fashion of someone with delirium and he did not recognize me. A cursory examination (I do not generally examine my own family) revealed to me that he was markedly dehydrated with lax skin, dry tongue and mouth, and sunken eyes. I could not believe what I saw. I walked to the nurse's station and asked if there were any recent laboratory values on my father to reflect his kidney function — or something I could use to determine whether my clinical hunch was right. There had not been any such blood tests in over a week. I asked the nurse if he had been eating and drinking and she said from the chart it seemed that although not completing all of his meals he was taking in "sufficient" amounts. She said the intravenous had been removed when he was transferred from the surgical floor the week before.

We were called into the team meeting where gradually as each team member spoke I wondered whether any of them had actually examined my father. As the team expressed concerns about his rehabilitation potential I could not hold myself back. "Are you aware that he is actively delirious at present and I suspect severely dehydrated? I would not be surprised if he has been drifting that way since he came here. How could you expect him to participate in rehabilitation in the state that he is in?" There was a pause as the attending physician shuffled some papers, searching for some laboratory results which I knew where not there as I had asked about them. "We will look into things and decide what to do." Sometime later Diti and I were informed that he was given intravenous fluids and that his therapy was put on hold until his hydration improved, which it did over the next few days.

There was, however, no great improvement in his function although there was some. His therapy period was extended when it became clear that his supplementary insurance covered him longer than Medicare payments alone, which is an issue with American health care funding, even for the elderly who have some government-sponsored health care insurance. Finally, it became clear to us that he was not going to make major headway and we had to decide on where he was to be discharged. We decided to bring him back to his apartment in the retirement home and through the network of personal care workers that looked after some patients in the hospital who also worked for some in the retirement home we were told that someone called Mario would be available about the time that my father would be going home. He came to meet him, addressed him as Max and it appeared that he was the kind of person my father needed to care for him in a decent, loving, and humane fashion. Our assessment was correct.

Max went home to the Oak Park Arms, with Mario as his full time attendant — sleeping in the small alcove which became in essence his bedroom. On those occasions when he was "off" he always found someone else from the close-knit Philippine personal care network to fill in for the day or two that care had to be provided. It always worked and over the next number of years Max always had wonderful people looking after him, including from time to time Mario's wife who also was a personal care worker who became very attached to Max when she visited, and sometimes on weekends would cook special Philippine dishes for him, which he loved.

Things seemed to progress gradually but attempts to mobilize my father following the fracture were not very successful. He could manage to walk short distances with his walker but need lots of supervision, which Mario with his great devotion provided. Gradually less and less ambulation occurred and increasingly Max was dependent on the wheelchair to get around. His personal care was provided increasingly by Mario — with the course of events following a very common scenario in a person with underlying cognitive impairment/dementia which was the case with Max. It is always hard for children to accept the decline of their parents, which was the case with Diti and myself even though I knew from long-standing professional experience that the course of events was one that should not be surprising.

Max's cognitive function continued to decline very gradually and at times almost imperceptibly with windows of lucidity combined with great areas of absence of immediate recall. On two occasions he inadvertently had the medication he was taking for his cognitive impairment discontinued and that resulted in a fairly rapid decline which, when noted and the medication was re-instated, he managed to recoup from — something I have seen often in my practice, although sometimes the recouping is not all that good. The symptoms of the loss of cognition were not so much "memory" as engagement, or as Diti once put it, "He is not as there as before".

During this period of gradual decline, but mostly maintenance of the status quo, he had a number of events that set him back and were a bit threatening to his well-being. One was an infection that resulted in his hospitalization where it was felt that he might be suffering from *aspira-tion pneumonia*, a condition in which a person, often with brain disease such as a stroke, or at times dementia, cannot swallow food properly and inhales it into the windpipe leading to an infection. In worse cases it is not even food that is the problem but the ordinary secretions that all people produce which we normally clear that are inhaled and cause the lung infection. Because the physician suspected that this might be the case with Max he ordered that he not be given any food by mouth until a special *swallowing study* be performed which would determine whether he could swallow safely or not. We waited a few days with Max expressing increased desire to eat because of "hunger" only to be told that the study was being postponed because of some sort of holiday long weekend. When Diti asked the doctor what was going on he told her, "We have to wait for the study because if he is aspirating we will have to put in a feeding tube to be safe."

Diti was shocked as the mention of a feeding tube never came up as an optional outcome of the swallowing study. A feeding tube was some-thing Diti and I and Max had discussed in great detail in the past when he indicated to us what in essence his verbal advance directive was that a feeding tube was categorically rejected as an option. Diti told that to the doctor whose response was, "Well if that's the case, you might as well take your chances and feed him." Diti agreed, not telling the doctor that for the previous two days in response to Max's persistent request for food she had been giving him small amounts of yogurt with fruit which he seemed to manage to swallow quite safely. With the cancellation of the prohibi-tion to eat we started feeding him and shortly after were able to take him back to his apartment. On my next visit shortly after, in keeping with a long-standing tradition I brought a box of my wife Gilda's homemade honey cake, a typically Jewish baked good served during Rosh Hoshanna (the Jewish New Year). He was delighted to receive the gift and while eating it I took a picture of him safely eating it and enjoying it — I had suggested sending it to his doctor but was not sure if that was ever done — it would have been a good lesson in respecting patient autonomy.

There were a number of illnesses peppering Max's later years, but he was looked after with great care by Diti and Mario, with me acting as the long-distance caring son and brother and when necessary the medical advisor. I came down whenever I could for a visit and usually Max could remember who I was and usually would say my name even when he was not spontaneously conversing any more. He would watch television but we weren't sure if he absorbed much of what he saw. Nevertheless, he was played his favorite movies over and over again. When the weather was good Mario took him out for walks in the wheelchair and Max seemed to enjoy those outings and seemed to notice his surroundings.

During what were to be the last few months of his life, Diti reported that he was not that responsive to her but seemed to recognize her and Mario and could no longer eat food other than what was pureed for him in a blender, which Mario did with great care. He seemed to continue to enjoy the tastes. For what turned out to be his last birthday we ordered his favorite Chinese dish, which was Pepper Steak and Onions (something he ordered every time we went to a Chinese restaurant for as long as I could remember). It was pureed for him and he seemed to relish the taste even in its rather mushy consistency. After that birthday there were a series of incidents, which in retrospect seemed to be the prologue to the end. This is something I have witnessed often in my own geriatric medicine and palliative care practice: the dwindling of life and the withdrawal from the ability to participate in the ordinary activities of the day — or as Diti continued to say, "Not being there."

I was in Vermont for the second last week in August. It was our time-share in Stowe that we had been going to since Talia was an infant, having purchased while she was *in utero*. Even though for the previous few years I had been going on my own for a week of cycling, writing, and just relaxing on my own, Talia offered to visit from Montreal where she was at university and was there prior to the new term starting. Stowe was a place she loved so much as a child and we had a lovely weekend of reminiscing and looking at the night sky and stars, while I told her the children's story I had made up for her and her brother Eytan when they were both small.

The Thursday before I left for Vermont, Diti called to tell me Max was not well and she thought it was a return of his previously experienced urinary tract infection, so while waiting to hear from the doctor she started him on the leftover supply of antibiotics that he had been prescribed previously. On the Friday she thought he was managing but was concerned that he was not drinking enough, despite Mario's best efforts, and she was concerned about his becoming dehydrated from the infection and lack of fluid intake. She tried to arrange for some homecare prior to the weekend beginning, but because the doctor was apparently away she could not succeed and the weekend started with Mario trying to force fluids into my father as he took the antibiotics.

I arrived at the time-share with Talia arriving later that evening and despite the worrying news from Chicago we had a lovely reunion, especially sitting outside the time-share and looking up at the night sky. Each day I called, sometimes twice in a day, it sounded like things were not getting better and Mario was becoming very upset that he could not give Max enough fluids. Diti and I were determined to not send him to the hospital — we wanted him to be able to be cared for in his own home. On the Monday Talia left back for Montreal after a lovely weekend, although negatively colored by my concern over my father which she shared as she loved him dearly. On Monday Diti tried to get some home care arranged and thought it was going to be implemented that day when she discovered a foolish glitch in the arrangements revealing that it was booked for the following day instead. That night Diti called in a panic. "Daddy's not responding and not taking anything by mouth." I wanted to tell her that this was what he had wanted, to be allowed to die in his own home, and in my mind I knew that this is what was happening. But Diti seemed so distraught and Mario was beside himself — his care wishes and fierce dedication to Max could not be fulfilled. I said with some reluctance in my heart, "There is nothing to do other than call 911 and they will likely take him to the hospital".

That is exactly what happened. The ambulance came, started fluid resuscitation of Max, brought him to the emergency room where he was investigated and received more fluids and antibiotics intravenously, and plans were made to move him to the Intensive Care Unit (ICU). Exactly what I was hoping to avoid but acute care hospitals have a way of carrying things along based on the assumption that if the patient or family wanted something else they wouldn't have called 911. Had there been a home care nurse in the apartment, someone we could confer with, and had the doctor been available maybe this could have been avoided, but in the world of life and medicine one can never reconstruct the past.

I spoke to Diti as they were planning to move our father to the ICU. She asked me what to do, "They asked if he should have a Do Not Resuscitate (DNR) order. I told Diti, "Daddy has always said he did not want CPR in such a situation and you know from reading so much of what I have written in the past years that in situations like Daddy's, CPR just doesn't work — if anything I really think it is a cruel and inhuman last medical rite. Please give them a DNR order — it is what he would want, please." She agreed. I could hear a sadness and sense of despondency in her voice.

I got the call early the next morning from Diti, "They told me to come to the hospital. Here is the number to the ICU." She gave me the name of his nurse. I called and introduced myself as the son, a doctor, and one of his powers of attorney. The nurse told me he had died earlier that morning. "Did he suffer at all? I knew this to be a terrible question to ask, but a very common one from loving family members. I also know that nurses and doctors are in the habit professionally of expressing the gentleness of death if this is at all possible, as that is what families need to hear. "Did he get CPR?" I asked. "No she said, he had a DNR order and never recovered consciousness. He just gently stopped breathing and died." I thanked her and in my mind thanked Diti profusely.

I left Vermont later that day to drive to Toronto to get a plane to Chicago so that we could plan a memorial service for Max. He had always indicated that he wanted to be cremated and we determined by calling the cemetery that his cremated remains could be buried in the plot that he owned next to our mother Roz. Although not highly acknowledged in the Jewish community, it is done and for him was the right thing to do. We had the service in Diti's synagogue with her daughter Ashley, friends, and neighbors in attendance. We both spoke to his memory — to the profound and wonderful person he was and the many humorous anecdotes that together helped make the two of us the people that we were. We arranged for the cremation as he wanted and I returned to Toronto — with the end of the Max and Roslyn saga having run its last chapter, or so I thought at the time.

The final chapter of the Roz and Max saga occurred in the spring of 2012, over a year and half after Max's death. Talia was visiting friends in Brooklyn when I received a phone call, "Daddy I want to visit the old house in Brooklyn. How do I get there?" She had been to the house only when she was very small but she said she remembered and wanted to see it and the neighborhood where I grew up. I have some wonderful pictures of her with her grandfather at a park near the house — they appear to be having a grand time and as I recall the afternoon when looking at the pictures, I remember just how much joy there was shared between the two of them. Talia was around four years old.

Since I no longer knew the New York subway system that well I asked her to confirm from her Brooklyn friend which train took her to Brighton Beach, which she did. I told her to call when she got there and I would instruct her where to go. When she called I instructed her with pauses between calls as she followed my instructions how to do the walk I had done hundreds if not more times in my life. As she rounded the corner from Brighton Beach Avenue, the main thoroughfare on which I had grown and walked to school in my younger years, and to the streetcar and subway in my junior high, high school, and sometimes college years, I told her to keep walking about 50 yards, passing the Italian restaurant that had been there for years, the small Korean grocery stores from which my father got his *New York Times* and an occasional bagel when he could not get on to "the Avenue" to visit one of the many Russian specialty stores and bakeries. There he could get all of his favorite foods including bagels, real rye and pumpernickel bread, herring with onions (with or without the sour cream), and all the delicacies that came with that part of the world, which shared so many similarities to the Bensonhurst Brooklyn he grew up in, and where I used to visit his parents when they were still living.

As she got close to the house I told her the landmarks to watch out for. "Daddy, it is not there. There is a building site where the house is supposed to be. I don't believe it. It's not there." She seemed very disappointed. I asked her if the house to its right was there and she answered yes. I told her to ring the doorbell and either a man or his wife would answer and she should tell them that she is the granddaughter of Max and

Roz. She did so while on the phone with me. She then said, "A woman just answered so I'm going to speak to her, goodbye."

Later she told me that the husband was not home but the wife shrieked with joy on meeting Talia and, despite her relatively poor English and thick Russian accent, welcomed her into the house and offered her food and drink and went on and on about how lovely her grandparents were as neighbors, how sorry she was when Max moved to Chicago, and how sad she was at his death. She was so sorry her husband was not home as he was the one who spent so much effort helping clear up the house when the move to Chicago was planned. Talia left with the woman giving her a big hug and she then called me and recounted the story. She was almost crying when she confessed she had really wanted to see the house for the last time but that at least she had shared some memories with people who knew her grandparents. The saga of Max and Roz and their bungalow in Brighton Beach was over. There would never be another reason to visit again and whoever would move into the house on that lot would never know the wonderful legacy of these two wonderful people — Max and Roz.

LESSONS LEARNED

The experiences I had with my mother taught me a number of lessons that I was able to use in helping my father, and my experiences with both of them have taught me lessons that have helped me in my clinical geriatric practice. I can now understand the predicaments of patients and their families, not only from a professional perspective, but also from the personal vantage point.

The experiences with my mother led me to do my best to make sure that I had the conversation with my father about his values and wishes should he fall ill and not be able to make decisions. I realized that sitting down and putting together a written living will was not going to happen, so I told him what I thought the important values were in his life and how I would make decisions if he were to become ill in a manner similar to my mother's experiences. When he confirmed these values and principles, I communicated them to my sister so that we were both party to his wishes and expectations. This proved to be very useful when it came time for him to agree to his cardiac surgery. All he had to do was reiterate that he would want to be "left alone" if he did not make a good recovery, which was enough for us to understand his wishes. The fact that Diti and I had the opportunity to have a face-to-face and heart-to-heart discussion about these issues again a few years later helped us to confirm our understanding of my father's deep-seated wishes and values, which were of great value when the difficult times came in his later years.

I learned from my mother's illness that children often find it difficult to accept bad outcomes and take it upon themselves to try to rectify the situation, especially in institutional settings. This is very reasonable and when done properly can lead to some improvements in care. It is useful to understand what clinical options make sense and to try to act on them. It is important not to allow others to make decisions that are very important to a family member. And while well-meaning others may provide advice and input, ultimately it is the family who has to decide what is right. However, once that decision is made, it is important not to revert to "what if" scenarios, but rather to accept that whatever decision was made was the right one. I use this concept with my patients and families who struggle with decisions. I try to help them understand that there are rarely "right" answers to difficult decisions — they can only do the best they can, and they must live with their decision as the best they could have made under the circumstances.

One of the important lessons I learned from caring for my father is knowing that timing is often critical in decision-making. It is not possible or proper to force a situation when the parent is not ready for that decision to be made. It becomes counterproductive to keep badgering a parent to make a decision that he or she is not yet prepared to make. I saw this in terms of my father's reluctance to move from his home until it was clear that he was in danger, and also in terms of his hearing aid — when he was ready, that was the only time to act. On the other hand, I also learned and now use in my practice the idea that sometimes waiting until someone is ready may be dangerous and result in acting too late. I try to help patients and their families make difficult decisions by outlining the implications of waiting too long to make a necessary move.

Another important lesson I have learned is that you *can* teach an old dog new tricks, meaning the opportunities to grow and develop can continue at every age. It is not necessarily the case that moving from one's own home to a facility is the beginning of the end; rather, it may be the beginning of a new era of interaction and enjoyment. I have seen this in my practice, but most important, I have now experienced it with my father. He had been transformed from a near-hermit, deteriorating physically and mentally, to a vibrant, active person who participated in social activities, including dancing and exercise programs. To see him greeted by his buddies at the retirement home lunch program was very satisfying for me, as I knew that once again my father was a *somebody*.

Another very important lesson is that helping one's parents can be very challenging, trying, and time-consuming. If possible, share the responsibility with other siblings, and if that is not possible, at least acknowledge and support the siblings who are carrying the main part of the responsibility. I am lucky that I have a wonderful sister who became the primary caregiver to my father. I had to remind myself how fortunate my father and I were to have her in Chicago. On the other hand, both my sister and I were fortunate to have had our parents, and caring for them in their later years was a small way of returning to them what they were able to provide for us and of promoting the values that they instilled in us.

My father had a number of acute hospitalizations during his stay in Chicago. They were complex ones but he managed to return home from all but one, in which case the illness was fatal. The lesson learned from these two hospitalizations is that family members are very important as advocates and supporters of their loved ones during a hospitalization. The challenge is to be on top of what is going on and not be afraid to ask the right questions and challenge decisions, but in a manner that is not threatening or aggressive. The staff has to understand that family members are loving allies of their patients, and also recognize that they have to act responsibly because there is a caring advocate observing and commenting on what is happening. The cover story of the May 1, 2006, issue of *Time* magazine, entitled "Q: What Scares Doctors? A: Being the Patient," confirms the importance of vigilance and support by family advocates as one of the ways to assure as good an outcome as possible for those we love. Diti and I certainly learned that during our father's hospitalizations.

Expressing gratitude in the care and acknowledging it when it is good opens the doors to questions about care and to *suggestions* when you feel something might be altered in terms of care approaches.

When you make plans for discharge from a hospital setting, explore carefully all the options before making a decision. Get input from knowledgeable people but also remember that you likely know your parent's wishes, needs, and desires better than anyone else.

Any discharge decision can in all likelihood be changed if it does not work, so it is important to have a "plan B" that can be implemented if the first one does not work. Sometimes there are administrative pressures to make plans on short notice, but always explore them and challenge within reason if they are not working to your loved one's advantage.

Any decision made due to administrative reasons can be challenged even if you are told that "this is the way it has to be based on … policy etc.). Find out the basis of the rule and if it seems to be in conflict with your loved one's long-term needs find out who is ultimately responsible and explore other options with that person. Rarely does one have to pursue more onerous approaches to solve what in essence are "person-centered decisions," which are usually written somewhere in the mission statement of the health care facilities — you can always refer to them when discussing alternatives to what has been recommended if the latter is contrary to your loved one's best interests and wishes.

Even when advance directives have been developed, it can be very challenging for children to adhere to them when facing the end. Therefore, those who will fill that role have to always remember that their duty is to follow the wishes of their loved one, if they know what those wishes are, no matter how difficult that may seem. In most jurisdictions that is the law, but even with that in mind it can be very hard for loving family members to fulfill the expectations and, in essence, "let go" of the person they so love.

A WEEK OF TRAUMA SETS THE STAGE FOR HURT, HOPE, AND ENDINGS

by Bart Mindszenthy

What follows is a chronicle of a terrible week when my mother very unexpectedly and completely imploded. It's all about what happens when a parent is undergoing rapidly advancing dementia that is suspected to be the dreaded Alzheimer's disease. There's nothing nice about any of this. It's painful for all involved. I feel a huge amount of love for both my mother, who succumbed to the "twilight zone" of her older age, and my father, who had to witness his wife of nearly six decades change before his non-seeing eyes into someone totally different in the time they had left together.

We hoped that in some way we'd manage to work through this dire challenge and be able to help and support my mother, to make her as comfortable as possible, and to somehow let her know how much we loved her and cared about her well-being. And we hoped my father would be able to cope with the fact that we couldn't ever go back to where we were: that nothing would ever be sure or safe or right again.

But the reality was that our worlds were changed forever. My mother ultimately had to be placed into a nursing home to eventually die there. My father reached a point where he didn't want to live any longer. And as the only child, I was the driving family caregiver to them both, through it all. Because that's how it works. On the face of it, it's a portion of life none of us is prepared to — or wants to — face. However, it's there, and for each of us it's there in a different way and form.

JULY 24

Dementia, my parents' doctor tells me, cuts a broad swath through the mind and behavior of the elderly. *Dementia* is a single word that seemingly means so little and yet affects so much. It ranges across a spectrum from pre-dementia to mild to moderate through to severe, and then to the end stage. Bottom line: cognitive capabilities — memory, judgment, insight, and reason — decline. Which is a nice way of saying that the mind is no longer able to do the work it once did, and that step by step a new mind-set enters that is confusing, difficult to accept, and eventually impossible to understand for all those who have to deal with it.

Dementia means many different things to many people, but what it means most to all of us who have a parent experiencing it is that there is a growing gap between what we used to experience with a parent and what is happening now.

My parents' doctor has given my mother a carefully balanced set of medications to help her cope with her increasingly fragile mental state. She's been tested in just about every imaginable way. A geriatric assessment team has spent time with her twice in the past six months, and then there were the CT scans and the blood work and the neurologist's examination. All of it has resulted in little more than the conclusion that my mother is far more demented than she was six or twelve months ago, and that, in fact, she's now delusional.

This diagnosis is borne out by her most recent allegations that my father — nearing 96 — and one of the women who come in to help them (who's in her late thirties) are having a sexual relationship. The accusations started several weeks ago when my mother became agitated because the helper was stroking my father's arm, and it built from there.

Yesterday, my mother claimed that the helper was in bed with my father.

Just today, she maintained that the helper was nude in my father's room, then in bed with him. She also asserted that the helper was stealing things from the house and lying about what medication my mother is taking.

This afternoon, my mother actually physically attacked my father, hitting and slapping him, and tried to hit the helper with her cane.

I talked to my parents at least a dozen times today on the telephone because I'm away. The concern, worry, agony, fear, anger, and love are overwhelming as the stress of the situation courses through me. Each time we talk, I hear the beleaguered voice of my father, weak as it is, straining to be heard, telling me how concerned he is about my mother and how terrible he feels — how her imagination is getting the best of her. He asks how I can help, and I tell him that I just don't know, because I'm way beyond my competency in this situation. He wants me to come to their house; I ask what that will achieve, and he tells me probably nothing.

When my mother gets on the phone, she's full of venom. Her anger is awesome and overwhelming. She verbally attacks my father: How could he have sexual relations with this woman after so many years of marriage, all through which she's been faithful and so caring of him and me? And how can he deny his transgression? And then my mother sets in on me: How is it possible that I, her son, could possibly question her about what she's seen? How is it possible that I would doubt her word when she's always been there for me over these many years? It's a nasty conversation during which I sometimes lose control and verbally shoot back and sometimes try very hard to give her comfort.

The reason we have so many telephone sessions is that my mother keeps hanging up on me. After one such set of calls, I telephone my parents' doctor and leave a message, asking him to call me as soon as he can. Then, in the next call to my mother, she tells me that I've abandoned her, that I've sided with my father, that I've been brainwashed by others, and that I've fallen to the charms of this helper of theirs as well. Along the way, my mother hurls a host of personal insults that sting and tear into my own mind, to the point where I don't know what to do to help my parents or myself.

Somewhere through these conversations, their doctor returns my call, and I can hear in his voice concern for both my mother and my father. He does something very special: he tells me he's going to call my mother tonight to talk with her. And he's going to look at whether it might be best to get her admitted into our local hospital's geriatric ward for a break and an assessment.

Later that night, I talk on the phone again to my parents. My mother is totally illogical. I try very hard to cope and to find some common ground with her. My father sounds even weaker than usual and totally drained, telling me that my mother's mind is confused and that we need to help her. While I agree with him, I don't know what to do or how to do it best.

Rushing through my own mind is a mix of frustration, love, and doubt.

They're old, I tell myself. *Very old. What can I do for either and both of them?* Then my mother comes on the line, still passionate with her anger and hurt. I try very hard to be calm and cool and loving, and it's a challenge as she again rips into me for being selfish and siding with my father and being completely blinded by my hate for her.

I don't know how to handle this. My personal world is in chaos. On the one hand, I want to reach out and hug my mother and remind her that I'm her son and that I love her and will take care of her forever. On the other hand, I want to yell at her that she's not dealing with the real world and that her mind's playing tricks on her, pushing her further and further into a false reality created by her advancing dementia.

But I've learned enough working on eldercare issues to know that to challenge her right now would be wrong and of no use. My mother is off into another dimension and the best I can do is try to listen, absorb the hurt, and see if I can in some way generate a calming effect on her. And I fail at this. I'm into new territory, and I don't know how to manage.

Later that evening, my wife, Gail, provides an excellent reality check by asking me a series of questions over a subdued dinner.

What do I think I can really do for my mother by being logical when she's not? When did my mother begin to show signs of behaving this way? What did my father or I do to help her in the past? How much of this load do I think I can carry, and for how long? How long do I think my parents can manage this family crisis? The truth is that I don't know the answers to any of Gail's questions.

What I do know is that I'm mentally, emotionally, and physically drained by what's happened this long day. Late into the night, I'm conscious and worried about my mother and my father, hoping that both can and will sleep deep and well into tomorrow so that we might move on and get this mess behind us.

JULY 25

During the night, my mother stayed in my father's bed and talked all night. Once she hit him again, and another helper who spends nights with them tried to restrain her. The helper tells me that both of them are exhausted, yet my mother continues to verbally badger my father, like a tape running over and over again. I hear this when she calls to tell me I'd better come to help. We're staying at our country home for a few weeks, with me going into town every couple of days to check on them, shop for food they need, and get our mail. Gail also stopped by when she was in town last week.

So I rush to the city, and in the process I manage to get a hefty speeding ticket. En route I try to call my parents' geriatric specialist but can't get through. I leave an urgent message, which is never returned. Then I call their family doctor, who calls back quickly. I tell him what's happened and that my mother has apparently stopped taking her pills; it seems she's claiming that she doesn't know what she's taking or why, and so she's not taking anything. He urges me to bring her into the hospital — where he'll be later in the day — and says that it would be a good idea to keep her in for a couple of days to do assessments and get her on her medication. Plus, he says, this would give my father a rest. He also tells me that if I can't get her to come with me, I might have to ask for assistance from the police.

When I get to my parents' house, my mother is still going on about my father and his alleged infidelity. She then takes some well-aimed verbal shots at me. I ask her several times to come with me to the hospital, and she refuses. It's exasperating. Then, suddenly, she agrees to come. She dresses, and then when she's ready and eating their usual very late breakfast, she tells me she's not coming after all — there's nothing wrong with her if people would just leave her alone. Throughout, she keeps talking in a totally disjointed way, zigging this way and then zagging that way in her train of thought.

And there's a new behavior I notice for the first time: every time I look at my father, or go and do something in another room, or touch something that's hers, my mother immediately wants to know what I'm doing and if I'm taking something that's hers. Repeatedly she talks about people stealing things from her or from their house. She alleges that we're all in collusion against her. And, worst for me to hear, she tells me over and over that I'm a total disappointment because I'm working against her, believing others and not her. My mother demands to know how I could have changed so much for the worse and who is influencing me to turn against her.

On and on it goes. And like playing spin the bottle or the roulette wheel, where it stops, no one knows. But it doesn't stop at all. It just changes direction, her mind obviously churning myriad confused thoughts.

On the front porch of their house, where my mother can't hear us, I ask my father what he would like me to do, because it's clear that there's no way she'll voluntarily come with me to the hospital. We discuss options, and I tell him of my concern for both his well-being and hers.

He thinks about it, then says that calling the police to take her to the hospital would probably do more immediate harm than if we tried to get her to a calmer state for a day or two and then try again. I'm not convinced.

I ask him again to consider the pressure on him and on all of us. But he's thought about it and stands by his decision.

I acquiesce because I respect his mind, and because he is a psychologist by training. I know he's old, but my father is mentally strong, even if physically very weak.

When we go back in, my mother asks if my father and I remember that a while ago we all stood in the hallway, made the peace sign, and shook hands to agree that we'll all be all right again. I tell her that didn't happen at all. My father agrees with me. And my mother immediately starts on another harangue about how we're conspiring to work against her. A thought flashes through my mind — something co-author Michael Gordon told me in one of our early meetings. He'd said that sometimes, when an older person is demented and delusional, if she or he believes something that's not harmful, it may be all right to let it be real. So I backtrack and tell my mother I don't mean that it didn't happen, only that I don't remember. And I propel my father into the kitchen and whisper to him that he should remember we shook hands and agreed, which is precisely what he does as he walks back into the living room. My mother looks victorious; she tells me that this is a good example of my own forgetfulness and confusion. We get a tiny step ahead for the moment, although it wasn't easy.

Moments later, she starts again about why and how I'm not being supportive of her. I manage to inject into her newest outpouring of confused thoughts that I've got some errands to do and that I'll be back later.

So I leave them for a few hours to get our mail, stop for a brief meeting, and do some grocery shopping for them. Along the way, my eldest daughter, Andrea, calls me on the cellphone, wanting to know how I am and how her grandparents are and to tell me about what she's doing. I give her a fast update. She's shaken by her grandmother's decline and says she's going to call them and then call me back.

Andrea calls me back some ten minutes later to report that her grandmother indeed sounds very confused. She tells me that she's very worried by what she's heard and scared by what her grandmother said, which was, in essence, that things are not right and that I'm one of the main causes. Andrea also talked to her grandfather and told him she understands how traumatic this is for all of them, especially for him.

She asks if she should come to help. I'm moved and thank her, but say that there's nothing she can do to help right now.

When I return from errands and shopping, my parents are having supper. My mother tells me that while I was away, she and my father had a good talk and that they've agreed to put all this behind them, not talk about it anymore, and get on with their lives. I'm delighted, relieved, and hopeful that perhaps we might have gotten over this family crisis. I have a bit to eat with them. Then my mother says we need to have a discussion about how I feel. I tell her that there's nothing to discuss; if they've agreed to put "this" behind them, that's all I care about. I suggest that we should never talk about it again, but it's clear my mother wants to do just that.

By now I'm tired and thinking about the drive ahead. So I tell her that I'm concerned for both of them, and that for the sake of all of us, we should agree not to talk about this anymore.

We all agree, and I leave.

And so another intense episode passes. Where this leads, I don't know. I only know I'm very tired. I know I'm watching and experiencing another level of descent into the vortex of dementia and all the challenges it's presenting. How we'll deal with it is a mystery to me. What I do know is that I'm afraid for both my mother and my father — for what each must cope with while we find a way forward and for the strength they will need to face the next hurdle.

JULY 26

The phone rings early afternoon. In his strained, reedy voice, my father tells me my mother is again on a verbal binge. She's still stuck in the "how-could-you-do-this-to-me" mode, and he asks me to come back from the country, where I'm working on the first edition of this book, to help. I honestly don't want to. I'm terrified of where this is leading.

I can hear my mother in the background yelling at my father to give her the phone, and when he keeps talking to me, I hear her attack him.

It's terrifying. She comes on the line and continues her rant about my father's infidelity, about how I don't seem to care, and about her personal hurt and shame. This goes on for a few minutes, and then my father is back on, asking when I can be there. Although I had dedicated this day to writing, I tell him I'll come as soon as possible, but that I need to try to reach their family physician first. I try, but he's not in. I call the geriatric clinic and talk to one of the staff, who a month ago spent time with my parents in their home. She's very understanding and gives me some good options for getting immediate help. The best is to contact something called the Mobile Crisis Team, and that's what I do first.

The woman who answers the phone at the Mobile Crisis Team is wonderful, understanding, and ready to help once I explain the state of affairs. Heidi tells me a team can be at my parents' house when I get there, and that if they determine there is danger to my mother or father, they'll arrange to have my mother taken to the hospital, even if it means calling in the police. I call to tell my father I'm on my way, then I change, jump in the car, and head off.

When I'm about half an hour away from my parents', I call Heidi back. This time I get her partner, Leslie, who explains that they're on the way to another emergency visit, but to call when I get to my parents' house and they'll come as soon as possible.

I get to my parents' house and call Heidi and Leslie on the cell phone while sitting in the car in the driveway. They're busy helping someone else, but they tell me that as soon as they're done — and they're not too far away — they'll come to see us.

I take a deep breath and knock on my parents' front door. My father opens it, looking gaunt and drained. My mother is sitting in her usual chair in the living room. When she sees me, she begins to explain intensely all the wrongs done to her by this conspiracy of people. We talk, argue, back off, start talking some more, and keep going in circles that leave none of us feeling any better. This goes on for an hour.

We continue at the kitchen table while we eat dinner. Then my cell-phone rings: it's Leslie to say they're out in front of the house, and I tell them they're needed. When they come in, Heidi takes the lead and she's smooth: relaxed, easygoing, and non-confrontational. My mother, who for some time has been so vocal and emotional, suddenly is the epit-ome of sweetness and reason. I'm amazed by this transition. Meanwhile, Heidi just keeps talking and asking questions, and each time my mother gets her back up, Heidi backs down to give my mother more comfort space. For example, when Heidi first asks about what medications she's taking, my mother won't tell, yet five minutes later, she's showing Heidi all her bottles of pills. So it goes for the better part of half an hour, until Heidi asks my mother a series of questions that somehow gets my mother to drop the facade and revert to her behavior of the past weeks. She becomes more belligerent and aggressive and keeps questioning why anyone would possibly want to doubt her version of reality.

After also asking my father some questions, Heidi thanks my parents for their time and says goodbye and signals me to follow her out, where, on the front porch, Leslie is concluding a cellphone conversation with another family in distress. As we stand in the driveway, Heidi tells me they can't call the police or anyone else to take my mother into the hos-pital, because while they believe my mother is delusional and a danger to herself and my father — and even me — there's no observed behavior to support that contention.

So they give me more options. One is to have my parents' fam-ily doctor make a house call and convince my mother to go into the hospital for an assessment. Another is to go to a justice of the peace and plead my case for a ruling that would allow my mother to be forcefully taken to a hospital for an assessment and treatment plan. A third is to get my parents' family doctor or the geriatric specialist to sign a special form that would allow the police to take and have her admitted to the geriatric psychiatric section at the local hospital for 72 hours of assessment and treatment.

Some choices. I don't want any of them. Each is plagued with personal and family danger. This is not where I want to be. No matter what I do, I realize, I'm going to hurt someone — my mother, my father, me, my children, my wife, my parents' few remaining friends — which means that as far as my mother is concerned, I'm going to be the villain. That's a lot of weight to carry, I think. But then again, I realize that it's not like I have many workable choices. As my friend and colleague Harvey Silver, an organizational psychologist, likes to remind one and all, we always have choices; we just need to consider them and decide, since even doing nothing is a choice we make.

When I go back in to talk to my parents again, I convince my mother to see the geriatric specialist whom they'd seen some six months ago. I ask her if she'd come with me to see him so we can talk about what medications she should be taking and to review how she's doing.

My mother says she'll come as long as we can also go have a cappuccino together afterward, and I agree. I feel like a traitor, a Judas, because I've already arranged the appointment with the doctor, and I know he'll give her two choices: to voluntarily go straight to the hospital or to have him sign the special form and be taken in against her will.

It's on that note that I head for my house in the city to get some sleep. I'm depressed, tired, and confused; I tell myself I'm doing the right thing and then second-guess myself the next moment. I have this ongoing debate in my head about what to do and recognize that in this case, I simply must get her the kind of help she needs, because we're all self-destructing the way things are going.

JULY 27

I call the doctor's office in the morning and talk with the woman who's been my contact and who's met my parents. We discuss the options again, and she assures me that, given her own assessment of my parents about a month ago, we must get my mother into the hospital.

I call my mother and tell her she has to get up and get ready for a 10:45 a.m. session with the doctor and that she should bring all her medications. Then I get ready, drive to my parents' home, and collect my mother and her five bottles of pills. She's agitated, confused, and confusing.

The doctor's office is only a five-minute drive; we get there on time, and then — what else is new? — we wait. He's running behind.

Eventually, he comes to get us and take us to his office. He's not the epitome of warmth and charisma, but he's very good at what he does.

It's a tense meeting right from the get-go. He spends some minutes looking at what's now become a rather thick file and asks my mother some questions, many of which she doesn't understand; some, neither do I, but I translate as best I can.

The long and short of it is that the doctor asks her to voluntarily check into the hospital immediately. My mother tells him there's nothing wrong with her, and that, no, she won't do that. Then he tells her that if she won't agree to go with me to the hospital, he'll have to sign papers to have the police take her there. My mother is clearly devastated, but says, no, she won't go. She looks at me and asks how I could do this to her — her only child, turning on her like this. And on it goes for another five minutes, when the doctor asks us to wait in the reception area.

My mother and I sit there, and for the better part of an hour she assaults me with a host of allegations about my memory, my behavior, my lifestyle, and everything else she can think of. Added to it all are various threats about what she'll do to me and my reputation and threats about how my father will die if I go through with this. She argues, she pleads, and she verbally attacks me as we sit there; she stops people walking by and asks for help; and she eventually says she wants nothing to do with me ever again and gets up and moves four seats away from me.

I'm in a living hell — as I know she must be. I keep telling her this is not something I like or want to see happen, but that there just isn't any other choice. We argue, and we ignore each other.

Finally, a squad car with two police officers arrives. They walk over to us and talk with my mother, asking her to come with them. She says she won't. But they are very gentle and caring and amazingly patient.

They kid with her, and they compliment her, and eventually they get her to stand up and head for the door. Meanwhile, several staff are looking on, and some of them even come by and whisper to me that I mustn't take this personally and that I'm doing the right thing.

I'm close to tears. This is so hurtful and painful. It's real and it's happening, and it shouldn't be. I feel a huge amount of love and sorrow and anxiety and hurt. It's like the morning my first marriage died and I watched the faces of my children as I left. It's one of those experiences that will stay with me for a lifetime. All I know is that I don't want to be here, to be in this scene. However, it's still better happening this way, here, and not in my parents' home with my father there.

The police officers are considerate yet again. They suggest that my mother ride in my car rather than in the patrol car. My mother tells them I'm not her son anymore, and she doesn't care. But in the end she sits in the front seat beside me, with one of the officers in the back seat and the other in the patrol car following. While my mother tells me that I'm the bane of her life and a worthless son she never wants to see again, I, for some crazy reason, become very conscious of driving right at the speed limit and using my turn signal at every turn we make. And so we get to the hospital emergency room, which is flooded with people.

While the officers help my mother check in, I rush back to my parents' house to tell my father what is happening. He sits in stunned, sad silence. He sighs deeply several times. His ever so slightly Parkinson's-induced shaking hands are clutched together, and he looks at me with such sorrow that I want to cry again.

I ask him: What else could we do? I ask him: Isn't this going to help my mother — his wife of 58 years — get the help she needs? Won't this give him a break from the tension that's been hanging smog-like in their house for the past weeks? My father acknowledges that it's the right thing but says it hurts, and I see the quiver of his lips for the first time in my life. And I know how much pain he also is experiencing at this moment. He wants to know how long she'll be in the hospital, and I tell him I don't know, even though I do know it's at least four days. But I don't want to make him feel even worse. I keep telling him that it's for the best, and he just nods and tells me that's probably right.

I rush back to the emergency room reception area and wait there with my mother for two hours. The police officers are helpful and considerate beyond anything I'd have expected. Finally, my mother's name is called, and we're taken to a cubicle in the treatment area. That's where we'll spend the next six hours, locked in verbal combat. I don't want to argue; I keep telling my mother that we're here to get her the help she needs, and she keeps telling me that she's fine. We go around and around in circles of complex and confusing dialogue. A few times I manage to get out to call my father to give him an update and to call Gail, to tell her what's going on.

My mother has now decided that this is a jail or prison of some kind. I keep assuring her it's not. And just to add to the drama and trauma of this event, the police arrive with a stocky, barrel-chested man in leg shackles and handcuffs who's plunked on a bed two cubicles down from where we're sitting. Of course, this adds more fuel to my mother's mental fire. Now we are in a prison, and we're just waiting for her cell to be cleared. And so it goes. We talk nicely, we talk passionately, and we argue.

A woman who's been there for almost 24 hours with her aging, ill mother waiting for a bed comes by, and we strike up a conversation, which gives me a chance to run out and find a sandwich and juice for my mother and me to share.

Time passes. Finally, two women arrive. They introduce themselves, and I can't remember the name of either. They tell us they're the crisis team. They sit and talk with my mother for about three-quarters of an hour, asking her a lot of questions. My mother responds and does quite well with her broken English. I urge her to tell them what she's most upset about, and she does: about my father's affair with their helper, and what a shame this is, and how terrible it all is, and how she's over that now, but how it hurts. The two women thank my mother for her time and tell her that soon she'll be moved upstairs.

Then we're alone again for another hour. My mother gives me several ultimatums that are essentially the same: get her out of here and take her home so she can care for my father or he'll probably die.

Yet another hour passes, and finally a cheerful orderly arrives with a wheelchair, only to discover we've already got one. So he picks ours and helps my mother into it, while she continues to tell me I've got one final chance to repent and relent and take her home. I keep telling her that I can't do anything right now and that we've got to get her the help she needs.

Upstairs, on the seventh floor, we are buzzed into the geriatric psychiatry wing. I read the sign and watch the procedure, and I'm on the edge of tears again. I can't believe I'm doing this: that my mother is here and so am I.

A bubbly nurse emerges from the locked nursing station and we wheel my mother into a private room with a large glass window in the door and its own bathroom. Then we tour the self-contained area while some woman with an accent almost as good as my mother's sings in a loud voice somewhere down the hall. As we walk to the communal dining room, hearing a few other people yelling and seeing others walking up and down the hallway, I keep thinking about the amazing book and movie, *One Flew Over the Cuckoo's Nest*. I just can't believe we're here, or that we have to be here. There is something totally terrifying about this, and yet I honestly believe that if we're to save my parents' lives for a while longer, this is what we must do.

Back in my mother's room — her cell, as she calls it — I try to get her as comfortable as possible. She's cold, and we get some extra covers, but the fact is hospitals are cold all the time, and for the elderly this is another discomfort.

I tell her I'll bring her a bathrobe, some other clothes, and her toiletries. This is of small consolation to my mother. She wants to know again why I did this to her and how long she has to stay in this terrible place, which, I must admit, it is. She reminds me that I betrayed her and pledges that she won't last more than a day here. She says again that by doing this to her I'm killing her and my father, who can't last on his own.

There's not much I can say. I'm hurting. I feel guilty. I'm tired. I'm scared. I'm 55 years old and would much rather crawl in my mother's arms so we can just hug each other. Instead, I help her change into hospital garb and get her into the bed, and I assure her I'll be back in the morning. I leave, shaken to the core.

I go back to my parents' house and sit in the kitchen with my father, who's nursing a Scotch and looking so pale and so sad that I don't know what to do or say. We sit there awhile in silence, and I start telling him that things will be all right. I see that he's about to cry — this father of mine who's close to 96 years of age and who's always managed his emotions with perfection. Finally, he agrees that my mother needs the attention and care she'll get at the hospital. He tells me that he knows this is right, but that it's still so very traumatic.

We sit there at the kitchen table and chat for a while. He's also very tired. I go and find a small suitcase and pack up clothes and toiletries for my mother, and when I'm done, I tell him to get some sleep. We agree I'll go see her in the morning and take him in to see her in the early afternoon.

And so we hug and part and I drive to the house in the city, feeling totally empty inside.

JULY 28

I get to the hospital late in the morning after a night of restless sleep. I'm tired and stressed. I'm afraid of what condition my mother will be in when I get there. En route, I stop to buy her a sweatsuit, which I think will be comfortable and warm. I buy myself a muffin in the hospital lobby because I'm very hungry. And up I go — back to that seventh-floor prison. I buzz. I'm admitted. I go to the nursing station and meet and talk with the nurse who's looking after my mother, who is very nice and helpful.

When she looks at what I have brought, she tells me I can't give my mother any nightgowns, only the bathrobes. I can't give her the sweatsuit, but I can give her the toiletries kit, and yes, I was smart to take out the razor blades and substitute one of my electric shavers. She says that my mother's doing all right, but that she's somewhat delusional.

My mother is sitting on the bed. She wants to know if I've come to take her home. No, I tell her, not yet, because they have to do some tests.

She gets angry. She wants to know why more tests are needed. She says that she's peeing and pooping quite well and she wants to go home. And, she tells me, a doctor came in to see her and talk with her and he also said she was doing really well. I show her what I have brought — the bathrobes, socks, toiletries, slippers, and a few other things. Meanwhile, I dig out the muffin and share it with her while I listen to her tell me what a horrible night she's had.

We spend an hour talking, with my mother seeming more subdued but still very angry with me. I help her into the bathroom and onto the toilet and wait outside until she's done, and then I help her get organized again and into a chair when her lunch arrives. Then she starts again to verbally attack me for what I've done to her, and my personal guilt monitor soars at once. While I feel huge pity for my mother, concurrently there is also a sense of anger for these continuing attacks, and I try very hard to control my emotions and my tongue so I don't say something I'll regret and in the process exacerbate an already fragile situation. So I tell her I'm going to get my father to bring him for a visit.

When I wheel him into her room an hour later, she's instantly in tears. He slowly gets out of the wheelchair and she slowly stands, and they hug and kiss. It's both heartwarming and heartbreaking to watch.

I stay a bit, then leave them to run some errands. When I return, they're sitting and talking as quietly as is possible for two people who are hard of hearing.

We all chat a while longer and I can see that my father is tiring, so I suggest we leave. There are a lot more tears and hugs and kisses before I wheel him back to the car and drive him home and then head back to the country myself.

I'm really, truly tired, both physically and mentally. I've been dashing to their home most days for several weeks and always spending way more time than I'd anticipated. I'm behind in my client work. And I'm way behind on my parts of the book. Michael is being highly understanding and supportive because he knows what I'm going through on both the personal and professional level. However, I need to get my mind in gear, and it's difficult.

Tonight, I call my daughter Andrea and ask her if she'd give me a day off and go see my father tomorrow and take him to visit my mother. She says she would be pleased to, and that relieves me.

JULY 29

It's amazing how tired I am. I worked for a couple of hours on this chronicle of events last night and then fell into bed and woke up not long before noon. I walk around, numb and dumb, for an hour and decide that today for a few hours I need to do mindless work around the property, so I paint things and glue things and change some light fixtures and move slowly. I even have a short nap late in the afternoon.

Through it all, I am mulling over the events of the past days, relating them to the past months and trying to fit those all into the past years.

I try to figure out if there is a pattern we missed, or if there is some special event that may be important. I think there are some pieces that loosely fit, but I realize that I'm just speculating.

Then my father calls to say that he and Andrea had a good visit with my mother and that she seems much calmer overall, and that he misses her and would like her back at home. He also asks me to call her, which I was planning on doing anyway, and see what I think. Then my daughter calls to tell me that her grandmother was in pretty good shape from all she could see and hear. This is heartening news.

I call the geriatric psychiatry wing nursing station and ask how I can speak to my mother. There is one patient phone and it's busy, so the nurse takes pity on me and gets my mother to her phone so we can talk for a few minutes. She actually does sound much more subdued and generally calmer. I feel good about that, although part of me is worried that this may just be a false positive signal and that more bad things may come sooner than later. But even given that cautionary thought, I want to believe that we're on the path to some kind of stable footing for the good of all of us.

JULY 30

Early this afternoon, my mother's in-hospital doctor calls. He asks me several questions about how I see her state of mind and general condition now compared to last week and suggests we meet tomorrow morning. He tells me that he thinks she might be able to go home in the next day or so.

I call my father with this news, and I can just sense him perking up over the phone. I ask him to think about what's best for him and for her and tell him I'll pick him up in a few hours.

Driving into the city, I reflect on the complexity of being a family member dealing with a loved one who's demented. It's sort of like a Catch-22. If my mother thinks something that isn't real is real, how do we deal with that? My experience so far is that it's a no-win debate.

The people who are watching her witness all sorts of times she's imagined things. There are myriad instances when my mother simply denies reality and clings with passion to her point of view. My father and I have talked about this many times during these past months, and he just shakes his head and tells me sometimes we simply have to let go and let her reality be the one we go with. This troubles me greatly. Where do you draw the line? How do we help our parents find the truth so that we can deal with it? Yet as Michael has said to me, sometimes if the reality of a demented person isn't hurtful, maybe it's best to let it be their reality. If a demented person with Alzheimer's believes it's Tuesday, for example, but really it's Wednesday, and in the greater scheme of life that doesn't matter, then perhaps that's how we should leave it. I see the sense in all of this, but it's still hard to practice.

By the time I think about all this and end up nowhere, I'm at my parents' house to take my father to see my mother. Today she's sitting in her chair in her hospital room, and she lights up like a birthday candle when I wheel him in. The hugs and kisses are sincere and laden with overwhelming affection. Again, I sit around and talk for a little while and then leave to let them have time alone. And again, when I return, my mother tells me that there's nothing wrong with her mind and demands to know why I am subjecting her to this humiliation and personal pain.

Even as she says this, she's confusing things and alleging things that just aren't so. But it is evident that she is much calmer overall, and that's somewhat reassuring.

She wants to know how long she has to stay. She explains that she met the doctor today and that he said she looked really well and all her tests were fine, and that it was up to me to get her home. We talk around this one for a little while, and my father injects that we should wait and see what the doctor has to say, and that being in the hospital is actually good for my mother, since it gives her a much-needed period of rest.

As I drive my father home, I ask him if he's really comfortable with the possibility of my mother coming home tomorrow. Can he cope? Will she cope? Will those who help them cope? I explain that I'm not just tired, but I need to do my work, and work on the book, and that while I love them dearly, I can't stop my world all the time to help, as selfish as that may seem to him. He understands and says that if the medications are right, it all should work out for the best. For how long, I ask, and he responds that the next critical stage will be another traumatic event that my mother will see as a threat to any one of us, but especially to herself.

He's very logical in his thinking, and I respect that.

So we part, and I tell him I'll either be reporting after seeing the doctor or be bringing my mother home. He says he hopes I'll be bringing her home now that he's rested and ready. He smiles and tells me that this part of his life sure isn't what he expected it to be.

JULY 31

This morning I get to the hospital early and wait for the resident psychiatric doctor at the nursing station. I sit around for a while and then look into my mother's room. She's sitting on the bed, sorting through some clothes. My strategy had been to avoid my mother and see the doctor, because I was frankly afraid of what I'd find or how things would go with her. But she looks up about the same time as I'm looking in, and she smiles and calls for me. I go in and kiss her on the cheek as I usually do, and she's so happy for the moment. Then she tells me that even though she's totally fine, she was told she couldn't go home today. I say that as far as I know, she maybe can go home today, but that I'm waiting and watching for the doctor to arrive and I don't want to miss him.

My mother and I have this disjointed conversation that covers how bad the nurses are to how badly she slept to how good the food is to how well she slept to how some spies are being kept down the hall to how nice the nurses are, all in one long outpouring. But she is much calmer, and her eyes are clearer and more focused.

After a few minutes, I tell her that I should go back in the hall to wait for the doctor; she agrees, and that's what I do.

The doctor arrives in a flurry of energy and kindly intensity. After we shake hands he tells me to follow him to someone's office way down the hall. My mother sees this and calls out to me, tells me to help her get home, and I assure her that's first on my agenda.

In the office the doctor and I are joined by a really gentle and caring nurse and a social worker. We spend 45 minutes talking about my mother's condition, what safeguards she needs, how we need to deal with her condition, and what medications she will require. I learn that after all the many tests these past many months, and through a process of elimination, they have diagnosed my mother with Alzheimer's. She's at about mid-point, which is bad, I know, from reading the material Michael has given me and from the conversations he and I have had.

In fact, the doctor tells me, most people in the same condition are institutionalized, but because my parents have care in the home and because my mother is responding to medications, her remaining at home is a viable option.

Then I collect my mother so she can talk with him for a few minutes as he explains the medications he's assigned for her. I want him to do that to avoid her suggesting again that medicines are sent to her without explanation.

The doctor also asks my mother how she is doing, and she assures him that she feels fine and that she appreciates the help she's been given, and she tells him how she's done so well in demonstrating her mental agility through all the tests she's taken. It's a sad moment for me. Almost as an afterthought — but a good one — the doctor suggests that he give my mother an overnight pass and that we come back tomorrow for a short meeting to see how my mother's doing before she's discharged. We all agree.

Back in her room, we pack her things and wait for the nurse to bring the medications my mother needs to take until her return visit. My mother is suspicious, wondering if they will really let her leave now or if they are going to keep her again when we come back tomorrow. I assure her that everything will be just fine.

With overnight bag in hand and pill packets in my pocket, we leave the wing, but only after a long battle with the armed door, because the staff person presses the wrong button and the door won't open, which reinforces my mother's impression that she's been confined in a jail of some kind. We head home. Along the way, we stop at a convenience store and I get a few cans of her favorite soft drink. My real motive is to use my cell phone while I'm in the store to call my father and alert him about my mother's condition and what that requires of all of us.

When we arrive at my parents' house, my father is at the front door, all smiles, standing wobbly but proud and happy. My mother works her way up the front porch steps and across the porch, and they hug and kiss.

Another heart-melting moment for me, as surely it is for them.

For the next hour, we talk about my mother's experiences in the hospital, which she still thinks was a prison of some kind with the spies, the too-cold air conditioning, the lack of help, the tests, and on and on. My mother says things that surprise and stun me, but I think I've learned to accept her world without too much challenge and debate. It's not easy or realistic or practical, but it's very necessary. As Michael and the psychiatric doctor both have said to me, it's important not to agitate a demented person, because that only serves as a trigger to another more intense irrational reaction.

On my drive home, I think about how we baby boomers all over are facing the same kind of crisis. We're worrying about our children and we're needing to care for our parents. Some call it the sandwich generation. Whatever you call it, the fact is that we're stuck carrying a lot of baggage, a lot of worry, and a whole lot of responsibility. And guess what? It's not fun.

But then again, maybe it's not a crisis at all. Maybe it's just one more rock to roll up the hill as Sisyphus did in Greek mythology: a test of ourselves and of our patience, endurance, commitment, and depth of our love for family. And if we're to pass that test, we've got to be a bit selfish. We've got to recognize that we won't be able to help our aging parents or our children if we don't take time out for ourselves. Easier said than done, yes, but critically important. As I talk and work with doctors and nurses and caregivers who are much more experienced and wiser than I am, they have one clear and consistent message: I'm the one who's delivering for my parents, and if I can't, it won't happen.

So what does that mean? It means, quite simply, that if I drop the ball, it's game over for all of us, because I'll be of no use to anyone, and my parents won't get the level and range of help they need and deserve. And I will certainly drop the ball if I get too stressed out or, worse, sick. Michael has talked a lot about the need to bear this in mind and to deal with it.

As I think about this, it seems to me that for those of us who, by design or default, end up as primary caregivers to our parents there are three serious challenges to face: managing the physical demands of time and stress, managing the mental drain of focusing so hard on their needs, and managing the frustration and guilt we feel as matters worsen.

To face the physical demands we have to arrange our priorities in such a way that we don't compromise the other parts of our lives. From my own experience in the past half-year especially, it's obvious that if we take on the task of helping our parents, the demands for time and attention will grow rapidly. In order not to jeopardize our other family commitments and our vocational expectations, we have to create some level of balance and set priorities. For example, I've talked to all three of my children and explained that right now I'm in a very difficult and demanding time with their grandparents, and so, for a while at least, they need to understand that I'll have less time for them. I have explained that this doesn't reflect a lack of love for them, but that it's a balancing act I hope they understand. I think they do.

On the work side, it's a matter of ensuring "the job" gets done. In my case, I'm fortunate that we have our own business and can juggle client work between Gail and me. It's also fortunate that as I'm deep into this especially trying time, we're not that busy — although that's a double-edged sword, because not being very busy also means not generating the level of income we need. Others I know who are engulfed in parental caregiving and who work tell me that managing their work lives has become very difficult, as they need to ask for more and more time off — with consequences.

And there's one more element to the physical demands of time and stress: not losing play and rest time. We all need to relax. Everyone needs to set aside some time each week to just go and do what it is they like to do best. To stop all playtime is to become vulnerable to fatigue, burnout, and illness.

Managing the mental drain of focusing so hard on our parents' needs is the second challenge. And that drain is real, even if we don't notice it. It's an unwelcome but constant companion. It eats at us and affects the soundness of our judgment and expected behavior. A tired, cluttered brain isn't one that's going to make sensible, logical decisions. It is one, however, that'll lead us into trouble faster than almost anything else.

For example, I know that I'm not as tolerant right now as I should be — with almost anyone. That bothers me, and I tell myself that I've got to watch it, but it's hard. I find I'm talking too much to too many people about what I'm experiencing. On one hand, it's probably therapeutic for me; on the other hand, I can imagine that in some cases I'm wearing out my welcome. People have their own problems and challenges to face, and clients have their own needs. So by dousing them with a stream of my personal woes, I'm not doing them any favors.

The key, it seems to me, is to understand and acknowledge the mental drain that comes with more involved caregiving, especially when a parent is suffering from physical or emotional problems. When the mental drain level soars, it's critical to take a break somehow — perhaps a quiet day, a short trip, or some kind of change to give the head and heart a break from the tension and pressure.

The third challenge — managing the frustration and guilt we feel as matters worsen — is a tough one. Feeling frustration and guilt is a natural part of caring for and loving our parents. But when either or both is physically or mentally ill, there's only so much we can do, and it's important to recognize and come to terms with that fact. While we can be supportive, while we can spend a lot of time and energy to help them, we can't turn back the clock and we can't fix the unfixable. We can be responsive and responsible, but we can't blame ourselves for what isn't our doing.

I know I'm battling frustration and guilt right now. I'm busy second-guessing what I should have done in the past couple of years and brooding over what else I could be doing right now. But when I look at it dispassionately, there really isn't much. I give, on all levels, as much as I can, and I have to accept that there's no more I can do, short of giving up my life and focusing totally on theirs. And that's not what a parent-child relationship is all about. Rather, I keep reminding myself, that relationship is supposed to be about our parents helping to rear and nurture us to a point where we launch into our own world and seek our own course.

That's why all of us who strive to help our parents must acknowledge that we will do the best we can, but we will not suffer guilt trips. I'm learning this the hard way because my mother is trying to induce guilt right now. Demented or not, Alzheimer's or not, she's really working me over. For a long time, I didn't understand or recognize that. Now I do. That doesn't mean I love her any less; it only means I'm finally getting smarter and learning how to deal with it better.

As I near my destination, I conclude that the three challenges we face are real and threats to all of us. I've learned so much, the hard way, over the past few months. I know I've got to manage as best I can, and with the help of Gail and my children and our ever-expanding number of medical and social worker specialists, I will. But I do have to be selfish to the extent that I manage my priorities and give myself permission to look after me.

It's as simple and as complex as that.

AUGUST 1

Today is my mother's birthday. She's 87.

This morning, Gail and I drive into the city, she for appointments and I to take my mother to her noon appointment with the psychiatric doctor. I arrive a few minutes early to pick her up and find her tense and apprehensive. I assure her all will be right, and she snaps back that this is her birthday. My father tells me he's tired, and my mother complains that no one's called to wish her a happy birthday. I remind her that their friends know not to call before early afternoon, but this doesn't wash with her. She's clearly miffed that her birthday isn't being celebrated as she thinks it should be.

We pack up my mother and her walker and I take her back to the hospital, arriving at the geriatric psychiatry wing right on time. On the way I had to listen to my mother tell me how I was late to pick her up, and how Gail says I'm always late for everything, and how it seems I can't manage my time very well, and more. After waiting a while, the doctor arrives in his usual breeze of energy, does a few things, and asks me to come to the same office I went to yesterday to talk about how my mother coped over the past 24 hours. I tell him I'm not sure, since I wasn't there, and I call my father to ask. He tells me in Hungarian, and I tell the doctor in English, that she was pretty tired and calm and, all things considered, everything worked out rather well.

After my report, he asks me to get my mother, which I do. He then asks her how she feels and a lot of other questions that, as I listen, make it clear he's probing to determine how mentally lucid she is. He explains again to her what medication to take and gives her a list and a prescription for one new pill (to help her relax more and sleep better). He says he's arranged for a nurse to see my mother twice a week and he wants me to make an appointment for her to see a geriatric psychiatrist next week. Finally, he says he's signing a discharge order and that my mother is free to go.

My mother is reasonably calm through the meeting, saying that she understands everything and is delighted to do everything. We all smile a lot and shake hands, and my mother and I head back down the long hall to the security door. And as we walk down the hall, she pushing her walker and me walking next to her, she tells me again how all that's happened has been a set-up — a conspiracy — organized to do something I don't quite understand.

Once I get her back into the car, we stop at the pharmacy to drop off the prescription, and I tell her we'll have a birthday lunch. She says that would be nice and that she'd like a bowl of hot soup, but she doesn't want to go anyplace where anyone will recognize her because she can't handle the shame. I ignore this and take her to a nice suburban mall restaurant she knows. We study the menu, and my mother says she doesn't want any soup. We study the menu some more, and she says she doesn't want any kind of chicken dish, of which there are a lot. I suggest a spinach salad, and she agrees. We order and talk and it's nice and comfortable.

I tell her stories about our friends, and she asks a lot of questions.

Lunch arrives, and my mother digs in and eats like she hasn't seen food in a long time. Bits and pieces stick to her chin and some fall in her lap, but I say nothing.

We have a very nice time, and I'm thankful and pleased. Then I lead her to a bench in one of the mall hallways and ask her to wait while I charge off to buy a few grocery items they need. When I get back, laden with bags, she's agitated. She needs toothpaste, she tells me — toothpaste she's asked me to get but I haven't. So I rush off to do that. When I get back, she tells me that she's tired and wants to go home because my father must surely be missing her and needing her attention. After all, my mother tells me, he's so fragile and wonderful, but she does wish he'd stop behaving so badly.

It's very hot out. We load into the car, crank up the air conditioning, and set off. We stop to pick up her new prescription and then drive to my parents' house. When we get inside, all hell breaks loose. She's suddenly very agitated and abusive. Everything is wrong. No one cares about her. It's her birthday and no one's called. She's ashamed to talk to anyone because she's been in a place that's locked up and her friends all know that. Where is the surprise party I said I'd arranged? And on it goes. Then she tries on her birthday present — a new sweatsuit — and it doesn't fit right, and that sets her off some more. My mother tells me with quite some intensity that she's got a lot of clothes, but none that fit right, and all of them are old and worn. She sternly scolds their helper for holding her arm as she walks, telling her that she'll call for help when she needs it.

My father looks wan again. Sitting in the living room, he tells me how tired he is and that he's taken some Aspirin (ASA) because he can feel pressure on his heart.

I just want out of there. It gets worse when my mother asks why I'm holding a container of her pills. I tell her it's one that's been replaced by what we just picked up and that we should throw it away, but she wants to study it and hold it as "evidence." I make the serious mistake of pulling it out of her hands and tossing it into the wastepaper basket. This leads to a major confrontation with her saying that she doesn't need her pills anyway, that her diabetes has been cured, and that no one is calling to wish her a happy birthday.

I backtrack, but it's not enough, and so I improvise as best I can. But the damage is done, and I did it, and so I tell her I'm going downtown to pick up Gail and her other birthday surprises, and we'll be back.

Two hours later my father answers the door, looking even paler than he was earlier in the day. He says my mother is in her bedroom. Gail and I go to see her, and Gail wishes my mother a happy birthday. My mother says she's tired and wants to rest and tells us to go away. Gail shows her the flower arrangement she brought and the cake with my mother's name inscribed. My mother wants to know why Gail didn't call her during the past week. And so we go again in a futile circle of senseless and unsatisfying conversation.

Gail tells my mother she'll put the flowers in a vase, and she leaves the room while I sit by her and talk nicely about our day. My mother, though, is focused on my father — how he's being so mean to her while she's being so forgiving. We talk about this for a few minutes, and my mother says that what she needs is to hear my father say that he loves her and that he's sorry about what he's done. Of course, he's said this a number of times over the past days, but she needs to hear it again, so I go to my father, who's sitting in the living room, and explain that he has to do it again. He's tired and wants to rest, but he props himself up, shuffles down the hall to her bedroom, and says it all one more time. I ask her to stand and for them to hug and kiss, which they do. And then my mother starts again about how my father refuses to confess his bad behavior. As I look at him, I feel a pang in my heart because I can see the hurt and the weariness on his face.

We all head back to the living room where Gail's sitting. For the next half-hour, we try to make pleasant conversation about nothing in particular and admire the flower arrangement. My mother keeps delving into the most recent black hole in her mind, but she seems to be more subdued. Finally, Gail and I hug and kiss my mother and father and leave.

In the car, I call a couple of my parents' friends who understand my mother's condition. I remind them it's her birthday and ask them to call her.

And that's the way the day closes.

Tonight, I dread the thought of the phone ringing. I don't want to hear any news. I'm tired. I'm dejected. I'm worried. I'm lost. I don't know what comes next, but whatever it is, I fear it.

On that note I'm going to head off to sleep, convinced that tomorrow another chapter will unfold in the drama of our lives — a chapter that, if we're all fortunate, will be calmer — but who knows for sure?

SEPTEMBER 12

I took my mother to the geriatric psychiatrist who's now seeing her for the second time since I brought her home from the hospital six weeks ago. They had a wonderful visit. My mother seems at ease and sharp as a tack.

My mother talks about her memory — how she'd like to improve her ability to remember especially near-term events and issues. The doctor then asks if she'd mind taking the same test she's taken four times in the past two years, which measures her cognitive abilities. My mother agrees.

The results genuinely surprise the doctor. Two years ago, on a scale that tops at 30 points, she scored about 24. The next time she scored 22, the third time she slipped to 18, and on the fourth test, some six months later, she was at a dangerous 14. The lower the number, the greater the short-term memory loss, and at 14, she was in serious trouble of having little retention and much confusion. And today her score is 25 — an amazing turnaround.

In fact, the doctor tells my mother that there's no need for him to see her for two months now, because he feels she's so much better and that her mind seems so much sharper. This is good news all around.

On the drive home, I tell my mother how proud I am of her and her progress. I explain that all the trauma of the past months is regrettable: having to take her to the hospital, having her tested, and living through all the personal emotional turmoil we all experienced. She tells me that she understands and that she knows she's for the moment better, both physically and emotionally.

I have dinner with my parents and go for a short walk with my father, who next week marks his ninety-sixth birthday. And then I head home with the profound hope that we've stabilized and that, God willing, things can be calm and all right for a time.

Yet there's always the nagging reality that both my mother and father are old and at risk, and we just don't know what tomorrow will bring.

MAY 2, THREE YEARS LATER

My father died during the night. Alone. At home, in his bedroom. At peace with himself, I fervently hope.

But let me backtrack.

It's now been nearly three years since we wrote the first edition of this book; since then there has been a second revised edition and an American version. When we started, I was living in fear and confusion because of my mother's condition and eventual forced hospitalization.

My mother did improve for a while. For nearly a year, she was reasonably well. And then she started a steep downward slide again.

A year and a half after the forced hospitalization she was totally immobile. We rented a Hoyer Lift to get her in and out of bed and used a travel wheelchair to move her around the house. My mother seemed to decline by the day, to the point where her words were intelligible, she was totally incontinent, and she had to be spoon-fed by my parents' caregivers.

It was painful to watch, and we were again into a new crisis.

She demanded to sleep with my father but would wake him at all hours to talk or to demand in no uncertain terms that they get dressed to go somewhere — to catch a train, escape, or whatever strange thought crossed her troubled mind.

Their family physician had decided to leave his practice some months before, and we had a new family physician in place: Dr. Gregory Gelman, a young man who had started his practice just a year earlier. From the first visit onward, he was as patient and caring as the day is long. He always made time for my parents when I took them for appointments. But he also was concerned about my mother.

He recommended yet another assessment for my mother by our local geriatric assessment team. He booked examinations. And given all the results — which reconfirmed that my mother was indeed suffering from Alzheimer's disease — he finally urged that we get her into a facility where a sound, longer term assessment and observation could be conducted.

So we got her on a wait-list for the neurological unit at the Baycrest Centre for Geriatric Care. After some weeks of waiting, the call came: get her in the next day and expect her to stay for at least a few weeks.

This time my mother didn't resist. We arranged for an ambulance, which was to arrive at eight o'clock, and it finally got there at eleven o'clock. I was at Baycrest, waiting at the unit for her arrival.

She was confused and afraid: that was obvious.

From mid-September through late December, my mother was a resident at Baycrest's amazing neurological unit. Week by week, there was a steady improvement in her overall condition. At least once a week, I took my father to visit her for an hour or two. I arranged for some of her friends to see her from time to time and for her to get her hair done weekly. I visited almost every day, wheeling her around, talking with her, just being there for her as best I could. Gail went to see her as often as she could, too.

Eventually, she was walking again, with the aid of a walker and loads of physiotherapy. She was feeding herself. She was no longer as incontinent. Her speech was much more normal. In short, she was in remarkably better shape than she had been in when she entered Baycrest.

Meanwhile, my father continued living at home, in reasonably good health, with around-the-clock support. But he was depressed. That was obvious. His continuously failing eyesight troubled him hugely, and my mother's hospitalization was a hurtful forced separation that gnawed at him. It was like he felt guilty about being in the comfort of his home while my mother was hospitalized.

Just before Christmas, she was released on the condition that if things didn't work out well at home she would be re-admitted. But things did work out reasonably well — for a few months. Part of the condition of her being at home was that she get up at a regular time, take her medications at given times, and be active; she was to join a senior's center for regular activities and exercise daily.

However, by early spring my mother refused to get up until at least early afternoon, often refused to take her medications on time, and definitely refused to go to any seniors' center, let alone exercise. She began haranguing my father again, moving into his bed and staying there, often not wanting to get up at all. She wouldn't let my father sleep at night, and even during the day she would wake him from a nap to talk. And she kept pointing out that this was her house, her domain, and that all others had to follow her wishes.

She was, more often than not, agitated and verbally combative.

My father clearly was suffering from the stress and strain of it all. He finally asked me do something to relieve the tension he was feeling. Although it was obviously a huge moral dilemma for him, by April my father asked me to see if we could get my mother back into Baycrest. It took a while, but we got my mother re-admitted a month later.

And the whole cycle started again. The visits: me often, Gail as often as possible, my father at least weekly. The treatments. The jiggling and juggling of medications. New CT scans. And while my mother responded somewhat, it was not the same as before. There was progress and improvement yet again, but not to the same extent as the first time.

The long and short of it was that the medical team recommended that for her own good and safety my mother should not return home again, but instead should be placed in a nursing home.

More conversations with my father. He understood intellectually, but it obviously troubled him emotionally. Me, too. It's the one place they both said they never wanted to be.

I then began a torrid round of reconnaissance visits to nursing homes that were in reasonable proximity to my parents' house. Most

of what I saw, I didn't like. Some places were just too big, too imper-
sonal. Some places looked nice, bright and new, but there was a feeling
missing from the staff: to me, they were just putting in time, and the
connection with residents was limited to the least that had to be done.
Some places smelled of urine, and I was startled to the core by the
dozens of elderly people I saw with heads lolling, strapped into wheelchairs, just existing — no, barely subsisting, with little dignity and even
less respect.

If I had to have my mother in a nursing home, I wanted it to be a
good one.

And I finally found one, recommended by a person who works out of
Baycrest. She said there might be an opening at a place called Thompson
House, actually very near my parents' house. She gave me a name and a
number, and I called and hurried to visit.

Thompson House is a small facility, home to about a hundred elderly
people who live on three levels, reflecting the need for relatively independent living, assisted living, and full-care living. My mother was a
full-care candidate.

I got the tour — yet another one. But this place felt good, smelled
good. The staff seemed to be caring. They knew the names of all who
lived there and had a good word, a smile, a pat, and patience for all. By
now I knew what to look for, and I found it at Thompson House.

I rushed to tell my father. He wasn't happy about it, but he concurred
this might be best.

So, in mid-July my mother was moved to Thompson House, her new
and final home.

My mother chose to dislike the place from the start. Yet for several
years to follow she was in better shape than she had been since our odys-
sey began in earnest.

The staff was genuine: the caring, the attention, and the ambiance
were real. Yes, the place was small and tight for space, she had to share
a room, and there was too much TV time, but my mother's condition
stabilized and with her new medication regimen her near-term memory was better. Friends visited her. And she's made a few new friends at
Thompson House.

But her complaints never ceased. In her mind she was just fine; it was only all the other residents there who were in some way mentally or physically unwell.

From her move to Thompson House through to Christmas, I took my father at least once a week to see my mother. But by November he was frailer, more agitated, and more restless. I took him for another visit to his geriatric psychiatrist, who prescribed a new antidepressant medication. The medication seemed to work at first, but the agitation and depression kept building. In early December the psychiatrist said we should increase the dosage, which we did, with no positive results.

By early January, my father seemed to be in worse shape. His caregiver was worried about him, as were we. But we were assured the medication would help and advised to give him yet more tablets at night.

Then, in early March, he just didn't want to get out of bed one morning.

And that was the beginning of the end.

I talked with Dr. Gelman, who made a house call to see him. He had tests conducted. The results: his system was strong, but he had a bladder infection.

Meanwhile, my daughter, Andrea, who at the time worked for a pharmaceutical company, started to worry yet more about her grandfather and did an in-depth search of the antidepressant medication he was given. Her conclusion: the higher dosage we were told was acceptable to give him actually conflicted with the drugs for his Parkinson's disease. I called our pharmacist, who checked with a pharmacological database and concurred that the dosage was way too high.

I checked with Dr. Gelman. He agreed, and immediately put him on another drug. I called and emailed the information to the geriatric psychiatrist who'd prescribed the drug in the first place, left another message some months later, but never heard back from him.

So whether it was the medication, the bladder infection — which in the elderly can cause numerous unwanted side effects, such as delusion — his decision that his life had lasted long enough, or a combination of these factors, my father started on his personal journey to death.

He ate less and less. He rejected all help. He remained in bed, sometimes quite lucid, but more often in some faraway place only he understood. He was on a daily sodium chloride drip and had a condom catheter attached to him.

Dr. Gelman came to see him weekly. He and I spoke numerous times about the options: to be aggressive (hospitalization) or passive (keep him at home and make him as comfortable as possible). I opted for keeping my father at home. In his lucid periods, when I asked, my father said he wanted to stay at home. I agreed with him. There was nothing they could have done in a hospital to make him better; he wouldn't walk again, let alone dance or think any better or do much of anything again.

Dr. Gelman and I also discussed the option of tube feeding. Aside from the discomfort of the process, I had real trouble grasping what benefit that might offer, other than making him live longer than he might wish. Keeping him alive would have been mainly for my benefit, not for his; to tube feed him really would have been an act of selfishness on my part. Tube feeding begs the debate of the quantity of life versus the quality of life, given any significant recovery was highly unlikely.

As he faded more and more, I shared memories from my childhood of fun and meaningful experiences together, in the hope of giving him some pleasurable mental moments and a sense of satisfaction. I often rubbed his neck and back and massaged his feet and legs, which he'd always enjoyed greatly.

In my heart, I so wanted him to be better, but in my head I knew he wouldn't be.

I reported on his condition to my mother on my regular visits. My mother clearly had mixed emotions, but as often as not she was remarkably astute given her condition. She observed that her husband was old, that he had lived a long life, and that he should not suffer.

A few weeks before his death, I arranged for my mother to have a visit home so they could share some time together. The next visit was scheduled for the day my father died. There was no sense in my mother seeing him dead.

Watching him wilt away, listening to him ramble on about people and events from his distant past or some terrible event imagined in his mind, and feeling him ever so slowly but surely sliding toward the personal conclusion of his life was an agonizing experience for me.

And I knew I must accept that he would die in the near future.

My profound hope was that he would die at peace with himself, in the knowledge that he did so many wonderful things and that he was respected and loved by those of us near to him.

And I hoped I would have the strength and resolve to grieve as I must, to celebrate all we shared, to carry the good memories, and to march on; because that's the way of the real world, like it or not.

So now my father is dead. He hasn't "left us" or "moved to the beyond" or "passed on," or anything like that. He is simply dead, and if there is an afterlife, his soul is bound to be there, and I guess and hope he'll know how much he meant to me and always will. And I look at his ashen face and kiss his cold forehead, and I cry, because crying is good when the pain is deep. I am alone with his body in his bedroom, and this is a safe and sure place full of flooding memories.

FEBRUARY 19, 2011

On this day, my mother died at dawn, six months shy of her ninety-seventh birthday.

For the past number of years, she'd lived in ever-quieter solitude, even though we were all around her.

Month by month and year by year, my mother slowly but surely regressed yet further into someplace in her confused and confusing mind. Conversations inevitably became jumbled phrases, needing ever fewer words. Her recollections grew generally inaccurate when she expressed them, but I'd learned, finally, to let them be what they were and to let the conversations go where they would. I stopped contradicting or correcting my mother, because all that created was angst and anger on her part.

I spent time with her almost every day when I wasn't out of town. Not too long — sometimes 15 minutes, sometimes an hour. I found that after an hour or so, she got tired and didn't mind at all that I left.

During her entire life in the nursing home, I had a series of women who were of Hungarian origin come to spend time with her every day — five hours a day the first few years and eight hours a day the final four years. It helped my mother feel engaged. And I know on some level she felt that she was being cared for and that she was valued. That was also why I arranged for my mother to have her hair done weekly and to have clothing that was colorful.

I also arranged to have a geriatrician examine my mother about three times a year. I knew and respected the Thompson House visiting physicians, but I also know that a good geriatrician will take a deep and long look at how an elderly person is doing with medications, with mindset, and with physical challenges. And I wanted that extra look for my mother.

But latterly, my mother suffered a series of mini strokes, all of which collectively took their toll. She had frequent bladder infections. She battled through bouts of pneumonia twice during her last three years, and those experiences seriously weakened my mother. As well, medical tests seemed to indicate that she may well have had an emerging case of stomach cancer. But short of having her hospitalized for serious testing, we didn't know for sure.

What we did know for sure, though, was that my mother had become just about completely insular. She did not want to eat most of the time, and would tolerate only a few spoonfuls of mashed food. She did not speak at all. She stared straight ahead most of the time. She didn't move a muscle all day, or all night. There was no interaction at all with her, whether it was her great-granddaughter visiting or me, or if we played music, showed pictures, or anything. Sadly but truly, it was like watching a shell; the body was there, but no one lived there anymore.

The consensus of the nursing staff, the physicians, and the geriatrician was that she would never improve, but could potentially live for some time in this condition. I consulted with my wife and two daughters and sadly decided that we should let her die with dignity. That meant stopping all her medications, and offering food only if she was willing to take it. She wasn't.

We kept my mother hydrated and up during the daytime. We kept close watch over her. And we watched her wilt away.

She lived for some weeks. Near what we knew was the end, she was given morphine patches to ensure there was little or no pain. A second cousin of mine, Apor, who has a lovely voice and sings in choirs, came and softly sang Hungarian hymns and recited soothing Gregorian chants.

Just before she died, I wrote this as I headed into my period of grief:

Hello, goodbye.
Don't fret, don't cry.
There's nothing much left now, but to die.
Hello, goodbye,
Take a deep sigh.
There's no tomorrow, no doubting for why
We're hugging hello and weeping goodbye:
'Cause we've come to an ending, come now to die.

And I think that said it all, along with the many tears that flowed freely, because there are times when crying is a very healthy thing.

LESSONS LEARNED

Friend, colleague, and co-author with me of another book, Dr. Harvey Silver, always talks about the difference between tender loving care and tough loving care. An organizational psychologist, Harvey likes to explain that tender loving care is easy: we just give what's wanted, do what's expected, and keep opting out of the difficult decisions that make us all accountable leaders in the truest sense. On the other hand, tough loving care demands making hard decisions that take us out of our zones of comfort. Tough loving care means that while we respect a person, we don't accept that person's problem behaviors and attitudes.

When I apply those concepts to my own experience with my parents — and in particular to my mother's problems — I think the biggest, most valuable lesson I learned is that we must abide by our parents' wishes, but only so long as they don't harm themselves or each other or anyone else. There comes a critical point in time when we have to take control and do the unthinkable: we have to bite the bullet and make decisions that hurt, but that will, in fact, help. Had I not taken the painful steps of having my mother hospitalized against her wishes, we may well have had a family crisis that could have cost us more emotionally than we could have managed. Had I not agreed that my mother was best off in a nursing home, I think my parents would have suffered immensely under any other option. And had I not listened to my father's wishes about wanting to remain at home during his final days, I think I would have done him a disservice and made those days much more trying and painful.

I have also learned that tolerance is golden. In the case of my mother, I needed to accept her concerns and fears. I didn't do that very well for a long time, and as a result I probably caused more mutual pain than was necessary. But I don't think I understood that as well at the outset of her difficulties as I did latterly.

It's a delicate balancing act to exercise tough loving care. It's knowing when to intervene and where to draw the line. Common sense should have told me that, but in retrospect I see there just wasn't much common sense evident when the emotions of the moment tended to overwhelm good reasoning.

Another lesson I learned was to better understand what the doctors were and weren't saying. They're trying to do the best they can, and I was touched by their genuine concern and by the eagerness of most to find the best possible ways to help my mother and father. But because they have their own pressures, and because many well-intentioned doctors can't seem to explain things in a calm, clear way, too often we don't understand what we hear. I learned to keep asking, to seek further clarification, to, as they say, drill down. I think I became somewhat of a pest with my persistent questioning, yet it was only because I kept asking questions that I got a better picture of what we were facing.

I also learned to slow down with my parents and to try to talk more slowly and more clearly. The more intense I'd become, the more agitated they'd become, and we'd end up in confrontational situations. While what I was saying to my parents was clear to me, I was operating in my paradigm, not theirs, which I found frustrating — but for too long I didn't understand that. So the more calmly I spoke, the more receptive they became. It's such a simple lesson, but one that I've learned the hard way.

A rather bitter and belated lesson struck home at the time of my father's death: one must be very careful about the caregivers one engages. For several years, we had a procession of people in and out of my parents' home, some from agencies and others we recruited. I never thought too much about it, but I discovered during the process of cleaning out their home and moving everything that a number of valuable items were missing. Most painful was the realization that my mother's diamond ring, worth quite a bit of money, was gone. I don't know how to guard against such situations, let alone prevent them. The fact is that when there are so many caregivers involved over a longer period of time, chances are there will be one who doesn't live up to your expectations of trustworthy behavior.

After my father's death, I discovered that I was no longer seized with fear when any of our phones rang. For several years, starting with my mother's initial outburst, I lived in constant concern every time the home, office, or especially my cell phone rang. I never knew who would be calling but always automatically assumed it was the caregiver, the nurse, a doctor, or someone who was about to tell me something I didn't want to hear or know. That, of course, was further reinforced when my mother died.

And I've learned that there was only so much I could do for my parents. I did my best to help make them safe and comfortable. I worked hard to ensure their financial matters were in order. I was there for them as often as I could. But I couldn't live their lives or abdicate my life for them. I sometimes may have wanted to, but it wouldn't have worked or helped.

Guilt plays such a large part in the process of caring for our parents. I know now that guilt only dissipates focus, energy, and ability. Yet guilt about whether or not I'd been doing the best I could dominated my thinking for too long. So perhaps the most important lesson of all was to manage my sense of guilt and not let it overwhelm me. If I could honestly say that I was doing the best I could for my parents, while maintaining some good measure of a personal and professional life, then I should not feel guilty at all, because I was helping make my parents' lives as full and rich as possible. And that meets their expectations (whether they acknowledge it or not) and fulfills my sense of love and responsibility. Looking back on it all, learning how to understand and deal with guilt wasn't easy and it took me some time — but I got there, overcame it, and moved on.

TOOLS TO HELP YOU

VULNERABILITY INDEX:
How Are Your Parents Right Now?

This is an inventory of the state of your parents' (or other elderly loved one's) health, mindset, and observed behavior right now. While this Vulnerability Index may seem to be difficult to complete because of the kinds of assessments you are being asked to make, please be objective and honest. Input answers based on what you know and what you can best assume. The end result is a profile of each of your parents (or other elderly loved ones) that will help you assess their current level of vulnerability.

Note: Be aware this is a completely subjective assessment, but it should give you a broad, high-level indication of their vulnerability. It isn't scientific; it is, though, a helpful early warning guide for your use and to provide you with a likely sense of immediate and longer term challenges you and your parents may be facing.

HOW TO WORK THE VULNERABILITY INDEX

Select the **one best response** for each of the 27 following statements about each person you're assessing. Each response has a numeric value, ranging from six (in good shape) to zero (you don't know). Please circle the appropriate number opposite the response you select for each statement. Note that in some cases the same numeric value is given to more than one of the response options, and in some cases, the numeric choices aren't in sequential order. This is intentional, since some options merit the same value because of the implications, and some options offer more severe implications.

Your score will be explained at the end of this section.

Example:

	Father	Mother
Age		
65–77	6	(6)
78–84	(5)	5
85–91	4	4
92–96	3	3
97+	2	2

	Father	**Mother**
1. Age:		
65–77	6	6
78–84	5	5
85–91	4	4
92–96	3	3
97+	2	2
2. Current Health:		
Good	6	6
Stable	5	5
Questionable	4	4
Eroding	3	3
Not good	2	2
Poor	1	1
I don't know, but need to find out	0	0
3. To the best of my knowledge, the doctor thinks my parent:		
Is doing well for this age	6	6
Has some minor problems	5	5
Has at least one major problem	3	3

	Father	Mother
Has very serious problems	1	1
I don't know, but need to find out	0	0

4. **Mentally/cognitively my parent seems:**

Sound/astute	6	6
Gets confused now and then	4	4
Gets confused often	2	2
Very confused	1	1
I don't know, but need to find out	0	0

5. **Physically, my parent is:**

Independent and mobile	6	6
Relatively balanced and steady	5	5
Steady but at times unsure on different surfaces	4	4
Safer with a cane or walker	3	3
Restricted to using a walker	2	2
Very limited; uses a wheelchair	1	1
I don't know, but need to find out	0	0

6. **When eating, my parent:**

Has a very good, consistent appetite	6	6
Eats a healthy balance of foods	6	6
Eats only what he or she likes/wants	4	4
Picks at the food, leaves a lot	2	2
Eats less than two full meals a day; there is food spoiling in the fridge	1	1
I don't know, but need to find out	0	0

7. **With prescription medication my parent:**

Is consistent and reliable	6	6
Sometimes forgets	5	5
Often forgets; needs reminders	3	3

	Father	Mother
Must be given pre-packaged doses	2	2
Must be administered medications	1	1
I don't know, but need to find out	0	0

8. **Socially, my parent is generally:**

	Father	Mother
Active, friendly, hospitable	6	6
Moderately active; welcomes at least some family/visitors	5	5
A bit passive; doesn't initiate communication	4	4
Passive; takes no initiatives to be social	2	2
Reclusive; withdrawn	1	1
I don't know, but need to find out	0	0

9. **With each other, my parents are:**

	Father	Mother
Supportive; gentle, patient, helpful	6	6
Moderately supportive; try to help to the best of his/her ability	5	5
Not very supportive; impatient, critical, anxious	4	4
Passive; takes no initiatives, indifferent	3	3
Unsupportive; refuses to help, impatient	2	2
Verbally and/or physically aggressive	1	1
I don't know, but need to find out	0	0

10. **With me, my parent is:**

	Father	Mother
Very pleasant, comfortable, honest, open	6	6
Somewhat pleasant, comfortable, honest, open	5	5
Not very pleasant, comfortable, honest, open	3	3
Somewhat restless, withdrawn	2	2
Very restless, agitated, non-communicative	1	1
Verbally and/or physically aggressive	0	0

	Father	Mother

11. With my spouse, my parent is:

	Father	Mother
Very comfortable/engaged; communicates openly	6	6
Somewhat comfortable; smiles, welcoming	5	5
Not very comfortable; remote, withdrawn	4	4
Somewhat restless; withdrawn	3	3
Very restless, agitated, non-communicative	2	2
Verbally and/or physically aggressive	1	1
Not really sure, but need to find out	0	0

12. With my children, my parent is:

	Father	Mother
Kind, caring, smiles, involved, communicative	6	6
Less involved; restrained, few communications	4	4
Mostly flat; uninvolved, closed, non-communicative	2	2
Totally uninvolved; closed, non-communicative	1	1
Not really sure, but need to find out	0	0

13. With other immediate family, my parent is:

	Father	Mother
Very comfortable, engaged, communicative	6	6
Somewhat comfortable; smiles, restrained, minimal communication	5	5
Not very comfortable; quiet, remote/withdrawn	4	4
Somewhat impatient; distant, uninterested	3	3
Very restless; closed, refusing contact	2	2
Verbally and/or physically aggressive	1	1
I don't know, but need to find out	0	0

14. My family would likely characterize my parent as:

	Father	Mother
Nice to be with most of the time	6	6
Nice to be with for shorter periods of time	4	4
Tolerable to be with occasionally	2	2
Unpleasant to be with	1	1

	Father	Mother
I don't know, but need to find out	0	0

15. Usually in appearance, my parent generally:

	Father	Mother
Is neatly groomed	6	6
Wears clean but mismatched clothes; unshaven	5	5
Wears the same clothes for multiple days	3	3
Is regularly disheveled; refuses to bathe, doesn't comb hair; sleeps in day clothing	1	1
I don't know, but need to find out	0	0

16. My parent participates in group activities and/or hobbies such as curling, playing cards, knitting, building model cars, photography, etc.:

	Father	Mother
Frequently	6	6
Regularly	6	6
Occasionally	4	4
Never	1	1
I don't know, but need to find out	0	0

17. My parent has:

	Father	Mother
Regular contact with at least a few friends	6	6
Regular contact with one friend	5	5
Infrequent contact with a few friends	3	3
No regular contact with friends	1	1
I don't know, but need to find out	0	0

18. My parent gets out of the home:

	Father	Mother
Frequently; two or more times a week	6	6
From time to time; once a week	4	4
Infrequently; once or twice a month	2	2
Rarely; only on special occasions	2	2
Never	1	1
I don't know, but I need to find out	0	0

	Father	Mother

19. My parent drives a car:

	Father	Mother
All the time (or does not drive)	6	6
At least once or twice a week	5	5
At least two/three times a month	2	2
License suspended recently	1	1
I don't know, but need to find out	0	0

20. When driving, my parent:

Drives safely; observes all rules of the road	6	6
Occasionally gets lost	5	5
Frequently gets lost	2	2
Often loses car in parking lot; misplaces keys	2	2
Drives unsafely, erratically; has minor accidents	1	1
Don't know, but need to find out	0	0

21. Concerning alcoholic beverages, my parent:

Never drinks	6	6
Tolerates drinking consistent with past use	5	5
Is drinking more than usual	3	3
Loses track of the amount consumed	2	2
I don't know, but need to find out	0	0

22. My parent's handling of money matters seems:

Responsible	6	6
Inconsistent but still reasonable	5	5
Erratic; impulsive	3	3
Irresponsible; unreasonable	1	1
I don't know, but need to find out	0	0

23. With regard to charitable solicitations, my parent:

Donates in keeping with past habits and considers new requests carefully	6	6

	Father	Mother
Loses track of donations made	4	4
Has made recent uncharacteristic donations	2	2
I don't know, but need to find out	1	1

24. My parent has:

A current will	6	6
A will written/updated in the past five years	5	5
A will written more than five years ago	3	3
No will	1	1
I don't know, but need to find out	0	0

25. My parent has a living will:

That is current	6	6
Written or updated in the past three years	5	5
Written more than three years ago	3	3
Does not have a living will	1	1
I don't know, but need to find out	0	0

26. My parent has given power of attorney for property and money to:

Me or my sibling	6	6
Another person _____	5	5
My other parent	4	4
I don't know, but need to find out	0	0

27. My parent has given legal authority for personal and health care decisions to:

Me or my sibling	6	6
Another person _____	5	5
My other parent	4	4
I don't know, but need to find out	0	0

Total Scores: _____ _____

INTERPRETING THE SCORES

162 to 108 points

If **both** of your parents scored in this range, then it would seem that right now each one is fairly stable. They appear to be relatively independent and operating safely on their own. This is actually an excellent time to start having a series of sincere and serious conversations with them, together and separately, to understand their wishes going forward and plan on how to ensure the best possible quality of life for them.

Specific actions to consider:

- Ask if they'll work with you to plan for their future wishes and needs.
- Talk with siblings and other close family members about what care issues may arise and how you could manage them together.
- Find ways to keep your parents mentally and physically active; look for and help them engage in activities they would like to do on a regular basis.
- If you're not already doing it, start calling and/or seeing them more regularly so you'll know firsthand how they're doing.

107 to 81 points

If **either** of your parents scored in this range, there would seem to be a definite trend toward changes beginning to happen or likely looming on the horizon. Your parent is becoming more vulnerable, and the potential for negative experiences is growing. Now is an important time to take a closer look at his or her capabilities and needs, and start planning for what kind of added assistance will be needed.

Specific actions to consider:

- Start keeping a closer watch on your parent's lifestyle, activities, and perceived health. Pay attention to their physical and cognitive capabilities.
- Ask more frequently and probe gently but more deeply about how they feel in general, what they're most often thinking about in terms of their health and lifestyle.
- Introduce the importance of planning ahead while they are well, so that their interests can be protected and their wishes respected.
- Keep them as socially, mentally, and physically active as possible.

80 points or less

If **either** of your parents scored in this range, you may well be on the brink of, or already in, a critical period in his or her advancing years. **Now is the time to act** promptly and decisively. Get sound medical advice and work at planning for next steps in securing added support for her or him, or both of them. The key point here is that *failure to act* could endanger your parents' wellbeing.

Specific actions to consider:

- Find a way to accompany your parents for an appointment with their family physician and get to know the doctor.
- See how you can get a geriatrician involved with assessing and examining them on a regular basis.
- Gently and respectfully enlist their cooperation in building a list of their important documentation: pension, insurance and health plans, banking, etc.
- If not already in hand, ask for powers of attorney for health and general issues.
- If they're still driving a car, determine whether they can do so safely.

Seven or more zeros

If **you scored seven zeros or more** for either parent, then you are probably out of touch with him or her. So now is the time to take a deep look inside and determine your willingness to help them and be more actively supportive, or at least help drive a process that will provide them with the safeguards and help they need or will soon need. You may wish to enlist the active support of siblings, other family members, or outside services. But please **take action now.**

Specific actions to consider:

- Identify a family member close to your parents who is willing to take the lead role in protecting their overall wellbeing.
- Think through, and make it clear to all those engaged in your parents' wellbeing, precisely what you can or are willing to do to support them, and also what you cannot or are not willing to do, so that you are engaged only as appropriate.
- Or, decide to get more active and engaged, and if you do, then please complete this Vulnerability Index assessment again and see if what you've done and learned will give a more accurate score and provide you with a better knowledge of your parents needs.

THE FINANCIAL CONSIDERATIONS:
What You Need to Know

If you're going to help your parents evaluate their financial situation, or if you have to make financial decisions for them, there are some key steps to take and considerations to bear in mind.

To accurately determine your parents' financial status, you should first create two statements: a Net Worth Statement and an Income and Expenses Statement. Your parents' accountant should be helpful in this exercise.

When completed, the Net Worth Statement will show the current value of your parents' estate. Assets such as homes, investments, Registered Retirement Savings Plans (RRSPs), and pensions in Canada and IRAs and 401 plans in the United States, should be listed in this section. This statement also should show current liabilities, such as any mortgages or loans. Assets minus liabilities result in net worth. Taxes may have to be taken into consideration in the event that investments are sold. At the end of the calculation, you should know your parents' net worth if you need to liquidate some or all of their holdings in order to provide for their care.

The Income and Expenses Statement will show your parents' sources of income and current expenses. This may include government benefits, such as Canada Pension Plan/Quebec Pension Plan benefits, Old Age Security benefits, and other provincial or federal income that your parents may be qualified to receive in Canada; or, in the United States, Social Security; and in both, investments such as CDs, stocks, bonds, mutual funds, annuity payments, or employer pension plans, and other benefits. Registered Retirement Income Fund (RRIF) payments also should be included, as well as income from bonds, Guaranteed Investment Certificates (GICs), or other investments. Once again, bear in mind that the income may be reduced by taxes. You should always have a copy of your parents' income tax return from the previous year. It will outline all of their sources of income.

It's also a good idea to have copies of statements of your parents' investments. These statements will show the name of the company, the contract number, the name of the contact person or representative, and a list of the investments. Having copies of these at hand will save you a lot of trouble. Just make sure they're updated annually.

Many elderly people are in a high marginal tax bracket. This is because they generally invest in passive investments such as GICs or bonds that attract high tax rates.

Variable annuities may be appropriate for individuals who want their principal to be protected but would like the opportunity for growth through market participation. Variable annuities are invested in the market and can be volatile; however, many have guaranteed death benefits for the heirs. In other words, if an individual dies while holding a variable annuity, his or her original investment, less any withdrawals, is protected, subject to the terms of the VA contract, which vary.

In cases of contract annuitization or the purchasing of an immediate annuity, both parents and children may be concerned with relinquishing control of the principal to the insurance company that issues annuities. However, an arrangement can often be structured whereby a parent receives income for life in a tax-efficient manner and if any balance of principal remains upon their death; it is returned tax-free to his or her heirs in the form of instalment payments or a lump sum.

Many elderly individuals invest in mutual funds. It's important for your parents' financial advisor to accurately measure their risk tolerance and their understanding of the volatility of the market. Unfortunately, many a nest egg has been lost because of misunderstanding and misinformation. If your parents aren't investment savvy, you may want to take an interest in their portfolio and sit in on the meetings with their advisors.

INVESTMENTS

If your parents are concerned that they're paying too much in taxes, and if they have funds invested in GICs, there may be other financial vehicles that are more tax efficient and will generate income for them on a guaranteed basis. Financial instruments such as prescribed annuities generate income that is tax favorable, continues for life, and is guaranteed. The tax efficient prescribed annuity can also reduce the amount of old age security claw-back, while increasing income, depending on your parents' jurisdiction.

Segregated funds may also be appropriate for older individuals who want their capital to be protected. The capital of these funds is protected under federal regulation. Investments are varied and can be volatile; however, the segregated funds have a guaranteed death benefit. In other words, if an individual dies while holding a segregated fund, his or her capital is protected.

In some cases, both parents and children are concerned with relinquishing control of the capital to a company that issues annuities. However, an arrangement can be structured where a parent receives income for life in a tax efficient manner and then the capital is returned tax-free to his or her estate upon death.

Many elderly individuals invest in mutual funds. It's important for your parents' financial advisor to accurately measure their risk tolerance and their understanding of the volatility of the market. Unfortunately, many a nest egg has been lost because of misunderstanding and misinformation. If your parents aren't investment savvy, you may want to take an interest in their portfolio and sit in on the meetings with their advisors.

LONG-TERM CARE INSURANCE

Long-term care insurance is available in both the United States and Canada. This form of insurance is becoming increasingly popular as the population ages. It's generally available to people until the age of 80. A pre-existing health condition doesn't automatically exclude an individual from qualifying for this kind of insurance.

The long-term care insurance plan provides for either a daily or a monthly benefit to be used to supplement care needed at home or in a long-term care facility. In order to qualify for long-term care insurance, an individual must be unable to perform at least two out of the six daily living activities or be cognitively impaired.

This type of insurance plan can be designed to fit a person's ability to pay the premium. Benefits may be received for a designated number of years or for a lifetime, and the level of the monthly benefit can vary to suit an individual's needs and cash flow.

According to "A Shopper's Guide to Long-term Care Insurance," which is produced by the National Association of Insurance Commissioners, whether you should buy a long-term care insurance policy will depend on your age, health status, overall retirement goals, income, and assets. You should not buy long-term care insurance if you can't afford the premiums, if you have limited assets, if your only source of income is a Social Security benefit or Supplemental Security Income, if you are currently on Medicaid, or if you often have trouble paying for utilities, food, medicine, or other important needs. You should consider buying long-term care insurance if you have significant assets and income, if you want to protect some of your assets and income, if you can pay premiums (including possible premium increases) without financial difficulty, if you want to stay independent of the support of others, or you want to have the flexibility of choosing care in the setting you prefer or will be most comfortable in.

Today, many parents and their children are jointly subscribing for long-term care plans. By having a long-term care insurance plan in place, parents are ensured that they'll receive the necessary funding to live out their lives in comfort and dignity. As important, their children won't have to feel guilty if they can't financially provide for their parents in their time of need.

REVERSE MORTGAGE

A reverse mortgage is a financial tool through which individuals can free up equity in their home in order to generate an income, without selling the property. The older the individual and the higher the value of the property, the more can be borrowed. At death, or when the home is sold, the loan and the interest are repaid.

Psychologically, many people might have problems with assuming a mortgage in their later years. Also, it's possible with a reverse mortgage that when the house is sold, 100% of the proceeds will be needed to pay off the loan. This may marginalize or even wipe out any inheritance for heirs.

LIFE INSURANCE

Many older people never had, or have canceled, their life insurance contract. This is unfortunate but it's not surprising. Years ago, the main purpose of life insurance was to protect the family if the wage earner died prematurely. It was also used in the event of death to pay off a mortgage. However, as children grew, many people no longer saw the need for their life insurance plan. Even if a parent can't afford the premiums on an existing life insurance policy, the child should consider paying the premium on behalf of the parent, because many of these policies accumulate cash value that can be used as collateral for a loan or to help generate income. As well, many older policies have tax efficient advantages, and the cash in the policies continues to grow in a tax-sheltered environment.

If, as a child, you need to provide financial support to your parents, a life insurance policy could be used to replace some of the money spent for care.

Even if your parents don't want to designate a child or their estate as beneficiary of the insurance policies, those policies still can be used in a tax efficient way by designating a charity as beneficiary. On death, the charity receives the cash benefit, and the estate receives a tax credit that can be used in the year of death or in the previous year to offset other taxes.

CRITICAL ILLNESS INSURANCE

Critical Illness Insurance still is a relatively new insurance product. The plan insures an individual for a predetermined amount; depending on the insurer, up to $2 million. If the person contracts one of the listed critical illnesses (there are generally about 22 illnesses covered in most contracts) and survives 30 days, the lump sum is paid to the survivor.

In most plans, if the insured dies without collecting a claim, all the premiums paid into the plan are refunded. The funds received from a critical illness insurance plan may be used to seek medical care, renovate a home, or take a vacation. How the money is used is not restricted in any way.

The cost of critical illness plans varies based on age of the client, amount of coverage, and the plan design.

EMPLOYER BENEFITS AND RETIREMENT INCOME

Most employer health plans don't provide retirement benefits. However, some do on a limited basis, while others might be more extensive. If your parents worked for a large company or for a government agency, they may have retirement benefits, including chronic care benefits. If they do, they're among the lucky few. Ask your parents if they have a copy of the Employee Health Benefit Booklet. If they don't have a copy, contact their past employers and check with the plan administrator.

Most pension plans pay out their employees in the form of a life or joint life annuity. This means a payment will continue for as long as either the employee and/or the spouse lives. There may be a guarantee period, defining the number of years that the payments are received. If the annuity is a joint life annuity, it'll continue for as long as either of your parents is alive. It's important that you know where the documents are located.

There are other forms of income that your parents may be receiving aside from annuities. Some are more flexible, in that the owner can determine the amount received and the nature of the investment. The cash flow may be increased in some cases (such as in a critical or palliative care situation), or decreased to preserve the capital and lower income tax. It's important that the family has a clear understanding of these contracts and their flexibility.

TRAVEL INSURANCE

It's critical for the elderly to have travel insurance, especially if they plan to travel outside of their jurisdiction. The cost of medical care in the event of an emergency out of province or state can be astronomical. Before your parents travel outside of their jurisdiction, especially abroad, you should be sure that they have appropriate protection in case of a health emergency. And remind them to carry their travel insurance certificate with them when traveling, while also leaving a copy with you or in a place to which you have easy access.

In addition, ensure that whenever your parents apply for travel insurance they answer all questions absolutely correctly. An error could void the policy: potentially a very expensive mistake.

It's usually best to buy travel insurance from one of the large and reputable senior's organizations, such as American Association of Retired Persons in the United States and Canadian Association of Retired Persons in Canada.

AMERICANS LIVING ABROAD

If your parents are American citizens or dual citizens living in Canada, Mexico, or any other country, they must annually file a statement of all foreign bank and financial accounts aside from their tax returns. It's called the Report of Foreign Bank and Financial Accounts, and it is filed with the Department of the Treasury at its Detroit, Michigan office. The form in use as of 2013 is TD F 90-22.1 and can be found online. There are hefty fines for not filing, and the filing has been largely ignored until the past two years, so take it seriously.

PICK THE RIGHT FINANCIAL PLANNER AND BE PREPARED

First and foremost, don't wait until it's too late. The sooner a family meets and plans together with their aging parents, the better. It's not easy, but if you think the time has come to become involved in your parents' financial planning, it probably has. Meet with them and find out if they've worked with a qualified financial planner. If they haven't, seek out a planner who has a proven understanding of — and experience in — the senior market. Ask around. A chartered financial consultant, a chartered life underwriter, a specialist in eldercare planning, or a chartered accountant who is part of Prime Plus will be able to help you and your parents.

If and when you meet a qualified financial planner, come prepared. Bring your parents' last will and testament, the power of attorney, a list of bank accounts, a list of investments, last year's income tax return, their accountant's and lawyer's names, addresses, and phone numbers, and the names of any other advisors.

Ask the planner to project the amount of income your parents would receive if they turn all their assets into income-generating investments. Discuss their investment risk tolerance. Review their health plan. Ask about tax efficient plans specifically designed for the elderly. Find out what is available from the government. Discuss long-term care plans.

Be prepared, be informed, and plan not for what might happen, but for what's likely to happen.

RESOURCE DIRECTORY

One of the most difficult and time-consuming tasks you'll face when dealing with aging parents is identifying and finding the right resources to get the information, help, and support that your parents need — and that *you'll* need in order to help them. The hardest part is knowing how to locate those resources and figuring out which ones offer which services or support mechanisms.

This high-level resource directory is in three sections: eldercare-focused health care and social service professionals in both the United States and Canada, and then organizations listed by each country that offer the range and scope of information and services that will be most helpful in the process of eldercare in your family. In short, this is your guide to major national and state/provincial contacts for advice and help.

There are an amazing number of resources across the United States and Canada — many more, in fact, than there were when we originally started researching this subject. In the American and Canadian directories presented here, we have not listed the many retirement home, assisted living, and nursing home/complex care facilities that now operate in both countries. There are many and you will find them in many cases in some of the sites listed here, and in other cases a relatively simple online search will deliver the information you seek.

To identify and locate the myriad local support groups that exist, it's best to consult your regional, community, or municipal health authority or local hospital, or speak with your parents' physician or your own.

We've done the best we could to ensure the contact names, telephone numbers, email addresses in some instances, and websites listed in this book are as current and accurate as possible, as of early 2013. But as we've discovered, phone numbers and websites are always being changed, so we're sorry for any inconvenience should you find an error. It is usually easy to find the updated information through online searching or even using the old-fashioned phone book, many of which now have various sections including public and community services listed by category.

As the challenge of caring for elderly parents continues to mushroom, there also are a growing number of local qualified individuals and smaller organizations that can provide counsel and support. These are often former social workers, nurses, lawyers, and others who specialize in various aspects of eldercare support. Frankly, sometimes asking around is just about the best way to find them.

And finally, because so many of us are comfortable searching the Web for information and resources, a word of caution: beware of all those sites that freely offer advice and guidance; ensure that they are not only current and credible but also qualified. One must always be aware of potential scams especially when things are offered that are "too good to be true." That, of course, takes some time and assessment on your part. It's demanding, yes, but also critical to ensuring that what you embrace is correct and helpful to you and your parents.

Note: Some of these resources offered are in the form of PDF documents. You will need Adobe Acrobat Reader to view them. You can download it for free at: *http://get.adobe.com/reader/*.

YOUR GUIDE TO HEALTH PROFESSIONALS

When it comes to caring for your parents, you're not alone. There are many qualified health care professionals ready to help, each with his or her own special expertise. Here's a quick introduction to the health professionals you may encounter in your caregiving journey.

Occupational Therapist

Occupational therapists focus on helping people be as engaged as possible in activities and occupations that are meaningful to them, based on the individual's abilities, needs, and interests. As a person becomes more dependent, the occupational therapist will continue to work collaboratively with you and other caregivers. They'll help to develop a safe and supportive environment that encourages your parents to participate in their lives as much as they are able by identifying and recommending customized solutions that could include modifying tasks and/or environments and using assistive devices such as wheelchairs and bathroom equipment. The therapist may help you to identify strategies to make sure that you are looking after your needs as well, in your role as the caregiver.

For more information:
U.S.: Contact the American Occupational Therapy Association at
1-301-652-2682; TDD: 1-800-377-8555, or *www.aota.org.*
Canada: Contact the Canadian Association of Occupational Therapists,
1-800-434-2268, or *www.caot.ca.*

Physicians

Family Physician

Family physicians provide continuing and comprehensive general medical care,
health maintenance, and preventive services to individuals. They are involved in
coordinating medical care.

The family physician will know your parents' medical condition. Because of
their familiarity with their patients, family physicians are best qualified to serve as
an advocate in all health-related matters, including the appropriate use of consultants, health services, and community resources.

For more information:
U.S.: Contact the American Academy of Family Physicians at
1-800-274-2237 or *www.aafp.org*, and visit its website for patients at
http://familydoctor.org.
Canada: Contact The College of Family Physicians of Canada, 1-800-387-6197,
or *www.cfpc.ca.*

Geriatrician

A geriatrician is a physician specially trained in the health needs and problems
of the elderly. Most geriatricians are internists or family physicians certified in
geriatric medicine. Family physicians and local hospitals are your best sources
for finding the kind of geriatricians you may need.

For more information:
U.S.: Contact the American Geriatrics Society at 1-212-308-1414,
email info.amger@americangeriatrics.org or visit *www.americangeriatrics.org.*
Canada: Contact the Canadian Geriatrics Society at 1-866-247-0086, or
www.canadiangeriatrics.ca.

Neurologist

A neurologist is a physician with specialized training in diagnosing, treating, and managing disorders of the brain and nervous system, including Alzheimer's disease. A neurologist will diagnose the condition, determine the proper treatment, and work with the family physician and others in managing a patient's overall health.

For more information:
U.S.: Contact the American Academy of Neurology at 1-800-879-1960 or *www.aan.com.*
Canada: Contact the Canadian Neurological Sciences Federation at 403-229-9544, or *www.cnsfederation.org.*

Psychiatrist/Geriatric Psychiatrist

A psychiatrist is able to diagnose and treat behavioral and emotional challenges that result from any form of dementia that may be emerging or that may have been present for some time. Psychiatrists are medical doctors with extra training in psychiatry and are thus able to prescribe medication for treatment. A geriatric psychiatrist has training in addressing the issues of the elderly. Information for older adults, family members, and caregivers — including brochures, fact sheets, resources, and a find-a-geriatric-psychiatrist feature — can be found on the (American) Geriatric Mental Health Foundation's website, *www.gmhfonline.org.*

For more information
U.S.: Contact the American Association of Geriatric Psychiatrists at 1-301-654-7850 or *www.aagponline.org.*
Canada: Contact the Canadian Academy of Geriatric Psychiatry at (416) 921-5443 or 1-877-330-5443, email info@cagp.ca or visit at *www.cagp.ca.*

Physiotherapist

Physiotherapists, also known as physical therapists, are health care professionals trained in the study of rehabilitation who evaluate, restore, and maintain physical function. They have a detailed understanding of how the body works and are trained to assess and improve movement and function and to relieve associated pain.

For more information:

U.S.: Contact the American Physical Therapy Association at 1-800-999-2782 or *www.apta.org.*

Canada: Contact the Canadian Physiotherapy Association, 1-800-387-8679, email information@physiotherapy.ca or visit *www.physiotherapy.ca.*

Psychologist

Psychologists specialize in treating behavioral, emotional, and motivational problems. They can assess cognitive dysfunctions and recommend non-drug treatments and intervention programs.

Psychologists who work with clients are sometimes called clinical psychologists. Neuropsychologists specialize in the diagnosis of brain disorders.

For more information:

U.S.: Contact the American Psychological Association at 1-800-374-2721, TDD/TTY: 202-336-6123 or *www.apa.org.*

Canada: Contact the Canadian Psychological Association, 1-613-237-2144, Toll free (in Canada): 1-888-472-0657, or *www.cpa.ca.*

Registered Nurses/Registered Nursing Assistants

Registered nurses and registered nursing assistants are often involved in the care and treatment of persons with any health-related need. From providing direct clinical care in the home or hospital to providing information and counseling and helping to assess overall health needs, nursing professionals can help you to develop a comprehensive plan for care.

Nurses can help with medical and medication issues and can help you arrange for support services, such as home support, respite care, and day programs. Nurses work closely with physicians and are key members of the team. A registered nursing assistant or a home health aide may also provide in-home care under the direction of a registered nurse.

For more information:

U.S.: Contact the American Nurses Association at 1-800-274-4262, or *www.nursingworld.org.*

Canada: Contact the Canadian Nursing Association, 1-800-361-8404, or *www.cna-aiic.ca/en/*.

Social Workers

Social workers help individuals, families, groups, and communities to resolve problems that affect their well-being on an individual or collective basis. They focus on the relationships between people and their environments, helping to enhance problem-solving and coping capacities.

For individuals and families coping with the challenge of aging parents, social workers offer counseling for crisis intervention when health and safety are at risk and for loss and grief. As well, they are able to help caregivers to access support services.

For more information:
U.S.: Contact the National Association of Social Workers at 1-202-408-8600 or *www.naswdc.org*.
Canada: Contact the Canadian Association of Social Workers, 1-855-729- 2279, email casw@casw-acts.ca or visit *www.casw-acts.ca*.

Speech-Language Pathologists/Audiologists

These professionals specialize in speech, language, and hearing disorders. Speech-language pathologists help individuals overcome and prevent communication problems in language, speech, voice, and fluency. Audiologists assess the extent of any hearing loss, balance, and related disorders, and recommend appropriate treatment.

For more information:
U.S.: Contact the American Speech-Language-Hearing Association at 1-800-638-8255 or *www.asha.org*.
Canada: Contact the Canadian Association of Speech Language Pathologists and Audiologists, 1-800-259-8519, email caslpa@caslpa.ca or visit *www.caslpa.ca*.

HELPING CHILDREN COPE WITH DISABLING ILLNESS, DEMENTIA, AND DEATH

Children often require special attention and support when an aging loved one is unwell, declining, or has just died. Here are some helpful books geared specifically for children.

What My Grandma Means to Say
by JC Sulzenko
Ages 8 to 12, deals with Alzheimer's disease

Young readers share Jake's experience as he watches his grandma change from world traveller, expert birder, and best cookie baker to someone who forgets where she lives and cannot remember her name.

With answers to frequently asked questions and a list of key website where more information is available, the book allows families a way to discuss with their children what is happening in their lives and helps each member of the family develop his or her own strengths and strategies for supporting someone dear to them, who is affected by Alzheimer's or a related dementia.

Available for purchase from *Amazon.com* or your local bookseller.

Now One Foot, Now the Other
by Tomie dePaola
Ages 4 to 7, deals with the effect of strokes

The story is about how Bobby helps grandfather, Bob, after Bob has a stroke. Everyone in the family thinks Bob is unable to understand what is happening around him, but Bobby insists that his grandfather is responding to him. With patience and determination, he helps Bob regain motor control, leading him through all the same exercises that Bob once used to help him gain coordination as a baby.

Available for purchase from *Amazon.com* or your local bookseller.

As Big As It Gets: Supporting A Child When A Parent is Seriously Ill, 2nd Edition
by Diana Crossley
Published by Winston's Wish

This booklet aims to help families cope with the serious illness of a parent or child. It provides a range of ideas for parents or carers so that they may feel more able to explain to their children or teenagers what is happening. The booklet also includes some suggestions about what parents might say to them and how to offer support. The message throughout is that although life can be very different and difficult when someone is faced with a life-threatening illness, families can learn to cope with the uncertainties and stresses of their lives.

Available for purchase from *Amazon.com* or your local bookseller

Helping Children When Someone Close Dies
A very helpful pamphlet from the UK-based Marie Curie Cancer Care that explains how children from infancy to adolescence conceptualize and react to death and the coping behaviors they might display: Provides advice on helping children handle grief.

PDF document: *http://www.mariecurie.org.uk/Documents/PATIENTS-CARERS-FAMILIES/Updated-pdf/helping-children-when-someone-dies.pdf*

Activity Book for Child-Caregivers Aged 5–9
Download this friendly new activity book about frontotemporal dementia co-authored by Dr. Tiffany Chow and Gail Elliot. In this case, FTD stands for "Frank and Tess, Detectives!" who are trying to help their mother, who is affected with FTD. Also involves lots of coloring and puzzle activities that can involve the patient.

PDF Document: *www.esearch.baycrest.org/files/Frank-and-Tess-Detectives-.pdf*

When Dementia is in the House: for Child-Caregivers
Launched by the renowned Baycrest Geriatric Health Care System in Toronto and written by Dr. Tiffany Chow and Gail Elliot, this is the first phase of educational materials on FTD and caregiving for children living with someone who has dementia. The site features tips for parents and child caregivers based on focus groups conducted with children aged 12 to 19.

Website: *http://www.lifeandminds.ca/whendementiaisinthehouse*

YOUR GUIDE TO RELEVANT ELDERCARE AND SUPPORT SERVICES IN THE UNITED STATES

Caregiving Resources

Aging Parents and Elder Care
A resource for family caregivers during all stages of care featuring articles, comprehensive checklists, links to key resources, and a support group.

Website: *www.aging-parents-and-elder-care.com*

American Hospital Directory
Provides on-line data for over 6,000 hospitals. Free information includes hospital name, address, and phone number; may also have number of beds, type of ownership, Medicare provider identification number, accreditation, medical school affiliation, a list of services provided, utilization statistics, and a link to the hospital's website. Searchable by hospital name, city, state, zip code, area code, or combination of these. Additional information is available with paid subscription.

Website: *www.ahd.com*

American Red Cross
The "Senior Services" section provides helpful services to seniors and their families, including respite care, caregivers' education, and friendly visitors who stop by each week to share conversation with seniors needing company. Contact your local chapter to find out if Red Cross offers any of these services in your area.

Website: *http://www.redcross.org/find-your-local-chapter*

CareGuide
This searchable site offers eldercare resources including medical, legal, and safety information as well as guidance for choosing types of care and service providers. Topics include memory and aging, home care, living alternatives (such as hospice and respite care), and wills and estate planning. It is provided by a care

management company. This site also includes information about the company's fee-based services and a directory of providers in the company's network.

Website: *www.eldercare.com*

Children of Aging Parents

A non-profit, charitable organization dedicated to assisting America's caregivers of elderly or chronically ill parents or relatives: Provides reliable information, referrals, and support.

Website: *www.caps4caregivers.org*

Family Caregiver Alliance

A source for "caregivers of adults with Alzheimer's disease, stroke, traumatic brain injury, Parkinson's disease, ALS, and related brain disorders." The resource center includes care and services, work and eldercare, and related online ser-vices. There are fact sheets on a variety of diseases, diagnosis, and research, some in Chinese and Spanish. There are also statistics, public policy issues, read-ing lists, and links to related sites.

Website: *www.caregiver.org*

Hospital Compare

From the U.S. Department of Health and Human Services.

"This tool provides you with information on how well the hospitals in your area care for all their adult patients with certain medical conditions." Specific American hospitals are compared with national averages in their treatment of three medical conditions: heart attack, heart failure, and pneumonia. Hospitals are searchable by name or by location.

Website: *www.hospitalcompare.hhs.gov*

National Association of Geriatric Care Managers

This organization lists individuals with the requisite training and certification who are capable of taking on the role of assisting families in navigating the health and social service care systems. They can be especially helpful when there is no immediate family available to assure that the day to day undertakings are completed and in many ways can act as a surrogate for distant but concerned family members.

Website: *http://www.caremanager.org*

National Center on Elder Abuse
Contains "resources on elder abuse, neglect, and exploitation." Includes FAQs, statistics, publications, links to related websites, and more.

Website: *www.ncea.aoa.gov*

National Respite Locator Service
"Respite … is a service [that provides] temporary care to a child or adult with disabilities, or chronic or terminal illnesses, and to persons at risk of abuse and neglect." The service "helps parents, caregivers, and professionals find respite services in their state and local area." Browse by state or complete an online search form by checking the boxes listing the condition(s) that afflict the person requiring respite care.

Website: *www.archrespite.org/respitelocator*

Nursing Home Abuse and Neglect Resource Center
A general information website on the quality and selection of a proper nursing home. Topics include how to assess and pay for care, signs of abuse, medical issues, federal and state laws, patient rights, what you can do, a list of ombudsmen by state, and how to pursue legal action. Searchable by keyword and has links to other resources. From a legal firm that tries cases for victims of nursing home abuse.

Website: *www.nursinghomealert.com*

Senior HousingNet
Searchable guide to find senior housing in retirement communities, assisted living residences, nursing homes, and Alzheimer's facilities in the United States.

Listings include detailed descriptions, color photos, floor plans, and some virtual tours. Includes information on housing options for seniors, health and wellness, and financial considerations in paying for care.

Website: *www.seniorhousingnet.com*

Visiting Nurse Associations of America
The Visiting Nurse Associations of America (VNAA) is a national association that supports, promotes, and advocates for community-based, non-profit home health and hospice providers that care for all individuals regardless of complexity of condition or ability to pay.

Website: *www.vnaa.org*

Seniors and Driving

Older Adult Drivers
Fact sheet from the National Center for Injury Prevention and Control providing statistics on older drivers, information about national programs, research on senior driving, and a bibliography. From the Centers for Disease Control and Prevention.

Website: *http://www.cdc.gov/Motorvehiclesafety/Older_Adult_Drivers/
adult-drivers_factsheet.html*

Physician's Guide to Assessing and Counselling Older Drivers
This guide, developed by the American Medical Association in cooperation with the National Highway Traffic Safety Administration, contains information on assessing an older driver's medical fitness to drive, lists of medical conditions and medications that may impair driving, and related legal and medical information. Although this guide is intended for physicians, most of the material is easy to understand and useful to the general reader.

Website: *http://www.ama-assn.org/ama/pub/physician-resources/public-health/
promoting-healthy-lifestyles/geriatric-health/older-driver-safety/assessing-
counseling-older-drivers.page*

Safe Senior Citizen Driving
From Helpguide, a joint project of the Rotary Club of Santa Monica and the Center for Healthy Aging.

Describes risk factors for the senior citizen driver, warning signs that someone should stop driving, safety tips, and alternatives to driving. Includes related links.

Website: *http://www.helpguide.org/elder/senior_citizen_driving.htm*

When You Are Concerned
From the New York State Office for the Aging.

"Leaving the wheel can be a watershed event for an aging driver." This online "handbook for families, friends, and caregivers worried about the safety of an aging driver" covers such topics as monitoring driving habits, resources for help, safe driving tips, equipment, alternative transportation, and how to help the elderly cope with giving up driving.

Website: *http://www.aging.ny.gov/Transportation//OlderDriver/ DriverIntroduction.cfm*

Government Services

Administration on Aging
Part of the U.S. Department of Health and Human Services.

Includes resources for elders, families, and caregivers (Alzheimer's resources, disaster assistance, elders' rights, housing, nutrition, services); information for practitioners (civil rights, government poverty guidelines, statistics, transportation); and links to grant programs.

Website: *www.aoa.gov/*

Eldercare Locator: Community Assistance for Seniors
From the United States Administration on Aging.

A database consisting of "information and assistance resources for legal services, elder abuse prevention, health insurance counseling, prescription assistance, and the long term care ombudsman program." Searchable by city, county, and zip code. Includes a glossary of aging terms, related fact sheets, and links.

Website: *www.eldercare.gov*

FirstGov for Seniors
From the Office of Citizen Services and Communications, U.S. General Services Administration.

This site provides online access to government information and services of interest to seniors in the areas of: consumer protection; education, jobs, and volunteerism; federal and state agencies; health; laws and regulations; retirement and money; taxes; and travel and leisure.

Website: *www.firstgov.gov/Topics/Seniors.shtml*

GovBenefits
This site is a partnership of several federal agencies and organizations.

Use a simple three-step process to identify what government benefits you or your elderly loved one are entitled to. While "many benefit programs are not featured yet in the GovBenefits website," it is "expanding regularly to include more programs." Representative categories include seniors, veterans, disaster victims, farmers, ranchers, students, the unemployed, home owners, health professionals, and widows or widowers.

Website: *www.govbenefits.gov*

Social Security Administration
Extensive site that includes disability information, employment support for people with disabilities, Medicare information, benefit payments, forms, rules and regulations, laws and legislation, a kids' section, information in Spanish, FAQs, and all program publications.

Website: *www.ssa.gov*

Uncle Sam: Forms from the Feds
Maintained by librarians at the University of Memphis.

Links to the most requested downloadable electronic government forms. Among the agencies listed are the Copyright Office, Department of Health and Human Services, Department of Labor, Food and Drug Administration, Internal Revenue Service, National Science Foundation, U.S. Citizenship and Immigration Services, and Department of Veterans Affairs. A link to passport application forms is also provided.

Website: *http://www.memphis.edu/govpub/forms.php*

Medicare Services and Prescription Drugs

BenefitsCheckUp
From the National Council on the Aging.

A customizable site you can use to search for federal, state, and some local private and public benefits for those 55 and over. Identifies programs that seniors may be eligible to receive and provides detailed descriptions of the programs, local contacts for additional information, and assistance in applying for the programs.

Website: *www.benefitscheckup.org*

Centers for Medicare & Medicaid Services
Consumer information on Medicare, Medicaid, the Health Insurance Portability and Accountability Act of 1996 (HIPAA), and Clinical Laboratory Improvement Amendments (CLIA). Covers news, laws and regulations, and programs. Resources include a searchable directory of contact information, forms, and a glossary.

Website: *www.cms.gov*

Consumer Reports Best Buy Drugs
From Consumer Reports with research input from Oregon Health and Science University.

Collection of reports that evaluate prescription medicines used for common conditions such as high cholesterol, arthritis, and heartburn. The reports look at efficacy, safety, and price to recommend the best medicines. Reports also provide a general overview of the drugs and cost comparisons between generic and brand name drugs.

Website: *www.crbestbuydrugs.org*

Find a Medicare Prescription Drug Plan
From the U.S. Department of Health and Human Services.

"An interactive tool that allows you to narrow your search for a Medicare prescription drug plan [and also enroll] based on your personal preferences such as cost, coverage, and convenience." Includes an overview on how Medicare works, a glossary of related terms, and coverage information for individuals receiving prescription drug coverage through military retiree benefits (TRICARE), veterans' benefits (VA), or federal employee retiree benefits (FEHBP).

Website: *www.medicare.gov/find-a-plan/questions/home.aspx*

The Medicaid Resource Book
From the Kaiser Family Foundation.

This full-text guide is intended "to assist the public and policymakers in understanding the structure and operation of the Medicaid program." Describes program eligibility, benefits, financing, and administration. Also includes legislative history, resource bibliographies, and indexes to federal laws and regulations.

Website: *www.kff.org/medicaid/2236-index.cfm*

Medicare
This official site provides databases for comparing nursing homes, Medicare plans and providers, dialysis centers, hospitals, home health agencies, and health plan options. Explains eligibility, what Medicare covers, prescription drug programs, and billing. Also provides contact information and links, a glossary, a directory of medical equipment suppliers, and information about the Medicare

Prescription Drug Improvement and Modernization Act of 2003. Some material available in other languages.

Website: *www.medicare.gov*

Medicare Prescription Drug Coverage
From the Centers for Medicare and Medicaid Services, U.S. Department of Health and Human Services.

Official information from Medicare about its prescription drug plan and the Medicare prescription drug coverage (Medicare Plan D) effective January 1, 2006. Covers enrolment periods, local plans, and common coverage situations. Includes a prescription drug plan finder, a drug finder, online enrolment, and publications.

Website: *www.medicare.gov*

For detailed information about the Medicare prescription drug coverage, download *Your Guide to Medicare Prescription Drug Coverage* here:

http://www.medicare.gov/Pubs/pdf/11109.pdf

Partnership for Prescription Assistance (PPA)
Searchable directory of patient assistance programs (offering free and low-cost medicines). You can assess which programs you may be eligible for by answering questions and using the online application wizard. Also features information on assistance programs for caregivers and doctors. Site is sponsored by American pharmaceutical research companies.

Website: *www.pparx.org*

Associations and Non-profit Organizations

AARP
AARP is a non-profit, non-partisan membership organization for people aged 50 and over. The site contains information on insurance, health, travel, housing, investing, benefits, and more. Also available in Spanish.

Website: *www.aarp.org*

Alzheimer's Association
Searchable site contains information on the causes, warning signs, diagnosis, and treatment of Alzheimer's disease; statistics, fact sheets, and reports; a glossary; an index to clinical trials; resources for diverse communities (African American, Chinese, Hispanic/Latino, and Korean); and more. Also available in Spanish.

Website: *www.alz.org*

American Cancer Society
This site highlights recent research, statistics, publications, and prevention tips. Includes survivor stories and information about support for cancer patients and their families. Contains material available in Spanish, Chinese, and Vietnamese. Searchable.

Website: *www.cancer.org*

American Diabetes Association
Contains research news and treatment advances, legislative and advocacy updates, clinical practice recommendations, fact sheets and self-care tips for patients, information on Type 1 (juvenile) and Type 2 (adult onset) diabetes, articles, and a dictionary of related terms. Also features information about grants and research projects, groups affected by diabetes, and risk factors. Includes information in Spanish.

Website: *www.diabetes.org*

American Society on Aging
A site for the ASA, an umbrella organization focusing on professionals and organizations that serve older people. Includes information about conferences, training, publications, news, and special projects. The section on "Constituent Groups" offers information related to mental health, health care, religion and spirituality, gay and lesbian seniors, and business.

Website: *www.asaging.org*

Arthritis Foundation
Resources about arthritis and related conditions, including disease descriptions and treatments, news, advocacy, research, and other resources.

Website: *www.arthritis.org*

American Heart Association
This site includes information on heart attack, stroke, and cardiac arrest warning signs; information on heart diseases and conditions; tips for maintaining a healthy lifestyle; statistics; and more. Also available in Spanish.

Website: *www.americanheart.org*

National Association of the Deaf
The site provides news, information on legal rights and advocacy issues, tips on finding a lawyer and mental health care, and more.

Website: *www.nad.org*

National Cancer Institute
From the U.S. National Institutes of Health's National Cancer Institute.

Information at NCI is reviewed by oncology experts and is based on the results of current research. Find types of cancer; treatments; prevention tips; information on the role of genetics and causes, screening and testing, and coping with cancer; support resources; cancer literature; and Physician Data Query (PDQ), a database with the latest information about treatment, screening, prevention, genetics, care, and clinical trials.

Website: *www.cancer.gov*

National Council on the Aging
The NCOA is an umbrella association of "organizations and professionals dedicated to promoting the dignity, self-determination, and well being of older persons." It promotes "vital aging," preferring to think of older people as the aging, not the aged. Unlike commercial sites aimed at seniors, this one is free of ads and offers information, especially in the area of policy and legislative

updates. Among other topics, the site offers information on adult day services, health care, housing, and independent living.

Website: *www.ncoa.org*

Caregiver Action Network (formerly National Family Caregivers Association)
The association is dedicated to improving the overall quality of life for caregiving families. The mandate is to encourage the family caregiver to feel empowered and to have the will to take action. This site contains articles, tip sheets, a newsletter, and referrals to other sources.

Website: *www.caregiveraction.org*

National Institute of Arthritis and Musculoskeletal and Skin Diseases
From the National Institutes of Health.

The site provides information about diseases such as arthritis, autoimmune diseases, gout, and osteoporosis as well as information about training programs, patient research registries, news, and links to related sites. Searchable. Available in Spanish.

Website: *www.niams.nih.gov*

National Institute of Mental Health
From the National Institutes of Health.

This site is about mental health: depression, anxiety, and panic disorders, Alzheimer's disease, learning disabilities, autism, schizophrenia, and other illnesses. It contains information for researchers, practitioners, and the public. Information includes news, events, grants, contracts, committees, research, clinical trials, funding opportunities, and links to other NIMH programs. Searchable. Some information in "For the Public" is available in Spanish.

Website: *www.nimh.nih.gov*

Senior Sites

Listing of non-profit providers and national and state associations involved with senior housing, health care, and services. Search providers by zip code, selecting facilities up to a two-hundred-mile radius, or search for a facility with the desired services and amenities.

Website: *www.seniorsites.com*

USDA Center for Nutrition Policy and Promotion

This government site has the latest nutritional and dietary guidelines and news releases as well as recipes. Entering age and gender information into the Interactive Healthy Eating Index will compare your diet to the food pyramid and provide a score based on analysis of the foods and quantities given, as compared to recommended intake levels. Some of the files require Adobe Acrobat Reader.

Website: *www.usda.gov/cnpp*

Life Activities for Seniors

Gardens for Every Body

From the University of Missouri-Columbia.

Guide to design elements for a garden accessible to people with disabilities and physical limitations. Discusses container gardening, raised beds, pathways, trellises, health and safety, and adaptive, enabling, and ergonomic garden tools. Includes sections on gardening tips and techniques to prevent repetitive motion injuries, as well as for children with disabilities, seniors, and people with arthritis, back problems, visual impairments, and heart and lung problems. Provides related links.

Website: *www.agrability.missouri.edu/gardenweb*

Senior Corps

Provides information about this program, in which Americans aged 55 and older "share their time and talents to help solve local problems as Foster Grandparents serving one-on-one with young people with special needs; Senior Companions helping other seniors live independently in their homes; and volunteers with the Retired and Senior Volunteer Program (RSVP) meeting a wide range of community needs." The site tells how to become involved and has resources for those participating in the program.

Website: *www.seniorcorps.org*

SeniorJournal

A searchable website for active seniors covering breaking daily news and featuring articles on entertainment, finances, grandparenting, health care, hobbies, nutrition, retirement, and travel, among other subjects. The index item "Links — Senior" provides an annotated list of websites for senior citizens and baby boomers on aging, investing, government programs, politics, and other issues.

Website: *www.seniorjournal.com*

Resources for Seniors

SeniorLaw

Operated by a New York law firm.

This site contains links and a searchable database of information and resources on topics such as case law, Medicaid, Medicare, elder law attorneys, social security, wills and trusts, nursing home law, long-term care insurance, and elder abuse and neglect. Recent federal court decisions, statutes and regulations, and articles pertinent to the field of elder law are posted. Also contains links to general sites on eldercare and resources for seniors on the Web.

Website: *www.seniorlaw.com*

SeniorNet

A non-profit group of computer-using adults 50 and over that features technology news, research and conferences, online courses and tutorials, discussion forums, and guides covering such topics as health, finance, travel, and volunteering. Also promotes the SeniorNet Learning Center, offering low-cost computer classes. Searchable.

Website: *www.seniornet.org*

GENERAL HEALTH

Growing Stronger: Strength Training For Older Adults
From the Centers for Disease Control and Prevention.

This presentation describes the benefits of strengthening exercises for older adults and provides guidance in starting and maintaining a strength-training program. The "Exercises" section features step-by-step instructions and animated drawings for each of the exercises. Also includes a physical activity readiness questionnaire to help determine if you should check with your doctor before you start.

Website: *www.cdc.gov/nccdphp/dnpa/physical/growing_stronger*

The Merck Manual of Geriatrics
Online edition of print book of same title, providing "information of clinical relevance on geriatric care." Searchable and browsable by index.

Website: *www.merckmanuals.com/professional/geriatrics.html*

NIH Senior Health
From the National Institute on Aging and the National Library of Health, both part of the National Institutes of Health.

A site specially designed for seniors, with larger print and short, easy-to-read articles. A growing collection of topics includes Alzheimer's disease and exercise for seniors. There are captioned videos, FAQs, quizzes, and links to MEDLINEplus for more information.

Website: *http://nihseniorhealth.gov*

UpToDate Patient Information
This site provides articles with current information on a variety of medical conditions and topics. Searchable by topic (such as "general health") or by name of condition (such as "arthritis" or "cancer"). Information is written by physicians and "reviewed by multiple experts for accuracy."

Website: *http://www.uptodate.com/home/uptodate-benefits-patients*

Aging

Anti-aging Therapies: Too Good to be True?
From the Mayo Clinic.

This article provides an overview of substances that are commonly advertised as having anti-aging properties. Discusses antioxidants ("certain vitamins, minerals and enzymes that protect your body by neutralizing free radicals"), hormones (such as testosterone and melatonin), and general strategies that could lessen the effects of aging.

Website: *http://cgi.cnn.com/HEALTH/library/HQ/00233.html*

Infoaging.org
From the American Federation for Aging Research.

A searchable site presenting advances and news in aging research, focusing on aging-related diseases, biological causes of human aging, and a healthier lifestyle. The research spotlights cellular aging, telomeres, longevity, caloric restriction, stem cells, Alzheimer's findings, the food pyramid controversy, geriatrics, and more. Additionally, there are links to a number of general age-related websites and topics.

Website: *www.afar.org/infoaging*

Internet Resources on Aging
"Browse or search AARP's database … and find more than 500 of the best sites for people over 50." Topics include genealogy, computers and technology, Medicare and Social Security information, classic 1950s TV shows, chat rooms, and more. Also covers statistics, research, and other areas of interest to gerontology professionals.

Website: *www.aarp.org/research/internet_resources*

LGBT Aging Issues Network
This site "works to raise awareness about the concerns of lesbian, gay, bisexual, and transgender (LGBT) elders and about the unique barriers they encounter in gaining access to housing, health care, long-term care, and other needed services." Includes a newsletter and links to related websites.

Website: *www.asaging.org/lain*

Health & Aging Organizations Directory
From the National Institutes of Health National Institute on Aging.

This searchable database lists more than 350 national health and aging organizations, reviewed by NIA for relevance and accessibility. View the full list or find an organization by topic or organization name. You can also browse the database by subject area by selecting the "Browse by Category" tab.

Website: *www.nia.nih.gov/health/resources*

Specific Health Issues

Age-Related Macular Degeneration
This eye disease, which affects millions of people, attacks the macula, where sharpest vision occurs. The fastest growing type is age-related macular degeneration (AMD). This site by the Macular Degeneration Partnership provides information on diagnosis and treatment, current breakthroughs in research, a glossary, FAQs, articles, and links to related sites for persons with low vision.

Website: *www.amd.org*

Alzheimer's Association: Diverse Communities and Alzheimer's
Offers materials "on Alzheimer's disease, dementia care, and other dementia-related topics" for families, caregivers, and health practitioners serving ethnically diverse communities. The site includes culturally appropriate materials in other languages (including Chinese, Japanese, Vietnamese, Korean, and Spanish), and links to websites.

Website: *http://www.alz.org/diversity/overview.asp*

Alzheimer's Association: Kids and Teens
The Alzheimer's Association has created a page for children and teens that explains the disease and offers reviews of age-appropriate books and links to relevant websites. This is a useful resource for families dealing with a disease that can be very frightening for children.

Website: *www.alz.org/living_with_alzheimers_just_for_kids_and_teens.asp*

Alzheimer's Daily News
A daily electronic newsletter that will help caregivers stay up-to-date on the latest developments in Alzheimer's treatment, clinical drug trials, and research. Searchable.

Website: *http://www.medicalnewstoday.com/sections/alzheimers*

The Alzheimer Society Blog also offers numerous tips on caregiving and coping: *http://www.alzheimersblog.org*

Alzheimer's Disease Education and Referral Center
From the National Institutes of Health, National Institute on Aging.

Contains an overview of Alzheimer's disease that covers symptoms, diagnosis, and treatment; tips for caretakers; a database of clinical trials; publications; and more. Includes information in Spanish (see top navigation tabs.)

Website: *www.nia.nih.gov/alzheimers*

American Foundation for the Blind
This site provides information and resources for the blind or visually impaired, support organizations, and the general public on "blindness and low vision, Helen Keller, and such issues as advocacy, aging and vision loss, education, employment, literacy, technology, and Web accessibility." Visitors can browse the Helen Keller repositories and collections of her personal material, view message and job boards, subscribe to online journals, and visit an online bookstore with specialized material for the blind.

Website: *www.afb.org*

CancerNews: Directory
Hosted by Cancer News on the Net.

A collection of sites about breast, prostate, lung, leukemia, gynecologic, skin, and other cancers, as well as AIDS, general news, research, and support groups.

Website: *www.cancernews.com/directory/default.asp?LinksCategoriesID=26&Links SubCategoriesID=34*

Cancer Patients and Caregivers
Information for cancer patients and caregivers. Topics include caregiver and cancer-related fatigue, coping with chemotherapy, complementary and alternative medicine therapies, hospice, evaluating health information, health insurance and disability benefits, helping children understand cancer, nutrition, and communicating with your doctor. Browsable. From the Helen Diller Comprehensive Cancer Center at the University of California, San Francisco.

Website: *http://cancer.ucsf.edu/crc*

Cataracts
From the National Library of Medicine.

This tutorial takes patients through the process of diagnosing and treating cataracts, which affect at least half of the people aged 65 or older in the United States. It explains the anatomy and physiology, the surgical techniques, the decision-making process, and follow-up care.

Website: *www.nlm.nih.gov/medlineplus/tutorials/cataracts/htm/index.htm*

Epilepsy.com
The site features basic facts about epilepsy and seizures; an epilepsy timeline; information about diagnosing, treating, and living with epilepsy; seizure first aid suggestions; articles; news; a glossary; and more. Also includes information for children, teens, women, families, seniors, and professionals. Searchable.

Website: *www.epilepsy.com*

Epilepsy Foundation
This site provides comprehensive information on epilepsy treatment, medications, surgery, diet, nerve stimulation, seizure recognition, partial seizures, safety, driving, finances, employment and law, and insurance. Search by audience: adults, parents, women, seniors, teens, teachers, police/law enforcement, babysitters, and legal system. Chat and discussion forums are available, as well as links to services, news, research, and advocacy. Searchable. Some information is available in Spanish.

Website: *www.epilepsyfoundation.org*

The Forgetting: A Portrait of Alzheimer's
Companion to a PBS program "aimed at helping people better understand and cope with the fearsome disease of Alzheimer's." Discusses symptoms of the disease, the Alzheimer's experience, risk factors, coping with the disease, and activity ideas. Also includes news stories, a viewer's guide, and related resources.

Website: *www.pbs.org/theforgetting*

Glaucoma
From the U.S. National Library of Medicine.

Medline Plus provides links on glaucoma at other medical sites, a useful one-stop site for information from other authoritative sources. Links include overviews, diagnosis/symptoms, treatment, pictures/diagrams, alternative therapy, and disease management. Searchable for many other diseases and health issues.

Website: *www.nlm.nih.gov/medlineplus/glaucoma.html*

Hearing Loss
From the National Institute on Deafness and Other Communication Disorders, part of the National Institutes of Health.

Fact sheet on presbycusis, the loss of hearing that gradually occurs in most individuals as they grow older. Discusses symptoms, causes, prevention, hearing aids, communication tips, and related topics.

Website: *www.nidcd.nih.gov/health/hearing/presbycusis.asp*

Internet Stroke Center
From the Stroke Center at Barnes-Jewish Hospital and Washington University School of Medicine, St. Louis, Missouri.

Information includes illustrations, a glossary of neurological terms, treatment, and symptoms. Also includes links to related organizations, clinical trials, and treatment centers. Some information also available in Spanish.

Website: *www.strokecenter.org*

Macular Degeneration
From the U.S. National Library of Medicine.

Medline Plus provides links to macular degeneration on other medical sites, including the latest news, overviews, diagnosis/symptoms, treatment, prevention/screening, nutrition, and disease management. Searchable for many other diseases and health issues.

Website: *www.nlm.nih.gov/medlineplus/maculardegeneration.html*

Mental Health
Internet Mental Health is a free encyclopedia of mental health information created by psychiatrist Dr. Phillip Long.

Website: *www.mentalhealth.com*

Oral Health Information for the Public
From the American Academy of Periodontology.

Discusses types of gum disease (such as gingivitis and periodontitis), causes, prevention, and treatment. Includes fact sheets for women, children, seniors, and smokers.

Website: *www.perio.org/consumer/gum-disease.htm*

Osteoarthritis
From the U.S. National Library of Medicine.

Information about osteoarthritis, "one of the oldest and most common types of arthritis … characterized by the breakdown of the joint's cartilage." Find news, diagnoses, treatments, alternative treatments, specific conditions, disease management, representative research articles, and more.

Website: *www.nlm.nih.gov/medlineplus/osteoarthritis.html*

Osteoporosis and Bone Physiology
Maintained by a professor in the University of Washington Department of Medicine.

Originally created to "prepare trainees who come to work in … [a] bone clinic," this site provides basic information about topics such as osteoporosis, its prevention and treatment, bone density measurement, and osteomalacia. Also includes advice for patients, images, a bibliography, and educational material for children. Searchable.

Website: *http://courses.washington.edu/bonephys*

Aging Changes in the Senses
From MedlinePlus, a service of the U.S. National Library of Medicine, National Institutes of Health.

General information on age-related changes in the ears (earwax, itchy ears, decreased hearing, tinnitus), eyes (cataracts, macular degeneration, glare sensitivity, reduced peripheral vision, dry eyes), mouth and throat (decreased taste/smell, sore throat, cough), nose (aging rhinitis, bloody nose, allergic rhinitis), and sense of touch (decreased sensitivity to temperature, vibration, pain or pressure).

Website: *http://www.nlm.nih.gov/medlineplus/ency/article/004013.htm*

Prostate Cancer Foundation
Find information about the disease with statistics, treatments, resource links, the latest information on research, a section on living with prostate cancer (which includes survivor portraits), nutrition and exercise advice, and reading

recommendations. Features a clinical trials database and a database of cancer therapies. Searchable.

Website: *www.pcf.org*

Prostate Cancer Screening
From the Centers for Disease Control and Prevention.

Provides information aimed at helping men decide whether they need screening for prostate cancer. Includes basic information about prostate cancer, the main screening tools (digital rectal examination and prostate specific antigen test), and pros and cons from medical experts.

Website: *www.cdc.gov/cancer/prostate/basic_info/screening.htm*

End-of-Life Issues

Elisabeth Kübler-Ross
The official site about Dr. Kübler-Ross, whose breakthrough book, *On Death and Dying*, revolutionized modern attitudes toward aging and death. Includes a biography, selected quotes, a link to a hospice locator, a list of related organizations, advice for caregivers, and a bibliography. In six languages in addition to English.

Website: *www.elisabethkublerross.com*

End-of-Life Choices: Feeding Tubes and Ventilators
From the Family Caregiver Alliance.

This fact sheet discusses two common decisions facing families of chronically ill people: using feeding tubes when the person cannot swallow and using ventilators when the person cannot breathe on his or her own. Topics include artificial hydration, nutrition, pneumonia, and ventilators. Provides a link to the fact sheet "Holding On and Letting Go" as well as other related resources

Website: *www.caregiver.org/caregiver/jsp/content_node.jsp?nodeid=399*

WidowNet
Designed to help widows and widowers deal with grief, bereavement, and recovery. Provides demographic data, information on support groups, email and message board discussion forums, book reviews, helpful links, and true personal histories of a handful of widows and widowers.

Website: *www.widownet.org*

Financial Matters and Reverse Mortgages

Financial Facts Tool Kit
Produced by the Securities and Exchange Commission to better inform consumers about saving and investing. Included are tips on planning for retirement; advice on investing; guides to mutual funds, market risks, and corporate and municipal bonds; and workbooks such as "Get the Facts: The SEC's Roadmap to Saving and Investing." Also links to an interactive version of a ballpark estimate worksheet for calculating how much money should be saved for retirement.

Website: *www.sec.gov/investor/pubs/toolkit.htm*

Financial Planning and Retirement
From AARP.

Information about financial issues facing retirees. Topics include estate planning, financial advisors, insurance, investing and saving, and retirement income (such as individual retirement accounts, Social Security benefits, pensions, and annuities). Includes links to related information.

Website: *www.aarp.org/money/financial_planning*

Internal Revenue Service: Seniors & Retirees
Collection of IRS documents on tax topics of interest for older Americans and individuals planning for retirement. Includes relevant IRS publications and forms as well as information about the Tax Counseling for the Elderly (TCE) program, retirement plans, and other related subjects.

Website: *www.irs.gov/individuals/retirees*

Reverse Mortgage Calculator
From AARP.

The two loan programs used for the estimates are the federally insured Home Equity Conversion Mortgage (HECM), and the Home Keeper Mortgage from Fannie Mae. Calculations are based on the age of the homeowner and the value and location of the home. Includes links to additional material about reverse mortgages.

Website: *www.rmaarp.com*

Reverse Mortgages: Get the Facts before Cashing in On Your Home's Equity
From the U.S. Federal Trade Commission.

A fact sheet about reverse mortgages. Explains eligibility, the three main types (single-purpose, federally insured, and proprietary), what to watch out for during the loan process, and alternatives to reverse mortgages.

Website: *www.consumer.ftc.gov/articles/pdf-0058-reverse-mortgages.pdf*

Reverse Mortgages: Is One Right For You?
From the California Department of Real Estate.

Explains how reverse mortgages work, outlines advantages and disadvantages, warns against scams, and discusses alternatives to drawing down the equity of a home to supplement income.

Website: *http://www.dre.ca.gov/files/pdf/re52.pdf*

Home Equity Conversion Mortgages for Seniors
From the U.S. Department of Housing and Urban Development.

Includes basic facts and information about the Home Equity Conversion Mortgage (i.e. Reverse Mortgages) program from the U.S. Department of Housing and Urban Development (HUD), a list of HUD-approved HECM counsellors in each state, and related information. Also includes information for HECM lenders.

Website: *www.hud.gov/offices/hsg/sfh/hecm/hecmhome.cfm*

Social Security Online: Retirement Planner
From the Social Security Administration.

This site provides calculators, charts, and other information for determining Social Security retirement benefits. The "Near Retirement" section addresses full retirement age, delayed retirement, break-even points, and related topics. Some information also available in Spanish.

Website: *www.ssa.gov/retire2*

YOUR GUIDE TO RELEVANT ELDERCARE AND SUPPORT SERVICES IN CANADA

Federal Government

Reference Canada
A central source of information for all federal government programs and services. Telephone lines are staffed by information officers who will direct you to federal programs, information sources, and services.

Telephone: 1-800-622-6232; TTY: 1-800-926-9105
Website: *www.canada.gc.ca*

Guide for Seniors Available
The federal government's *Services for Seniors* covers everything from health, pensions, and taxes to recreation, volunteering, and the Internet. This document is available on demand in alternative formats such as large print, braille, audio cassette, CD, DAISY, and computer diskette.

Telephone: 1-800-622-6232; (TTY) 1-800-926-9105
To order PDF, visit: *www.seniors.gc.ca/content.jsp?contentid=100*.

Health Canada, Division of Aging and Seniors
Provides information on a broad range of health-related issues. To receive publications, visit the website, call 613-952-7606 or 1-866-225-0709, or send an email to seniors@hc-sc.gc.ca.

Telephone: 613-946-8043
Website: *www.hc-sc.gc.ca/hl-vs/seniors-aines/index-eng.php*

Human Resources and Skills Development Canada
HRSDC administers two income assistance programs for seniors (Canada Pension Plan and Old Age Security) through its Income Security Programs. For information, call the 1-800 number or visit the website.

Telephone: (English) 1-800-277-9914; (TTY) 1-800-255-4786
Website: *http://www.hrsdc.gc.ca/eng/home.shtml*

Canadian Seniors Policies and Programs Database
The SPPD is a very helpful Internet database of government policies and programs for which seniors are the primary beneficiaries. It was developed and is maintained by federal, provincial, and territorial governments. Select your province or territory from the menu.

Website: *http://www.canadabenefits.gc.ca/f.1.2ch.4m.2@.jsp?lang=eng*

Seniors Canada On-line
Seniors Canada On-line provides single-window access to Web-based information and services that are relevant to seniors 55+, their families, caregivers, and supporting service organizations. This is an exceptionally helpful website. Links are provided to information on a wide range of subjects such as safe driving courses, home care, health, housing, calculating Old Age Security payments, food and nutrition, and sexuality, as well as to the weather, Canada 411, and Canada Post's postal code lookup. Start your search for Web-based seniors' information here.

Website: *www.seniors.gc.ca*

Veterans Affairs Canada
The Veterans Independence Program provides special home care services to Canadian veterans. Services range from transportation, home adaptations, counseling, and health care to housecleaning and maintenance. There are income qualifications for specific services. Call the number above to find the regional office nearest you.

Telephone: (English) 1-866-522-2122; (French) 1-866-522-2022
Website: *www.veterans.gc.ca*; Email: information@vac-acc.gc.ca

General Resources

Alzheimer Society of Canada
The Alzheimer Society provides a nationwide network of support and helps people find programs and services (day and respite programs, home support, and help with the difficult transition to long-term care), administers a nationwide Alzheimer Wandering Registry, and offers many educational tools and resources for caregivers.

Telephone: 1-800-616-8816
Website: *www.alzheimer.ca*; Email: info@alzheimer.ca

Arthritis Society
A non-profit organization devoted to funding and promoting arthritis research, patient care, and public education. There are divisions in each province; see the provincial listings for details.

Telephone: 1-800-321-1433
Website: *www.arthritis.ca*
Canadian Cancer Society
The Canadian Cancer Society is a national, community-based organization of volunteers, whose mission is the eradication of cancer and the enhancement of the quality of life of people living with cancer. Each office provides various kinds of support and services. The toll-free line is a good entry point for those with questions and to learn the telephone number of your local divisional office. The website has a number of informative articles that you can download, as well as access to *The Canadian Cancer Encyclopedia*, a comprehensive, searchable

database of cancer information. Another useful feature is found by clicking on "Cancer Information" at the top of the page to read short definitions of many types of cancer.

Cancer Information Service: 1-888-939-3333; TTY 1 886 786-3934
Website: *www.cancer.ca*; Email: ccs@cancer.ca
For information about cancer: info@cis.cancer.ca

Canadian Council of the Blind
A national self-help consumer organization of people who are blind and deaf-blind. Contact the national office for services in your area.

Telephone: 613-567-0311 or 1-877-304-0968
Website: *www.ccbnational.net*; Email: ccb@national.net

Canadian Deafblind Association
Provides intervention services to deaf-blind and rubella handicapped people across Canada. To locate the provincial chapters, call the number above or visit the website.

Telephone: 1-866-229-5832
Website: *www.cdbanational.com*; Email: info@cdbanational.com
For information specifically about Rubella: *www.deafblindinternational.org*

Canadian Diabetes Association
With more than 150 branches across Canada, the Canadian Diabetes Association supports research, education, and advocacy for and on behalf of those with various levels of diabetes. Their helpful website provides information to patients and professionals; patient information is available in English and Chinese.

Telephone: 416-363-3373 or 1-800-BANTING (226-8464)
Website: *www.diabetes.ca*; Email: info@diabetes.ca

Canadian Hearing Society
The Canadian Hearing Society provides services and programs that encourage prevention of hearing loss and enhance the independence of deaf, deafened, and

hard of hearing people. Several programs are provided, including a hearing aid program to dispense and fit hearing aids and a hearing care counseling program for those 55 years and older. Call one of the numbers below or send an email to be referred to the office nearest you.

Telephone: 1-877-347-3427; (TTY) 1-877-216-7310
Website: *www.chs.ca*; Email: use the form on the "Contact Us" page

Canadian Home Care Association
The CHCA focuses on the advancement of quality home and community care nationally through information and knowledge sharing in order to facilitate best practices at all levels. On the website, the "Related Sites" tab has helpful links to several Canadian caregiver and health information websites.

Telephone: 289-290-4389
Website: *www.cdnhomecare.ca*

Canadian Mental Health Association
The CMHA focuses on combating mental health problems and emotional disorders through more than 10,000 volunteers and staff in 135 branches across Canada.

Website: *www.cmha.ca*

Canadian National Institute for the Blind
The CNIB is a national volunteer agency that provides a range of services to those suffering from varying degrees of loss of vision, with offices across Canada. It offers numerous resources, including counseling and referral, orientation and mobility training, sight enhancement, and technical aids.

Telephone: 1-800-563-2642
Website: *www.cnib.ca*

Canadian Red Cross Society
The Canadian Red Cross provides a number of home care services and equipment loans for eligible persons. One example is the Home Support Service: a

complete program of in-home care services. Services vary by region; call your regional office to find specific services offered in your area.

Telephone: 613-740-1900
Website: *www.redcross.ca*

The Complete Aging and Caregiving Resource Guide
Developed from the television program *Caregiving with June Callwood*, this is a very thorough listing of federal and provincial resources and services available to those who are providing care for a parent, spouse, or themselves. You will need Adobe Acrobat to view this document. You can download a free copy at: *http://get.adobe.com/reader/*.

Website: *www.caregiver.ca/resource.pdf*

Heart and Stroke Foundation of Canada
This organization has more than 250,000 volunteers dedicated to improving health by preventing and reducing disability and death from heart disease. To find a listing of local offices, click on "Contact Us" to find listings.

Telephone: 613-569-4361
Website: *www.heartandstroke.ca*

Meals on Wheels
This program provides hot meals delivered to seniors in their homes. There are hundreds of Meals on Wheels programs across Canada. To find the program nearest you, please check your local phone directory, ask your care coordinator or family physician, or visit *www.mealcall.org/canada/index.htm*.

Medbroadcast Corporation
This Vancouver-based company specializes in providing online consumer health and wellness information and services. Click on "Senior's Health" on the left side of the page. The website also contains very useful information on Canadian prescription drugs. Click on the "Drugs" tab at the top of the page.

Website: *www.medbroadcast.com*

Multiple Sclerosis Society of Canada
Undertakes research into the cause and cure of multiple sclerosis and works to educate the public about the condition.

Telephone: 416-922-6065
Website: *www.mssociety.ca*; Email:info@mssociety.ca

Internet Mental Health
Internet Mental Health is a free encyclopedia of mental health information created by Canadian psychiatrist Dr. Phillip Long.

Website: *www.mentalhealth.com*

Salvation Army
The Salvation Army provides pastoral care visits upon request. It also operates some long-term care facilities, respite care programs, and day-away programs in co-operation with local health care authorities. Services vary from region to region.

Telephone: 1-800-725-2769
Website: *www.salvationarmy.ca*

Nursing and Homemaking Agencies

Both non-profit and private nursing agencies provide nursing and support personnel to clients in their homes. A case manager/care coordinator from your regional health authority, local Community Care Access Centre, or Centres Locaux de Service Communitaires will provide a needs assessment to determine if funding is available.

A variety of funded services are available, including nursing, homemaking, respite, and personal care. For example, personal support workers are often provided for people with physical disabilities, advancing dementia, or Alzheimer's to help with household chores and/or personal care.

You can also purchase extra help by contacting a local nursing or homemaking agency directly and arranging to pay for the services you need to supplement those paid for by the government. Ask your health professional for names of local agencies to contact.

Victorian Order of Nurses (VON)
A non-profit agency. In addition to traditional nursing services, most provincial branches of the VON provide day-away programs for persons with dementia. These programs give caregivers a break while providing their clients with an opportunity to socialize and maintain their independence. Call the number below or visit the website to find the office nearest you.

Telephone: 613-233-5694 or 1-888-VON-CARE (866-2273)
Website: *www.von.ca*; Email: national@von.ca

Home Health Care Retailers, Home Safety, and Environment

A variety of home health care products and services are available from national retailers and also from your local pharmacy. Depending on your location, many stores offer in-home assessments, equipment trials, and rental programs for short-term needs.

Your health professional should be able to refer you to local stores, or you can call and ask one of the following national retailers for the location closest to your home.

As well, there are government support programs and a Canada Post alert program that are worth exploring as the need arises.

Canada Mortgage and Housing Corporation (CMHC)
CMHC's Home Adaptations for Seniors' Independence (HASI) program is designed to provide information about and fund home adaptations related to accessibility for seniors 65 and over. A forgivable loan of up to $3,500 is provided to qualified applicants (based on gross household income) for fixed items such as ramps, stair glides, and grab bars. Its Residential Rehabilitation Assistance Program (RRAP) offers differing levels of financial assistance for homeowners and landlords who are modifying dwellings for occupancy by low-income persons with disabilities.

The programs are administered on a provincial or municipal level depending on the region. In some areas, there is supplemental funding available from the province as well.

Telephone: 1-800-668-2642
Website: *www.cmhc.ca*; Email: chic@cmhc-schl.gc.ca

Canada Post's Letter Carriers Alert Program

Canada Post's letter carriers keep an eye on customers and report if they detect an unusual build-up of mail or newspapers at the customers' residences. This service is free in participating communities. Contact your local postmaster or call the toll-free number and ask a customer service representative if there is a program in your area.

Telephone: 1-800-267-1177

Canadian MedicAlert Foundation

The Canadian MedicAlert Foundation provides service and protection to Canadians with medical information and personal requests that should be known in the event of a medical emergency, including medical conditions, drug and food allergies, special needs, and medications.

Telephone: (English) 1-800-668-1507
Website: *www.medicalert.ca*

Lifecall of Canada

Lifecall is an emergency response service that provides immediate attention to seniors in need. It can offer peace of mind for caregivers and family members; however, seniors must remember to use the service. There is a fee.

Telephone: 1-800-661-5433
Website: *www.lifecall.ca*

Lifeline Systems Canada Inc.

Personal response service for people living alone or at risk. A portable alarm button is linked by telephone line to a central call center. A fee is charged.

Telephone: 1-866-784-1992
Website: *www.lifeline.ca*

MEDIchair

There are MEDIchair locations from coast to coast providing a full range of medical equipment for assisted daily living.

Telephone: 1-800-667-0087
Website: *www.medichair.com*

Motion Group
More than 30 specialized providers of seating, patient room equipment, mobility products, and assistive devices for persons with disabilities.

Telephone: 1-888-850-9188
Website: *www.vgmmobilitygroup.com/*

Shoppers HomeHealthCare
A network of specialized stores that offer a wide variety of home health care and wellness products for safety, comfort, and independence. Professionally trained staff work with you to assess your needs. Home visits are available without charge.

Telephone: 1-800-746-7737
Website: *www.shoppersdrugmart.ca/english/home_health_care/index.html*

Driving Capability Assessment for All Jurisdictions

In each province and territory, the Ministry of Transportation makes the official decision on when a person must stop driving. Your family physician is legally required to report any case in which someone's driving ability may be impaired due to the progression of age or any resulting condition. The physician must file his or her report with a medical review board, which may, based on research and interviews with key health care professionals, request a driving assessment to determine driving skills. Based on test results, a decision will be made on whether the individual will be allowed to continue to drive.

If you are concerned about your parents' ability to drive, you can request an independent assessment for one or both of them. Such assessments, which are provided by private companies for a fee, will help determine your parents' safety while on the road. For an assessment, please contact DriveAble. Fee for service.

Telephone: 1-855-365-3748

Website: *http://www.driveable.com/index.php/contact* (look for the "Find Your Assessment Centre" section below the contact form).

Financial Planning/Legal

The following organizations will refer you to trained professionals in your region who will assist you with general information you may need and on various aspects of estate and financial planning as well as protecting your rights.

Canada Revenue Agency
This is the government agency responsible for all tax matters within Canada. It maintains taxation records as well as information on the Canada Pension Plan.

Telephone: 1-800-959-8281
Website: *www.cra-arc.gc.ca*

Canadian Institute of Chartered Accountants
Provides a directory of accounting firms by geographical information and has a subsection called "Prime Plus" that designates firms and individual accountants that specialize in meeting the financial planning needs of the elderly. (Look in the 'Services Offered — Assurance, Advisory & Risk Management Services" box.)

Telephone: 416-977-3222 or 1-800-268-3793
Website: *www.cafirmdirectory.com*

Certified General Accountants Association of Canada
This group will refer you to your provincial association, which will, in turn, provide a list of accountants within a local area. Call the above number, send an email, or go to the website and click on "CGA Affiliates."

Telephone: 1-800-663-1529
Website: *www.cga-canada.org*; Email: public@cga-canada.org

Financial Advisors Association of Canada — Advocis
This organization represents professionals who can provide assistance with

overall financial planning. Look on the website to find a financial planner; click on "Find an Advisor" at the top of the page.

Telephone: 1-800-563-5822
Website: *www.advocis.ca*; Email: info@advocis.ca

Canadian Anti-Fraud Centre (formerly PhoneBusters)

Managed jointly by the Ontario Provincial Police, the RCMP and the Competition Bureau of Canada, the Canadian Anti-Fraud Centre is mandated to fight many variations of Mass Marketing Fraud. These frauds are essentially schemes that target many victims at the same time whether by telephone, facsimile, postal mail, or the internet, as well as identity theft and identity fraud. Offers free video information tapes and pamphlets. Available in French and English.

Telephone: 1-888-495-8501
Website: *www.antifraudcentre-centreantifraude.ca/english/home.html*;
Email: info@antifraudcentre.ca

Special Needs

The associations and foundations below offer a wealth of information and contacts on specific conditions other than dementia.

Aphasia Institute

The Aphasia Institute helps those with a language disorder resulting from an injury to the brain — most often a stroke. Offers direct services in the Greater Toronto Area but can help with training and communications resources across Canada.

Telephone: 416-226-3636
Website: *www.aphasia.ca*; Email: aphasia@aphasia.ca

Canadian Association of the Deaf

A national consumer group that provides a research and information center, a self-help society, and a community action organization. Available in French and English.

Telephone/ TTY: 613-565-2882
Website: *www.cad.ca*; Email: info@cad.ca

Canadian Continence Foundation

The Canadian Continence Foundation offers a wealth of information on incontinence management and treatment, including books, videos, audiotapes, and newsletters. The Foundation also will put you in touch with health care professionals who have expertise with urinary incontinence.

Telephone: 705-750-4600
Website: *www.canadiancontinence.ca*; Email: help@canadiancontinence.ca

Canadian Hard of Hearing Association

The CHHA provides information and brochures on improving communication skills and helping people deal with hearing loss. There is a page of helpful information for seniors here: *www.chha.ca/chha/projects-seniors.php*

Telephone: 1-800-263-8068
Website: *www.chha.ca*

Canadian National Society of the Deaf-Blind

The Society distributes information to help the deaf-blind and those who are caring for them.

Telephone: n/a; Fax: 416-730-1350
Website: *www.deafblindcanada.ca*; Email: info@deafblindcanada.ca

Canadian Hospice Palliative Care Association

The Association provides leadership in hospice palliative care, which is aimed at relief of suffering, loneliness, and grief for those who are approaching death.

Telephone: 1-800-668-2785; (Hospice Palliative Care Info Line) 1-877-203-4636
Website: *www.chpca.net*

Dieticians of Canada

Dieticians provide tips on nutrition and eating management. The organization doesn't provide names over the phone; however, you can visit the website to search for a dietician in your area.

Website: *www.dietitians.ca*; Email: centralinfo@dietitians.ca

Dying with Dignity
This organization educates caregivers on the rights of their loved ones as they near the end of life. They also provide counseling and information on living wills, advance health care directives, and power of attorney. They can refer caregivers to a local health care professional with specialized training in end-of-life care.

Telephone: 1-800-495-6156
Website: *www.dyingwithdignity.ca*

Osteoporosis Society of Canada
The Society assists people who have osteoporosis and those who are at risk. Services include free publications, a bilingual toll-free information line, educational programs, a South-Asian group of volunteers, and referrals to self-help groups and community resources. Visit the website or call the number below to find the chapter nearest you.

Telephone: (English) 1-800-463-6842; (French) 1-800-977-1778
Website: *www.osteoporosis.ca*

Tetra Society of North America
Tetra works with people with disabilities without regard to the reason for their disabilities. The Tetra Society matches community volunteers with people with special needs. These volunteers then create custom-designed assistive devices to help improve the individual's daily life. Visit the website or call the number below to find the chapter nearest you.

Telephone: 604-688-6464 or 1-877-688-8762
Website: *www.tetrasociety.org*; Email: info@tetrasociety.org

Caring for Yourself

CARP (Canada's Association for the Fifty-Plus)
A national association for those 50 and older that provides a range of services, including advice on health, travel, and finances. Links on the website take you to useful sites such as the Canada Pension Plan, Old Age Security, and the Passport Office. Free electronic newsletters are available on a variety of topics. Group savings are available on a range of benefits, including insurance, travel, and car rental. Membership is free.

Telephone: 416-363-8748 or 1-800-363-9736
Website: *www.carp.ca*; Email: support@carp.ca

The Canadian Caregiver Coalition
This is an alliance of individuals, groups, and organizations that promotes awareness and action to influence policy and address the needs of caregivers of all ages across Canada.

Telephone: 1-888-866-2273
Website: *www.ccc-ccan.ca*

Caregiver Network Inc. (CNI)
Although it is based in Toronto, the goal of CNI is to be a national single information source to make your life as a caregiver easier. The website has very helpful information on many topics of interest to caregivers, such as nutrition, support groups, driving, long-distance caregiving, and home care. There are also several useful links, for example, to the Alzheimer Society and the Canadian MedicAlert Foundation, as well as sites that will help you locate home care services and housing.

Telephone: 416-323-1090
Website: *www.caregiver.ca*; Email: karenh@ltcplanningnetwork.com

Family Caregiver Alliance
An American website with interesting information for family caregivers.

Telephone: 415-434-3388
Website: *www.caregiver.org*; Email: info@caregiver.org

Caregiver Solutions — a Boomer's Guide to Work and Life Balance
This magazine is published six times a year and positions itself as Canada's family guide to home health care and wellness. It provides readers with a host of tips and tactics on the challenges of caring for aging parents, as well as product and literature reviews.

Telephone: 1-866-290-2909; Toll-free 1-800-798-6282
Website: *www.solutions-online.ca*

ALBERTA

Government

Toll-Free Access to All Provincial Government Programs
You can contact any provincial government program toll-free from anywhere in the province by calling Alberta's RITE line telephone service. Simply dial 310-0000 and then enter the telephone number you need or press zero for RITE assistance. If you do not have a touch-tone telephone, stay on the line and an operator will help you place your call.

Alberta Seniors Information Line and Seniors Service Centres
The toll-free Alberta Seniors Information Line and Seniors Service Centres offer comprehensive information on programs and services for seniors in Alberta. Additional information is listed in the *Seniors Programs and Services Information Guide*. Go to *www.seniors.gov.ab.ca/publications* and click on the title. You need Adobe Acrobat to read this document; there is a link to a free copy of Acrobat on the website. You can also get a copy of the guide by contacting the Alberta Seniors Information Line at the numbers below.

Telephone: 1-877-644-9992; (Edmonton) 780-644-9992; TDD/TTY: Toll-free: 1-800-232-7215; Edmonton and area: 780-427-9999
Website: *www.seniors.gov.ab.ca*

Alberta Health Services

In Alberta, any one of the nine regional health authorities is a good point of entry to the health care system. Your local health authority will conduct an assessment and direct you to the resources you need. In addition, there are a number of independent associations and organizations (such as nursing agencies) that contract work through the health authority. You may be able to access these private services directly and pay for any additional care you require.

Telephone: for toll-free calling, dial 310-0000, then 780-427-1432
Website: *www.albertahealthservices.ca*
For information on provincial health services and departments related to seniors' home care, visit: *www.albertahealthservices.ca/4482.asp*

Alberta Seniors Housing Services Division
Facilitates the provision of adequate and affordable housing to seniors in need.

Telephone: Toll-free in Alberta: 1-877-644-9992; Edmonton area: 780-644-9992
Website: *www.seniors.gov.ab.ca/housing*

Long-Term Care Facilities

There are a number of facilities throughout the province that provide varying levels of care. Your local regional health authority has a complete list. Your care coordinator will be able to direct you to the proper facility based on the level of care your parents may need.

You also can contact the Alberta Continuing Care Association, whose members represent the public, private, and voluntary sectors in the province. Telephone: 780-435-0699 (Edmonton), or 1-888-212-4581
Website: *www.ab-cca.ca*; Email: info@ab-cca.ca

The Care Guide, Alberta Edition
Operated by CARE Planning Partners Inc., this site provides information on seniors' housing and care services. The site features provider search tools, community bulletin boards, and an online assessment tool. A print copy of its directory is available from the website or by calling the below number.

Telephone: 1-800-311-2273

Website: *www.thecareguide.com*

General Resources

Alberta Council on Aging
A province-wide charitable organization concerned with the process of aging.

Telephone: 780-423-9666 or 1-888-423-9666
Website: *http://www.acaging.ca*; Email: info@acaging.ca

Alberta Association for Community Living
This organization helps aging individuals with developmental disabilities. Support services and counseling are based on need.

Telephone: 1-800-252-7556 in Alberta; (Edmonton) 780-451-3055; (Calgary) 403-717-0361
Website: *www.aacl.org*; Email: mail@aacl.org

Financial Planning/Legal

ABCs of Fraud® Program
The Calgary Seniors' Resource Society offers this program to educate seniors about fraud, provide complimentary support materials, and provide referrals to additional resources.

To book a presentation in Calgary, call: 403-266-6200
Website: *http://www.calgaryseniors.org/fraud.php*

Public Trustee of Alberta
This office is responsible for protecting the financial rights of cognitively challenged people. The staff helps individuals make decisions on personal care and medical treatment. The office also advises family members on guardianship and on how to obtain the legal authority to make decisions on behalf of loved ones. The website is very useful for answering basic questions concerning trusteeship of dependent adults.

Telephone: 780-427-2744 (Edmonton) or 403-297-6541 (Calgary)
Website: *http://humanservices.alberta.ca/guardianship-trusteeship/office-of-the-public-trustee.html*

Alberta Transportation Alberta Traffic Safety Initiative
This department provides driver assessments to determine driving competence.

Telephone: 780-422-8839 or for toll-free, dial 310-0000, then 422-8830
Website: *http://www.saferoads.com/drivers/aging-drivers.html*

The Support Network: Edmonton's Crisis & Information Centre
A 24-hour, confidential, non-judgmental listening service that provides support and referrals for people experiencing difficulty in their lives. Help is also provided in suicidal and violent situations.

Distress Line: (Edmonton and area) 780-482-HELP (4357);
Northern Alberta: 1-800-232-7288

Senior Abuse Help Line
Offered by the Alberta Elder Abuse Awareness Network.

This is a 24-hour help line. Call for information about senior abuse or if you think a senior is being taken advantage of or abused.

Telephone: 780-454-8888 (Edmonton area)
Website: *www.albertaelderabuse.ca*

Caring for Yourself

Calgary Health Region Family Caregiver Centre
The center refers unpaid caregivers to information and support services in the health system and the community. There are also a number of resources available such as books, videos, articles, educational workshops, and personalized resource kits to fit your situation.

Telephone: 403-955-1674

Website: *www.albertahealthservices.ca/services.asp?pid=service&rid=1604*, or go to *www.albertahealthservices.ca* and enter "family caregivers" in the search box.

The Family Centre of Northern Alberta
A non-profit center offering homemaking services for in-home care and appointments. Family counseling and development workshops/seminars and interpreting services are offered. Charges a sliding scale fee for services.

Telephone: 780-423-2831
Website: *http://www.the-family-centre.com*; Email: info@the-family-centre.com

Local Information Centres
In addition to Public Health Services and Family and Community Support Services offices, many communities have local information centers that provide information on the services available in your community. Larger centers are as follows:

Calgary: Kerby Centre
Telephone: 403-265-0661
Website: *www.kerbycentre.com*; Email: information@kerbycentre.com

Calgary: Calgary Seniors Resource Society
Telephone: 403-266-6200
Website: *www.calgaryseniors.org*

Edmonton: The Support Network Community Referral Line
Telephone: 780-482-0198
Website: *www.thesupportnetwork.com*; Email: admin@thesupportnetwork.com

BRITISH COLUMBIA

Government

There are a variety of non-profit and private organizations contracted through British Columbia's regional health authorities that can provide home support services. They range from minimal home care to homemaking and full-time, live-in care. They also offer supervision, respite, and personal support for persons with dementia.

The B.C. Ministry of Health Services can direct you to the regional health authority in your area; call the ministry's information line at 1-800-465-4911 or visit its website at *www.healthservices.gov.bc.ca/socsec/contacts.html*. For the Seniors Health Care Support line, call 1-877-952-3181.

To contact BC's regional Health Authorities, visit *http://www.gov.bc.ca/health/*.

SeniorsBC
Responsible for informing the public on government policies and programs for seniors. The *Information for Seniors* guide is available in English, French, Chinese and Punjabi. Download a PDF version online at *www.gov.bc.ca/seniorsguide*, or call the Seniors Health Care Support line (1-877-952-3181) to order a printed copy. This is a comprehensive guide to programs and benefits in British Columbia.

Website: *www.seniorsbc.ca*

Long-Term Care Facilities

In British Columbia, long-term care is offered at extended care facilities throughout the province. Each facility has a specific number of multi-level care beds that offer varying levels of care. The first step is to call your local regional health authority and request an assessment. The assessment will help determine the level of care your parents require and any other needs. Admission to a facility is based on this assessment.

To locate your local regional health authority, call the B.C. Ministry of Health and Seniors Information Line at 1-800-465-4911 or go to *http://www.gov.bc.ca/health/*.

The Care Guide — British Columbia
Operated by CARE Planning Partners Inc., this site provides information on seniors' housing and care services. The site features provider search tools, community bulletin boards, and an online assessment tool. A print copy of its directory is available online or by calling the number below.

Telephone: 1-800-311-2273
Website: *www.thecareguide.com*

General Resources/Special Needs

Seniors Medication Information Line (BC Smile)
Operated by University of British Columbia licensed pharmacists, the line assists seniors and their caregivers with drug-related questions, especially those requiring extensive research (e.g., new medications, interactions, side effects, herbs, and vitamins).

Telephone: 1-800-668-6233
Email: smileubc@unixg.ubc.ca

Western Institute for the Deaf and Hard of Hearing

A non-profit information and service resource for people who are deaf and hard of hearing, as well as for concerned individuals and agencies. Registered Audiologists/Hearing Instrument Practitioners provide speech and hearing clinics and recommend hearing aid options that best meet your hearing needs, support network, and budget.

Telephone: 604-736-7391; (TTY/TDD) 604-736-2527
Website: *www.widhh.com*; Email: info@widhh.com

Financial Planning/Legal

ABCs of Fraud® Program
The Centre for Seniors Information provides presentations to groups of 10 or more, within a 2-hour drive of Kamloops, to educate seniors about fraud. The

organization distributes complimentary support materials and provides referrals to additional resources.

Telephone: 604-437-1940 or 1-866-437-1940
Website: *www.csikamloops.ca/fraud-awareness*; Email: jmcdona@telus.net

Community Legal Assistance Society
Provides free legal assistance, in particular to those who are physically, mentally, or economically disadvantaged throughout B.C.

Telephone: 604-685-3425; (TTY) 604-685-8295
Website: *www.orw.ca/source/legal/communit.htm*; Email: clas@vancouver.net

Legal Services Society
Non-profit organization providing legal services and information to people who cannot afford a lawyer, and legal education and information to the residents of B.C.

Telephone: 604-601-6000 (Greater Vancouver); Toll-free: 1-866-577-2525
Website: *www.lss.bc.ca*

Office of the Public Guardian and Trustee
This office is responsible for protecting the financial rights of cognitively challenged people. The staff helps individuals make decisions on personal care and medical treatment. The office also advises family members on guardianship and how to obtain the legal authority to make decisions on behalf of loved ones.

Telephone: 604-660-4444 (Vancouver); 250-387-6121 (Victoria);
Toll-free: 1-800-663-7867
Website: *www.trustee.bc.ca*; Email: mail@trustee.bc.ca

Support Agencies

Seniors Serving Seniors
Seniors Serving Seniors was incorporated in 1981 as a non-profit society to promote the well-being of seniors in the Greater Victoria Area. It operates a set of programs designed to encourage and maintain social activation and community support networks. Services are free and provided by approximately 100

volunteers and one employee. Information and referrals are provided to all of the non-medical emergency resources available in the region, as well as personalized advice and expertise on many issues, including financial assistance, government services, housing, legal, personal support services, etc.

Telephone: 250-382-4331
Website: *www.seniorsservingseniors.bc.ca*; Email: info@seniorsservingseniors.bc.ca

Caring for Yourself

PeerNetBC (formerly the Self-Help Resource Association of BC)
This association was formed to meet the needs of the self-help community; it facilitates the development of self-help groups, peer support initiatives, networks, and resources.

Telephone: 604-733-6186
Website: *www.peernetbc.com*; Email: info@peernetbc.com

MANITOBA

Government

The Manitoba Home Care Program (*www.gov.mb.ca/health/homecare*) is designed to help your parents live with dignity in their own home, for as long and as safely possible. The local home care office should be your first point of access in Manitoba. There are a number of home care offices throughout the province. They are all are operated by one of the 11 regional health authorities. To locate your local home care office, check your local phone directory, call the Winnipeg Regional Health Authority at 204-926-7000 or visit the website at *www.gov.mb.ca/health/rha/contact.html* to find contact information for each Regional Health Authority.

When you contact the local home care office, a health care professional will visit your parents and prepare a report, which will be forwarded to a panel of professionals who will review the application and determine the services and level of care required.

Manitoba Government Inquiry

Provides direct communication between Manitobans and the provincial government. If you have a question but are not sure of the appropriate government department or agency to approach, this service will refer you to the correct office.

Telephone: 1-866-626-4862 or 204-945-3744; (TTY) 204-945-4796
Email: mgi@gov.mb.ca

Manitoba Seniors and Healthy Aging Secretariat

A central point of contact for information and as a liaison with seniors, seniors' organizations, and government departments to ensure that government programs, policies, and legislation enhance the status of seniors.

Telephone: (Seniors' Information Line) 1-800-665-6565 or 204-945-6565
Website: *www.gov.mb.ca/shas/index.html*

Manitoba Health

The website provides information on health services in the province and contact information for the regional health authorities, which can direct you to services in your area. If you prefer, call Manitoba Government Inquiry.

Telephone: 204-945-3744 or 1-800-626-4862; (TY) 204-945-4796
Website: *www.gov.mb.ca/health*; Email mgi@gov.mb.ca

Pharmacare
Pharmacare is a drug benefit program for any Manitoban, regardless of age, whose income is seriously affected by high prescription drug costs.

Telephone: 1-800-297-8099 or 204-786-7141
Website: *www.gov.mb.ca/health/pharmacare*; Email: pharmacare@gov.mb.ca

The Seniors Abuse Help Line
A confidential information service aimed at providing seniors, caregivers, and

others with a one-stop information resource on elder abuse. There are useful publications available at the website.

24-hour Telephone Line: 1-888-896-7183 or 204-945-1884
Website: *http://www.gov.mb.ca/shas/elder_abuse/resources.html*

Long-Term Care Facilities

In Manitoba, there are two types of facilities that provide long-term care: supportive housing and personal care homes. Supportive housing provides light care; personal care homes provide a higher level of care.

An assessment is first conducted by a nurse to determine the person's needs. This assessment is then passed on to a central panel that decides what level of care is required. Based on this decision, a person may be referred to home support, respite care in the community, or a long-term care facility. For more information on assessments, contact your regional health authority or the Assisted Living department at 204-788-6648.

General Resources/Special Needs

A&O Support Services for Adults (formerly Age and Opportunity)
A community service agency that offers a broad range of services to promote the health and wellness of older adults throughout Winnipeg. In addition, it operates a number of senior centers.

Telephone: 204-956-6440
Website: *www.ageopportunity.mb.ca*; Email: info@ageopportunity.mb.ca

Creative Retirement Manitoba
Offers a number of learning programs and services for seniors.

Telephone: 204-949-2565
Website: *www.crm.mb.ca*; Email: info@crm.mb.ca

Association for Community Living, Manitoba
Advocates on behalf of people with intellectual disabilities to assist them in living

a quality lifestyle through the development of community living programs.

Telephone: 204-786-1607
Website: *www.aclmb.ca*; Email: aclmb@aclmb.ca

Contact Community Information

Refers Manitobans to social services and programs available through health, educational, cultural, and recreational resources in the province.

Telephone: 204-287-8827 or 1-866-266-4636
Website: *www.contactmb.org*; Email: alanna.palmer@volunteermanitoba.ca

Meals on Wheels of Winnipeg, Inc.
Provides nutritious meals delivered by volunteers to those in the community unable to prepare or otherwise obtain them.

Telephone: 204-956-7711
Website: *www.mealswinnipeg.com*; Email: info@mealswinnipeg.com

Financial Planning/Legal

Legal Aid Manitoba
Legal Aid Manitoba can fully or partially fund a lawyer to represent a person or group in a lawsuit. Individuals must complete an application and be found eligible. Legal Aid also offers informal drop-in services for simpler questions.

Telephone: 204-985-8500 or 1-800-261-2960
Website: *www.legalaid.mb.ca*

Office of the Vulnerable Persons' Commissioner
This office protects the rights of adults living with a mental disability, helps individuals make decisions on personal care and medical treatment, and advises family members on guardianship and on how to obtain the legal authority to make decisions on behalf of loved ones.

Telephone: 204-945-5039 or 1-800-757-9857
Website: *www.gov.mb.ca/fs/vpco/index.html*; Email: vpco@gov.mb.ca

The Driver Assessment & Management Program
Manitoba Public Insurance provides driver assessments to determine driving competence.

Telephone: 204-985-7000 (Winnipeg); Toll Free: 1-800-665-2410;
TTY/TDD: 204-985-8832

NEW BRUNSWICK

Government

In New Brunswick, home and community health care services are offered through the Department of Family and Community Service regional offices. The Department will conduct an assessment and financial evaluation to determine the level of care required. Based upon this evaluation, you will then be referred to the correct services your parents require. Whenever possible, individuals are expected to contribute financially to their care. To locate a Family and Community Service office near you, call 506-453-2001.

The *Seniors' Guide to Services and Programs* can be accessed on the Internet at *http://www2.gnb.ca/content/dam/gnb/Departments/sd-ds/pdf/Seniors/Seniors Guide-e.pdf*, by faxing a request to 506-453-2869, or by email: seniors@gnb.ca.

Social Development — Long-Term Care Services
This department offers long-term and in-home support services based on assessments and eligibility (depending on the level of needs of the individual). It also provides case management and referrals to various service providers.

Website: *www2.gnb.ca/content/gnb/en/services/services_renderer.10115.html*;
Email: sd-ds@gnb.ca

Prescription Drug Program
The Pharmaceutical Services Branch provides prescription drug benefits to

eligible residents of New Brunswick. The program is targeted to those with a demonstrated medical and financial need.

Telephone: 506-453-3983 or 1-800-332-3692
Website: *http://www.gnb.ca/0051/0212/index-e.asp*; Email: Health.Sante@gnb.ca

Service New Brunswick
Online link to over 200 government services, available in English and French.

Telephone: 506-684-7901 or 1-888-762-8600
Website: *www.snb.ca*

Long-Term Care Facilities

In New Brunswick, there are two types of long-term care facilities: special care homes and nursing homes. Special care homes are for people who can care for themselves; nursing homes provide a higher level of support and are for people who require 24-hour care.

Admission to either is based on a referral from a family physician or by contacting the Department of Family and Community Services (see "Government" below) to obtain information and start the process. Requires an assessment conducted by a public health nurse or social worker to determine the necessary level of care and funding required and any other needs. Admission is based on the assessment.

General Resources/Special Needs

The Blue Cross Seniors' Health Program
Provides access to the New Brunswick Drug Program for those residents of the province who are not otherwise eligible.

Telephone: 1-800-565-0065
Website: *www.medavie.bluecross.ca* — type "Senior" (not "seniors") in the Search box at the top right hand corner.

Easter Seals New Brunswick (formerly Canadian Rehabilitation Council for the Disabled, New Brunswick Branch)
Helps people of all ages who may have physical disabilities achieve maximum rehabilitation.

Telephone: 506-458-8739
Website: *www.easterseals.nb.ca*

Chimo Helpline (formerly Chimo Crisis Line)
A toll-free, 24-hour, province-wide telephone helpline for people who are experiencing a crisis.

Telephone: 1-800-667-5005
Website: *www.chimohelpline.ca*

Greater Saint John Seniors' Directory
A useful directory of a wide range of services for seniors in the Saint John area, including listings for counseling and support, elder abuse, housing, recreation, and respite services.

Telephone: 506-633-4636
Website: *www.town.grandbay-westfield.nb.ca/rec/senserv.htm*

New Brunswick Senior Citizens' Federation
Strives for awareness of the human community and its environment by exploring issues relevant to seniors.

Telephone: 506-857-8242
Website: *www.sjfn.nb.ca/community_hall/N/newb8242.html*

New Brunswick Association for Community Living
Works with people who have intellectual disabilities and their families to build inclusive communities where those with intellectual disabilities can live, learn, work, and actively participate in their communities as valued and contributing members.

Telephone: 506-453-4400 or 1-866-622-2548
Website: *www.nbacl.nb.ca*

Tele-Care
A bilingual, province-wide, 24-hour service for help with non-emergency medical problems.

Telephone: 811 TTY: 1-866-213-7920
Website: *www.gnb.ca/0217/Tele-Care-e.asp*

Volunteer Agencies

Senior Goodwill Ambassador Program
Part of a government project initiated in order to promote New Brunswick at home and abroad. Use the skills of volunteer retirees 65 years of age and older to make presentations to schools, community colleges, service clubs, and businesses on the positive aspects of New Brunswick.

Telephone: 506-457-6811
Website: *http://www2.gnb.ca/content/gnb/en/services/services_renderer.10095.Senior _Goodwill_Ambassador_Program.html*; Email: seniors@gnb.ca

FINANCIAL PLANNING/LEGAL

ABCs of Fraud® Program
The Saint John Volunteer Centre — generously sponsored by the New Brunswick Securities Commission — offers the ABCs OF Fraud® Awareness Program. This educational program is available for all groups and all ages, at no charge, and gives valuable information to protect us from becoming victims of fraud.

Telephone: (506) 658-1555 or Toll Free 1-877-332-1555
Website: *http://volunteersaintjohn.com/abcs-of-fraud*
French ABCs Program: vol.sjvc@nb.aibn.com
English ABCs Program: vol.training@nb.aibn.com

Department of Transportation and Infrastructure
This department provides driver assessments to determine driving competence.

Telephone: 506-453-3939
Email contact form: *www.gnb.ca/0113/sendmail-e.asp*

Vehicle Retrofitting and Accessible Vehicle Program
This program is designed to provide assistance for retrofitting vehicles with eligible accessibility features.

Telephone: 506-453-5818
Website: *www.gnb.ca/0113/Policy/vretro/veh-retrofit-e.asp*;
Email: claudette.mcallister@gnb.ca

NEWFOUNDLAND AND LABRADOR

Government

There are six health and community services boards in Newfoundland that look after home care and other related services for aging parents with special needs. Once you contact your local office, a health care professional will visit your parent and conduct an assessment. This assessment will help determine your parent's needs and the level of care that he or she may require. Call the Department of Health and Community Services at 709-729-4984 or email *healthinfo@gov.nl.ca* to locate the office nearest to you.

Long-Term Care Facilities

There are a number of facilities throughout the province that provide varying levels of care. Your local community health board has a complete list. Your care coordinator will be able to direct you to the proper facility based on the level of care that your parent requires.

General Resources

Seniors' Resource Centre
The center offers a number of programs for caregivers, including a free newsletter and a Friday friendship club, as well as friendly visiting and other community services. Operates a toll-free line for unpaid caregivers at 1-888-571-2273.

Telephone: 709-737-2333 or 1-800-563-5599
Website: *www.infornet.st-johns.ca/providers/seniors*;
Email: seniorsresource@ng.aibn.com

Financial Planning/Legal

Office of the Public Guardian and Trustee
This office is responsible for protecting the financial rights of cognitively challenged people. It helps individuals make decisions on personal care and medical treatment. The office also advises family members on guardianship and on how to obtain the legal authority to make decisions on behalf of loved ones.

Telephone: 709-729-0850
Email: karenelawlor@hotmail.com

NORTHWEST TERRITORIES

Government

The Department of Health and Social Services provides programs and services related to senior care, such as Extended Health Benefit Seniors Program, Home Care, Long Term Care, Seniors Home Heating Subsidy Program, and many others. Call 1-800-661-0830, visit the website (*www.hlthss.gov.nt.ca*), or email hsa@gov.nt.ca for details. Visit the Seniors Policies and Programs Database at *www.sppd.gc.ca* and click on the red "Benefits Finder" button for a comprehensive listing in one place.

General Resources

Financial Planning/Legal

Legal Services Board, Law Line

This board is responsible for ensuring that all eligible people in the Northwest Territories receive legal services. The board follows prescribed guidelines for determining if a person is eligible and oversees the operations of legal aid clinics situated in every administrative region of the N.W.T. If you require further information about legal aid, the legal system, or if you have a specific legal problem, you can call the Law Line and speak to a lawyer for free and in confidence.

Telephone: 1-867-873-3130
Email: lsb@gov.nt.ca

Office of the Public Guardian and Trustee

This office is responsible for protecting the financial rights of cognitively challenged people. It helps individuals make decisions on personal care and medical treatment. The office also advises family members on guardianship and on how to obtain the legal authority to make decisions on behalf of parents.

Telephone: 867-873-7464 or 1-866-535-0423
Website: *www.justice.gov.nt.ca/PublicTrustee/index.shtml*;
Email: larry_pontus@gov.nt.ca

Northwest Territories Transportation

This department provides driver assessments to determine driving competence.

Telephone: 867-873-7406

NUNAVUT

Government

Nunavut Department of Health and Social Services
This department provides information on provincial health services and departments related to home care and caring for aging parents.

Telephone: 867- 975-5766; Toll Free: 1-800-661-0833
Website: *www.hss.gov.nu.ca*

General Resources

Financial Planning/Legal

Office of the Public Guardian, Department of Health and Social Services
This office is responsible for protecting the financial rights of cognitively challenged people. It helps individuals make decisions on personal care and medical treatment. The office also advises family members on guardianship and on how to obtain the legal authority to make decisions on behalf of parents.

Telephone: 867-975-5700
Website: *www.hss.gov.nu.ca/en/CFS%20Guardianship.aspx*

Motor Vehicles Department
This department provides driver assessments to determine driving competence.

Telephone, Toll-free: 1-888-975-5999

NOVA SCOTIA

Government

Public Enquiries Officers respond to telephone enquiries about all provincial government services, programs, and initiatives. The service offers a province-wide toll-free telephone line at 1-800-670-4357; the local number is 902-424-5200.

Health care service delivery is provided through one of nine district health authorities. Each is responsible for delivering all care services to people in its particular region. In addition, the Nova Scotia Department of Health has established a toll-free number that will direct you to the closest facility. Call the Nova Scotia Department of Health and Wellness at 902-424-5815 or 1-800-387-6665. You can visit the website at *www.gov.ns.ca/health* for a list of programs and services and access to the websites of the district health authorities.

Nova Scotia Department of Health: Continuing Care Branch,
including Long-Term Care
This office serves people who need ongoing care outside of hospital, either on a long-term or short-term basis. Its services include home care, long-term care, and protection for vulnerable adults.

As of 2005, residents who live in nursing homes, residential care facilities, and community-based options under the Department of Health's mandate are no longer required to pay for their health care costs. As well, residents no longer have to use their assets to pay for their long term care accommodation costs. Comprehensive information about the programs and services available can be found at the website below.

Telephone: 1-800-225-7225 (if calling from out-of-province, please visit the website for a list of regional contacts.)
Website: *www.gov.ns.ca/health/ccs*

Senior Citizens' Secretariat and Seniors Information Line
A comprehensive listing of provincial government services for seniors. The publication *Programs for Seniors* is updated annually and is available online or as a booklet. The website offers some very useful links to information on topics such as health, safety, legal matters, and retirement/leisure.

Telephone: (Halifax/Dartmouth) 902-424-0065; 1-800-670-0065
Website: *www.gov.ns.ca/scs*; Email: seniors@gov.ns.ca

Long-Term Care Facilities

There are a number of facilities throughout the province that provide varying levels of care. Your local district health authority has a complete list. Your care coordinator will be able to direct you to the proper facility based on the level of care that your parent requires. For more information about home care and long-term care services, call 1-800-225-7225.

General Resources/Special Needs

Continuing Care Association of Nova Scotia
CCANS is a not-for-profit organization representing some 50 facilities and service providers that offer residential care or various support services for the elderly with special needs.

Telephone: 902-492-0681 – President, Marty Wexler
Website: *www.nsnet.org/ccans*; Email: ccans@eastlink.ca

Nova Scotia Association of Health Organizations
Represents more than 100 organizations, including nine district health authorities, 50 continuing care providers, and home care and home support agencies.
Telephone: 902-832-8500

Website: *www.healthassociation.ns.ca*; Email: alex.cross@healthassociation.ns.ca

Society of Deaf and Hard of Hearing Nova Scotians
Assists adult deaf, deafened, and hard of hearing Nova Scotians to gain access to existing public, private, and community services.

Halifax area and Mainland NS:
Telephone/TTY: 902-422-7130; Videophone: 902-422-7132
Email: sdhhns@ns.sympatico.ca

Cape Breton:
Telephone/videophone: 902- 564-0003; TTY: 902- 564-0486;
Toll-free within NS: 1-888-770-8555
Website: *www.sdhhns.org*; Email: cbdeaf@ns.sympatico.ca

Financial Planning/Legal

Legal Information Society of Nova Scotia
Provides information and resources about wills, family, power of attorney, and other legal matters.

Legal Information Line/Lawyer Referral Service: 902-455-3135 or 1-800-665-9779
Website: *www.legalinfo.org*

Nova Scotia Legal Aid
There are 13 regional offices and three sub-offices in the province. Legal aid may be provided to people on social assistance or in an equivalent financial position in certain areas of family and criminal law. Check the phone directory or visit the website below for the Nova Scotia Legal Aid office nearest you.

Website: *www.nslegalaid.ca*

Public Trustee of Nova Scotia
This office is responsible for protecting the financial rights of cognitively challenged people. It helps individuals make decisions on personal care and medical treatment and advises family members on guardianship and on how to obtain the legal authority to make decisions on behalf of loved ones. The Public Trustee also manages the estates of people who need services of a trustee, guardian, or attorney not readily available in the private sector.

Telephone: 902-424-7760
Website: *www.gov.ns.ca/just/pto*

Volunteer Agencies

Good Neighbours, Great Neighbourhoods
Encourages people to reach out and help one another and to create caring, sharing, and friendly communities. The website *myHRM.ca* is an online community for people who want to make a personal commitment to doing small but significant neighbourly acts that make their neougborhoods great places to live, work, and play.

Website: www.myhrm.ca; Email: myhrm@halifax.ca

Family Caregivers Association of Nova Scotia
This non-profit organization offers information and practical support for all caregivers, whether family, friends, or neighbors. It provides a newsletter and other resources and has a strong network with other caregiving groups throughout the province.

Telephone: 902-421-7390 or 1-877-488-7390
Website: *www.caregiversns.org*; Email: support@caregiversns.org

Volunteer Resource Centre — Sydney
Coordinates and administers Meals on Wheels, Each One Teach One, a friendly visiting service, transportation, and snow-shoveling. It is a non-profit organization and a member of the United Way of Cape Breton.

Telephone: 902-562-1245
Website: *www.newdawn.ca*; Email: jennifer@newdawn.ca

Registry of Motor Vehicles: Medical Section
This department provides driver assessments to determine driving competence. A voluntary assessment will require a fee; an assessment that is requested by a physician or the ministry is free of charge.

Telephone: 902-424-5732

Nova Scotia Safety Council — 55 Alive
A national mature driver refresher course. The course, free to those 65 years and over, consists of six hours of classroom instruction only, commonly offered over two mornings. There are no tests and no negative effects on the licence.

Telephone: 902-454-9621; Toll-Free: 1-866-511-2211

ONTARIO

Government

Fourteen Community Care Access Centres (CCAC) located throughout the province serve as the entry point to the Ontario community health care system. The local CCAC will conduct an assessment and direct you and your parents to the resources and services that are required.

In addition, you may be able to access private services (such as a nursing or homemaking agency) from independent associations and organizations through the local CCAC. The center also will provide you with information on other important caregiving resources such as support groups, crisis lines, related health care associations, and long-term care facilities.

To locate the Community Care Access Centre in your area, call 1-800-268-1154 (Ontario Ministry of Health) or the CCAC head office at 416-750-1720; or visit its website at *www.oaccac.on.ca.*

Assistive Devices and Home Oxygen Programs
These programs offer financial assistance for those who have a prescribed need for home care products such as wheelchairs, scooters, walkers, etc. It also provides home oxygen services.

Telephone: 416-327-8804; 1-800-268-6021; (TDD/TTY) 416-327-4282 or 1-800-387-5559
Website: *www.health.gov.on.ca/en/public/programs/adp/default.aspx*;
Email: adp@ontario.ca

Ministry of Health and Long Term Care: Health Information Centre
This provincial office is responsible for health care delivery within Ontario. The ministry provides referrals to provincial services (including Community Care Access Centres) that offer specific assistance for different kinds of needs. At its website, click on the menu selection "Home, Community, & Residential Care Services for Seniors" to go to the website that discusses care options.

Telephone: 1-800-268-1154
Website: *www.health.gov.on.ca*

Ontario Seniors' Secretariat
Provides access a variety of information of interest to seniors, their families, and those who work with seniors.

Telephone: 1-888-910-1999; TTY: 1-800-387-5559
Website: *www.seniors.gov.on.ca/en/index.php*; Email: Infoseniors@ontario.ca

Telehealth Ontario
Call to speak to a registered nurse about medical or health-related issues 24 hours a day, 7 days a week.

Telephone: 1-866-797-0000; TTY: 1-866-797-0007

Long-Term Care Facilities

There are a number of long-term care facilities throughout the province that provide varying levels of care. Your local Community Care Access Centre has a complete list of local facilities. Your care coordinator will be able to direct you to the proper facility based on the level of care that your loved one requires. In addition, there are numerous retirement homes that provide light, supportive care. The association listed below will help you find the proper facility.

The Care Guide
Operated by CARE Planning Partners Inc., this site provides information on seniors' housing and care services. The site features provider search tools, community bulletin boards, and an online assessment tool. A print copy of its directory is available online or by calling the number below, or you can order online here: *www.thecareguide.com/OrderTheGuide.aspx*

Telephone: 416-287-2273 or 1-800-311-2273
Website: *www.thecareguide.com*

General Resources/Special Needs

Ontario Home Care Association
An organization of home health and social care providers. The website has very useful links to current information about home health care in Ontario.

Telephone: 905-543-9474
Website: *www.homecareontario.ca*; Email: info@homecareontario.ca

St. Elizabeth Health Care
A non-profit nursing agency with a full range of nursing and homemaking services available throughout Ontario and consulting services to other agencies across Canada.

Telephone: 905-940-9655 or 1-877-625-5567
Website: *www.saintelizabeth.com*; Email: communications@saintelizabeth.com

Financial Planning/Legal

ABCs of Fraud® Program
The ABCs of Fraud® program gives group presentations concerning information and tips on identifying and preventing consumer fraud victimization, along with complimentary support materials and referrals to additional resources.

Ottawa:
Telephone: 613-564-5555
Website: *http://abcsfraudottawa.tripod.com*

In Toronto, contact Crime Prevention Association of Toronto at:
Telephone: 416-225-1102
Email: office@cpatoronto.org

Advocacy Centre for the Elderly
A legal clinic for low-income, 60+ seniors in the Greater Toronto Area. ACE offers one-on-one legal advice and provides updates on new legislation relevant to the rights of seniors. Most of the ACE services are provided free of charge.
Telephone: 416-598-2656

Website: *www.advocacycentreelderly.org*

Legal Aid Ontario

Legal aid is available to lower-income people for a variety of legal issues. Eligibility is based on financial need and the type of case. The applicant may pay nothing or a portion of the costs of the legal aid, depending on his or her financial situation. Once approved, a legal aid certificate entitles a person to retain the lawyer of his or her choice. The lawyer is then reimbursed by Legal Aid Ontario.

Telephone: 416-979-1446 or 1-800-668-8258 TTY: 416-598-8867 or Toll free: 1-866-641-8867
Website: *www.legalaid.on.ca*; Email: info@lao.on.ca

Legal Line

Provides free legal information to residents of Ontario through the Internet. The service will provide Ontario residents with sufficient legal information to know when the assistance of a lawyer is advisable and direct them to the Ontario Bar and other appropriate resources for further assistance.

Office of the Public Guardian and Trustee

For assistance with treatment decisions, call 416-314-2788 or 1-800-387-2127. To report a situation involving an adult whom you believe to be mentally incapable and suffering, or at risk of suffering or serious harm, contact 416-327-6348 or 1-800-366-0335. This office is responsible for protecting the financial rights of cognitively challenged people. It helps individuals make decisions on personal care and medical treatment. The office also advises family members on guardianship and on how to obtain the legal authority to make decisions on behalf of loved ones.

Ontario Ministry of Transportation

This department provides driver assessments to determine driving competency.

Telephone: 416-235-2999 or 1-800-387-3445

Caring for Yourself

Self Help Resource Centre
Provides listings of self-help groups across Ontario for family, friends, and caregivers looking after aging parents, and many other self-help categories.

Telephone: 416-487-4355 or 1-888-283-8806
Website: *www.selfhelp.on.ca*; Email: shrc@selfhelp.on.ca

Ontario Community Support Association
A good resource to connect to some 360 agencies across Ontario providing a host of services, including Meals on Wheels, many of which will be relevant to caregivers, including referrals to organizations that offer therapeutic counseling and relief from caregiving duties.

Telephone: 416-256-3010; 1-800-267-6272
Website: *www.ocsa.on.ca*

PRINCE EDWARD ISLAND

Government

In P.E.I., contacting your local regional health board is your first step in finding the home care resources you need. Each region has a Home Care Office that offers a variety of services. Upon contacting the local office, a health care professional will visit your home and conduct an assessment. This assessment will help the professional to determine your parent's needs and the level of care that he or she requires. To locate the Home Care Office nearest you, check your local phone directory or visit the comprehensive provincial website at *www.gov.pe.ca/seniors*.

PEI Department of Health and Social Services
This department provides information on provincial health services and departments related to home care.

Telephone: 902-368-4900
Website: *www.gov.pe.ca/hss*

Island Information: Seniors
The purpose of this website is to help seniors, their families, and those who work with seniors find information about programs, services, and areas of interest.

Website: *www.gov.pe.ca/infopei/seniors*

Long-Term Care Facilities

Nursing care is accessed by contacting a placement officer in one of the five health regions on P.E.I. There are a number of facilities throughout the province that provide varying levels of care. Your local Home Care Office has a complete list. Your care coordinator will be able to direct you to the proper facility based on the level of care that your loved one requires.

General Resources/Special Needs

Island Help Line
The Island Help Line is a 24-hour, free, confidential service providing information, support, and crisis counseling on family matters, child abuse, alcohol and drugs, parenting, and suicide.

Telephone: 1-800-218-2885

PEI Senior Citizens' Federation
The purpose of the federation is to further the interests and promote the happiness and welfare of senior citizens and pensioners in Prince Edward Island in every way possible. This chapter has its own newspaper, holds workshops across the Island, and advocates for seniors.

Telephone: 902-368-9008; Toll Free 1-877-368-9008
Website: *www.peiscf.com*; Email: peiscf@pei.aibn.com

Financial Planning/Legal

Office of the Public Guardian and Trustee
This office is responsible for protecting the financial rights of cognitively challenged people. It helps individuals make decisions on personal care and medical treatment. The office also advises family members on guardianship and on how to obtain the legal authority to make decisions on behalf of loved ones.

Public Guardian: 902-368-6506; Email: jaharper@gov.pe.ca
Deputy Public Trustee: 902-368-4561; Email: rllandry@gov.pe.ca
Website: *www.gov.pe.ca/jps/index.php3?number=1027626*

Volunteer Agencies

Charlottetown Meals on Wheels Inc.
Run by volunteers.

Provides nutritious meals and social contact to those who cannot obtain adequate nutrition on their own.

Telephone: 902-569-7700

PEI Transportation and Public Works
This department provides driver assessments to determine driving competence.

Telephone: 902-368-5100

Driver Refresher Course — 55 Alive
The 55 Alive/Mature Driver Refresher Course is a classroom course designed for mature drivers. It is offered by the PEI Senior Citizens' Federation in partnership with the PEI Department of Transportation and Infrastrucutre Renewal and the Department of Community Services and Seniors. This is a six hour course taught in a classroom. There is no testing at the end of the course. Drivers learn how to compensate for the physical changes of aging. The course provides opportunities for participants to identify individual problem areas, and improve their behavior as drivers.

Telephone: 902-368-9008 or 1-877-368-9008
Website: *www.peiscf.com/55_Alive_Course.html*

QUEBEC

Government

The Quebec government has a very centralized approach to providing information about its services. Services Québec: Citizens is its principal information portal, providing comprehensive lists and descriptions of services available. Call 1-877-644-4545 or visit the website to download the PDF guide to *Programs and Services for Seniors* at *http://www4.gouv.qc.ca/EN/Portail/Citoyens/Evenements/aines/Documents/guide_aines_anglais_2013_2014_web.pdf.*

Centres Locaux de Service Communitaires (CLSCs) are located throughout the province of Quebec and are your first contact for finding the health care services you need. Each CLSC provides a number of services, including nursing care, home care and domestic help, and referrals to outside agencies. You can find the closest CLSC by calling the Association des CLSC at 514-317-2683, by emailing info@indexsante.ca or by visiting their website at *www.indexsante.ca.*

Long-Term Care Facilities

There are a number of facilities throughout the province that provide varying levels of care. Your local CLSC has a complete list. Your care coordinator will be able to direct you to the proper facility based on the level of care that parent requires.

General Resources/Special Needs

Héma Québec
The Quebec equivalent of the Canadian Blood Services.

Telephone: 514-832-5000 or 1-888-666-4362
Website: *www.hema-quebec.qc.ca*; Email: info@hema-quebec.qc.ca

Financial Planning/Legal

Curateur public du Quebec (Public Trustee)
This office is responsible for protecting the financial rights of cognitively challenged people. It helps individuals make decisions on personal care and medical treatment, offers power of attorney kits and wills, and helps search for heirs and next-of-kin. The office also advises family members on guardianship and on how to obtain the legal authority to make decisions on behalf of loved ones. Telephone: 1-800-363-9020

Website: *www.curateur.gouv.qc.ca/cura/en/index.html*

Commission des services juridiques (Legal Aid)
Legal Aid offers economically disadvantaged people access to the courts, the professional services of an attorney or a notary, and the information they need regarding their rights and obligations. Eligibility for legal aid is based on several factors, including the applicant's family obligations, income, property, and liquid assets. People eligible are entitled to the services of a legal aid lawyer. They also are entitled to a lawyer in private practice if he or she accepts; however, not all services are covered.

Telephone: 514-873-3562
Website: *www.csj.qc.ca*; Email: info@csj.qc.ca

Ministère des Transports du Québec
This department provides driver assessments to determine driving competence.

Telephone: 511 (from anywhere in Québec); 1-888-355-0511 (from elsewhere in North America)
Website: *www.mtq.gouv.qc.ca*

SASKATCHEWAN

Government

In Saskatchewan, district health boards and one health authority in the north are responsible for all health care within the province. They are your first step to finding the services you need in your area. The health boards and health authority hire their own staff and do not contract work out to independent companies. Phone the Saskatchewan Health and Social Services Department of Community Care at 306-787-7239 for the district health board nearest you. Long-term care facilities are also referred through this system, or you can visit the website at *www.health.gov.sk.ca/community-care.*

Information is also available through 3sHealth — Shared Services of Saskatchewan.

Telephone: 306-347-5500
Website: *www.3shealth.ca*; Email: info@3shealth.ca

Social Services Saskatchewan
Saskatchewan has a number of housing programs to assist seniors including: Affordable Housing Rentals (seniors' rentals), Personal Care Home Benefit, and Saskatchewan Rental Housing Supplement, Seniors Income Plan, and the Social Housing Rental Program. Call the below number or visit the website for more information.

Website: *www.socialservices.gov.sk.ca/seniors*; Email contact form: www.socialservices.gov.sk.ca/Contact

Saskatchewan Aids to Independent Living
The program provides benefits for people whose long term disabilities or illnesses leave them unable to function fully. The aim is to assist people in leading more independent and active lifestyles.

Telephone: 306-787-7121
Website: *www.health.gov.sk.ca/sail*

Saskatchewan Health Community Care Branch
Helps develop and support community programs such as home care, safe driving, and special care (nursing) homes.

Telephone: 306-787-7239
Website: *www.health.gov.sk.ca/ph_br_community_care.html*

Long-Term Care Facilities

There are a number of facilities throughout the province that provide varying levels of care. Your local district health board has a complete list. Your care coordinator will be able to direct you to the proper facility based on the level of care that your loved one requires.

General Resources/Special Needs

Saskatchewan Association for Community Living (SACL)
Helps aging individuals with an intellectual disability. Support services and counseling are based on need. Call the number below or send an email to find the branch nearest you.

Telephone: 306-955-3344
Website: *www.sacl.org*; Email: sacl@sacl.org

Saskatchewan Deaf and Hard of Hearing Services Inc.
This non-profit organization serves deaf, hard of hearing, and late-deafened persons with a variety of support services. These include communication services, social work, and hearing aid battery sales

Regina:
Telephone: 306-352-3323 or 1-800-565-3323, Videophone 306-352-3322
Email: regina@sdhhs.com

Saskatoon:
Telephone: 306-665-6575 or 1-800-667-6575; Videophone 306-665-6578
Website: *www.sdhhs.com*; Email: saskatoon@sdhhs.com

Financial Planning/Legal

Office of the Public Guardian and Trustee
This office is responsible for protecting the property of people who do not have the capacity to manage their own financial affairs. It helps individuals make decisions on personal care and medical treatment and advises family members on guardianship and on how to obtain the legal authority to make decisions on behalf of loved ones.

Telephone: 306-787-5424 or 1-877-787-5424
Website: *www.justice.gov.sk.ca/pgt*; Email: pgt@gov.sk.ca

Saskatchewan Legal Aid Commission
Provides legal services to people who can't afford a lawyer. Call to find the office nearest you or email using the contact form.

Telephone: 306-933-5300 or 1-800-667-376
Website: *www.legalaid.sk.ca*

Saskatchewan Government Insurance, Medical Review Unit
Provides driver assessments to determine driving competence.

Telephone: (Regina) 775-6176; 1-800-667-8015 ext. 6176
Website: *www.sgi.sk.ca/individuals/medical/driveconditions/mru.html*;
Email: mruinquires@sgi.sk.ca

YUKON

Government

Home care and long-term care services are accessed throughout the territory by calling the government departments listed below or 1-800-661-0408 ext. 5774 or visit the website at *www.hss.gov.yk.ca/homecare.php*.

Extended Health Care Benefits for Seniors
Range of health services for elderly people who are not covered by private insurance.

Telephone: 867-667-5403; Toll free: 1-800-661-0408, local 5403 (Yukon only)
Website: *www.hss.gov.yk.ca/extended_care.php*

Home Care/Home Support Program
This government office will refer callers to numerous home care services such as occupational and physical therapy, nursing, and social work. It also provides home care services such as personal care, support activities, health and safety, and bathing.

Telephone: 867-667-5774
Website: *www.hss.gov.yk.ca/homecare.php*

Seniors Information Centre
Funded through Yukon Council on Aging, the center provides information on federal, territorial, municipal, and other programs for seniors. Publishes *Information Please: A Handbook for Yukon Seniors and Elders*, a helpful guide to seniors' services.

Telephone: 867-668-3383 or 1-866-582-9707
Website: *http://www.yukon-seniors-and-elders.org/yukoncouncil/yukoncouncil_ seniors_info_centre.htm*; Email: ycoa@yknet.yk.ca

General Resources

Alpine Health Supplies and Services
Provides a full line of medical supplies, ranging from wheelchairs to commodes, and all items an elderly person in need of special aids may require.
Telephone: 867-393-4967

Canada Mortgage and Housing Corporation,
British Columbia and Yukon Division
See the Canada-wide listing under "Home Health Care Retailers, Home Safety,

and Environment" for services offered. Call the number below or visit the website to find the office nearest you.

Telephone: 1-877-499-7245
Website: *www.cmhc.ca*

Financial Planning/Legal

Office of the Public Guardian and Trustee
This office is responsible for protecting the financial rights of cognitively challenged people. It helps individuals make decisions on personal care and medical treatment and advises family members on guardianship and on how to obtain the legal authority to make decisions on behalf of loved ones.

Telephone: 867-667-5366 or 1-800-661-0408 ext. 5366
Website: *www.publicguardianandtrustee.gov.yk.ca/index.html*;
Email: publicguardianandtrustee@gov.yk.ca

Yukon Community and Transportation Services,
Motor Vehicles and Driver Licensing
This department provides driver assessments to determine driving competence. Call to find the office nearest you.

Telephone: (Whitehorse) 867-667-5315 or 1-800-661-0408 ext. 5315
Website: *www.hpw.gov.yk.ca/mv/mvdrlic.html*; Email: motor.vehicles@gov.yk.ca

FURTHER READING

Some other books by the authors on aging and eldercare in the family:

Late-Stage Dementia, Promoting Comfort, Compassion and Care
by Dr. Michael Gordon with Natalie Baker
Available online at *chapters.indigo.ca, amazon.ca, barnesandnoble.com,* and *amazon.com.*

Moments that Matter: Cases in Ethical Eldercare: A Guide for Family Members
by Dr. Michael Gordon
Available online at *chapters.indigo.ca, amazon.ca, barnesandnoble.com,* and *amazon.com.*

The Family Eldercare Workbook & Planner
by *Bart* Mindszenthy
Available online at *http://www.familyeldercareworkbook.com/family-eldercare-workbook-planner/*

Aging Parents: 200+ Practical Support Tips from My Care Journey
by Bart Mindszenthy
Available online at *http://www.familyeldercareworkbook.com/aging-parents-200-tips/.*

OF RELATED INTEREST

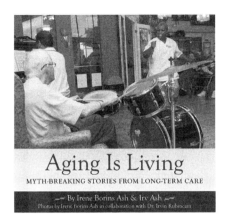

Aging is Living
Myth-Breaking Stories from Long-Term Care
by Irene Borins Ash
978-1550028836
$26.99

Through the inspirational, wise, and informative stories of the residents, either in their own words or based on interviews, and environmental photographs of each, this book focuses on various residents of long-term care facilities and especially on the positive facets of their life, their thoughts, and their feelings. The only issues that reach the media about nursing homes are the negative and unfortunate events that sometimes occur, but there is so much more to the story.

Most people are afraid of long-term care homes because they recognize that it is the last phase in their life — it is the step before death. But some people have years from the time they enter the home until they die. This book shows how many men and women make the best of their situation — often leaving a positive legacy for family and friends — and how these can be fulfilling and quality years.

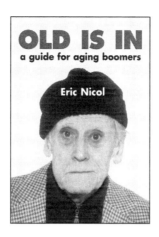

Old Is In
A Guide for Aging Boomers
by Eric Nicol
978-1550025248
$16.99

Is impotence contagious? At what age should a senior be surgically separated from his automobile, or obligated to donate his sex toys to the
Salvation Army?

These and other timely questions are among those not answered in
Eric Nicol's latest cure for serious reading, *Old Is In*. This palsied opus
responds to demographics warning that our Western society is about to
be engulfed by a tidal wave of seniors.

How to cope? Is stoicism the answer? Hell, no! The best way to relieve
the stiff upper lip is with a smile. And that prescription is filled, merrily,
by Eric Nicol's *Old Is In*.

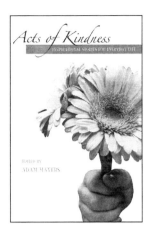

Acts of Kindness
Inspirational Stories for Everyday Life
by Adam Mayers
978-1554887491
$14.99

Small things can often mean a great deal. For the past five years readers of the *Toronto Star's* website have been telling each other that, as they shared their stories in a feature called "Acts of Kindness." The common thread is that a stranger helped when it was needed most, without thought of a reward and often without leaving a name.

Since its debut in December, 2004, "Acts of Kindness" has become a daily fixture at *thestar.com*. About four thousand stories have been submitted and two thousand have been published. *Acts of Kind*ness, the book, represents the best of the best — a collection of 200 of the most memorable tales.

The stories are a reminder that goodness is non-denominational, non-political, and transferable across race and language. They also remind us that although our lives are full of hard realities, the smallest gesture can raise a spirit or lift a heart, and the time to do it is now.

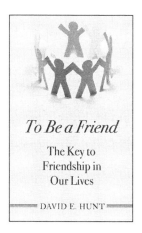

To Be a Friend
The Key to Friendship in Our Lives
by David E. Hunt
978-1554887514
$14.99

In today's busy world, we may fail to realize that our need for friendship is as vital and important as our basic needs for food, air, and water. However, thanks to the high-stress environments people currently live in, they are now starting to realize how important friendship is to a healthy and full life.

This book shows readers how to open the flow of friendship in their lives by learning to be friends. It offers activities that have proven helpful to participants in the author's workshops, exercises that prompt readers to examine their personal beliefs about friendship and apply them in daily life. By following these activities, readers discover how to be friends with themselves, how to be friends with others, and how to strengthen existing friendships. Author David Hunt also describes his experiences with learning how to be a friend, including his successes and failures.

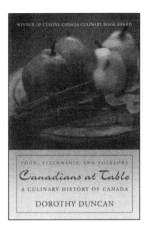

Canadians at Table
Food, Fellowship, and Folklore: A Culinary History of Canada
by Dorothy Duncan
978-1459700383
$24.99

In *Canadians at Table* we learn about lessons of survival from the First Nations, the foods that fuelled fur traders, and the adaptability of early settlers to their new environment. As communities developed and transportation improved, waves of newcomers arrived, bringing memories of foods, beverages, and traditions they had known, which were almost impossible to implement in their new homeland. They discovered instead how to use native plants for many of their needs. Community events and institutions developed to serve religious, social, and economic needs from agricultural and temperance societies to Womens' Institutes, from markets and fairs to community meals and celebrations.

Available at your favourite bookseller

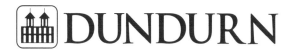

Visit us at
Dundurn.com
@dundurnpress
Facebook.com/dundurnpress
Pinterest.com/dundurnpress